Diagnosis and Treatment of Cardiovascular Disease

Diagnosis and Treatment of Cardiovascular Disease

Editor: Mia Dunn

AMERICAN
MEDICAL PUBLISHERS
www.americanmedicalpublishers.com

AMERICAN
MEDICAL PUBLISHERS
www.americanmedicalpublishers.com

Cataloging-in-Publication Data

Diagnosis and treatment of cardiovascular disease / edited by Mia Dunn.
p. cm.
Includes bibliographical references and index.
ISBN 978-1-63927-657-8
1. Cardiovascular system--Diseases. 2. Cardiovascular system--Diseases--Diagnosis.
3. Cardiovascular system--Diseases--Treatment. I. Dunn, Mia.
RC667 .D53 2023
616.1--dc23

American Medical Publishers,
41 Flatbush Avenue,
1st Floor, New York,
NY 11217, USA

ISBN 978-1-63927-657-8 (Hardback)

Contents

Preface

Cardiovascular disease (CVD) refers to a group of diseases that affect the blood vessels or the heart. CVDs include coronary artery diseases (CADs) such as myocardial infarction and angina. A few other CVDs include thromboembolic disease, abnormal heart rhythms, venous thrombosis, heart failure, valvular heart disease, hypertensive heart disease and peripheral artery disease. These diseases can be diagnosed through a variety of techniques such as blood tests, chest X-ray and EEG. They can also be diagnosed through CT scans, MRI scans and cardiac catheterization. CVDs can be treated by introducing major lifestyle and dietary changes such as exercising, limiting alcohol consumption, eating healthy, avoiding tobacco smoke and making lifestyle changes. These preventative measures are also effective in treating other risk factors including diabetes, high blood pressure and blood lipids. Since influenza increases the likelihood of CVDs; administering influenza vaccination can help in reducing the chances of cardiovascular events. This book provides significant information to help develop a good understanding of cardiovascular diseases and the latest advances with respect to their diagnosis and clinical management. It is appropriate for students seeking detailed information in this area as well as for experts.

Significant researches are present in this book. Intensive efforts have been employed by authors to make this book an outstanding discourse. This book contains the enlightening chapters which have been written on the basis of significant researches done by the experts.

Finally, I would also like to thank all the members involved in this book for being a team and meeting all the deadlines for the submission of their respective works. I would also like to thank my friends and family for being supportive in my efforts.

Editor

1

Probiotics, Prebiotics and Synbiotics—A Promising Strategy in Prevention and Treatment of Cardiovascular Diseases?

Beata Olas

Department of General Biochemistry, Faculty of Biology and Environmental Protection, University of Lodz, Pomorska 141/3, 90-236 Lodz, Poland; beata.olas@biol.uni.lodz.pl

Abstract: Recent evidence suggests that probiotics, prebiotics and synbiotics may serve as important dietary components in the prevention (especially) and treatment of cardiovascular diseases (CVD), but the recommendations for their use are often based on brief reports and small clinical studies. This review evaluates the current literature on the correlation between CVD and probiotics, prebiotics and synbiotics. Although research on probiotics, prebiotics and synbiotics has grown exponentially in recent years, particularly regarding the effect of probiotics on CVD, their mechanisms have not been clearly defined. It has been proposed that probiotics lower cholesterol levels, and may protect against CVD, by increasing bile salt synthesis and bile acid deconjugation. Similar effects have also been observed for prebiotics and synbiotics; however, probiotics also appear to have anti-oxidative, anti-platelet and anti-inflammatory properties. Importantly, probiotics not only have demonstrated effects in vitro and in animal models, but also in humans, where supplementation with probiotics decreases the risk factors of CVD. In addition, the properties of commercial probiotics, prebiotics and synbiotics remain undetermined, and further experimental research is needed before these substances can be used in the prevention and treatment of CVD. In particular, well-designed clinical trials are required to determine the influence of probiotics on trimethylamine-N-oxide (TMAO), which is believed to be a marker of CVDs, and to clarify the long-term effects, and action, of probiotic, prebiotic and synbiotic supplementation in combination with drug therapy (for example, aspirin). However, while it cannot be unequivocally stated whether such supplementation yields benefits in the prevention and treatment of CVDs, it is important to note that clinical studies performed to date have not identified any side-effects to use.

Keywords: probiotic; prebiotic; synbiotic; cardiovascular disease

---

1. Introduction

Cardiovascular diseases (CVD) are conditions that involve the heart or blood vessels, the most well-known being coronary artery diseases (angina and myocardial infarction), stroke, hypertensive heart diseases, cardiomyopathy, venous thrombosis, arrhythmia and thromboembolic disease. The underlying mechanisms vary depending on the disease. For example, coronary artery disease, peripheral artery disease, and stroke involve atherosclerosis [1,2]. They may be associated with various lifestyle factors such as poor diet or smoking, and are characterized by high blood pressure, high cholesterol levels, obesity and hyperactivation of blood platelets [1]. CVDs are believed to have been responsible for about 18 million deaths worldwide (about 32%) in 2015 [2].

CVD management does not necessarily require therapeutic intervention or prophylaxis. For example, it is known that a diet high in fruits and vegetables can decrease the risk of CVD via various mechanisms, including reducing plasma cholesterol level and inhibiting blood platelet activation. However, such dietary modification can also result in changes in the microbial and metabolic composition of the intestines, which themselves are known to be characteristic of a range of physiological and pathological states, including CVD; the composition of the gut microbiota has been found to be associated with atherogenesis, thrombosis, chronic heart conditions and arterial hypertension [3–7], and this correlation has also been noted in a recent meta-analysis [8].

Dietary supplements, often termed functional foods, can bestow beneficial effects against various risk factors associated with cardiovascular diseases. However, little, if anything, is known about the role of probiotic, prebiotic and symbiotic supplements as important dietary components in the prevention and treatment of CVD. For example, in a review paper, Vascquez et al. [9] indicated that probiotics may decrease the production of reactive oxygen species, and reduce oxidative stress. Nevertheless, some brief reports and small clinical studies have been conducted, and these may nevertheless offer new directions in treatment; in addition, the body of research regarding these supplements, particularly concerning the effect of probiotics on cardiovascular diseases, has recently grown exponentially. For example, 201 articles were published during 2014–2020, and 63 were published on "probiotics and cardiovascular diseases" during 2009–2013 (PubMed June, 2020). Therefore, the aim of this review is to discuss the roles of probiotics, prebiotics and synbiotics in the prevention and treatment of cardiovascular diseases based on data from journals recorded in international databases, including *inter alia* PubMed and Scopus.

2. Probiotics

Belief in the beneficial effects of certain types of bacteria on the human body dates back to ancient times. It is known that Plinius the Elder advocated drinking beverages made from fermented milk to alleviate stomach troubles [10].

The term *probiotic* is derived from the Greek *pro bios*, meaning *for life*. It was introduced in 1965 by Lilly and Stillwell, who identified a probiotic as "an organism or substance that affects the balance of intestinal microflora". In 1989, Fuller saw the benefits of probiotics and described them as a "live, microbiological food supplement" [10]. In 2002, the Food and Agriculture Organization/World Health Organization (WHO) defined probiotics as "live micro-organisms which when present in adequate amounts, confer benefits to the body of the host" [11].

In the early twentieth century, research on probiotics chiefly focused on the species of *Lactobacillus* found in dairy products, for example *Lactobacillus casei* (the first probiotic strain isolated in Japan), and on its Western equivalent *Lactobacillus acidophilus*. In 1970, Ilyich Metchnikoff (who is usually considered the founder of probiotics) reported that the quantity of *Lactobacilli* in the gastrointestinal tract has an influence on the health of the host [12]. *Lactobacillus* is one of the main genera of probiotic microorganisms with a long history of safe use; it is recognized by the US Food and Drug Administration (FDA) for consumption, and is approved for use in dairy products [10,13].

Probiotic bacteria are constantly present in humans and are naturally present in the digestive tract and the mouth; they are consumed around the world along with traditional food products. They have also been widely used to preserve the freshness of foods such as salami, cheese, soy sauce or sauerkraut for hundreds, or even thousands, of years [10].

Probiotics are believed to adhere to intestinal epithelial cells, preventing the development of harmful microorganisms by producing anti-bacterial substances including bacteriocins and organic acids. The quantitative share of bacteria in the digestive tract is variable, with the number of *Bifidobacteria* in the human colon ranging from 8×10^4 to 2.5×10^{13} cells (mean 1.6×10^{10} cells), and the number *Lactobacillus* bacteria ranging from 4×10^4 to 3.2×10^{12} (mean 4×10^9 cells). Twelve species of *Bifidobacteria* are known to occur in humans, particularly *B. longum*, *B. pseudolongum*, *B. animalis* and *B. bifidum*; *Bifidobacteria* is one of the first genera of microorganisms to colonize the sterile digestive tracts of newborns, and is believed to constitute the largest group of intestinal microflora, representing up to 95% of the total microbial population during breast feeding [10].

WHO regulations state that the number of living cells in probiotic foods at the time of human consumption may not be lower than 10^6 cells per 1 mL or 1 g of product, while the therapeutic dose is 10^8–10^9 cells in 1 mL or 1 g of product. Given that the microorganism must remain viable and should not be killed by passing through the gastrointestinal tract, the probiotic must be resistant to the action of gastric juice and bile salts. After passing through this chemical barrier, probiotics should adhere to the surface of the intestine, where their health-promoting functions can be realized. In addition, if probiotic microorganisms do not colonize the intestine, the repeated consumption of probiotic products may be necessary [10].

Probiotics can enhance the nonspecific cellular immune response through the activation of natural killer cells, macrophages and the release of various cytokines. They can also improve the gut mucosal immune system by increasing the number of IgA(+) cells [14,15]. In addition, probiotics can also aid the process of digestion and the breakdown of lactose, improve the absorption of minerals such as calcium, zinc, iron and manganese, and improve the synthesis of many vitamins, including thiamin, riboflavin, niacin, pantothenic acid and vitamin K. Probiotics play an important role in the treatment of various diseases, such as hepatic disease, diarrhea and gastroenteritis. Probiotics have also been shown to have anti-proliferative, pro-apoptotic and anti-oxidative properties [14,15].

Probiotics and CVDs

Probiotics may support the prevention and treatment of some cardiovascular diseases by reducing elevated cholesterol levels [10,16,17]. Unfortunately, most studies on the effects of probiotics on cardiovascular diseases have been performed in vitro. While some in vivo studies have examined the effect of probiotic supplementation on risk factors of CVDs in people and animals, the number of commercial probiotic supplements is too limited to unequivocally demonstrate that such probiotics have a beneficial effect on the cardiovascular system.

Probiotics may reduce cholesterol levels by several mechanisms [18]. Most *Bifidobacteria* bacteria demonstrate higher choliloglicin hydrolase activity than other microorganisms. This enzyme hydrolyzes the amide bonds conjugated with taurine or glycine in bile acids, resulting in the release of primary bile acids; these are easily precipitated at low pH, resulting in their expulsion from the gastrointestinal tract. As these are not reabsorbed from the intestine, they must be replaced by bile produced in the liver from blood cholesterol. Alternatively, *Bifidobacteria*-driven cholesterol assimilation, or precipitation in the acidic environment of the gut, can also reduce plasma cholesterol level by slowing its absorption from food into the blood [10].

A recent meta-analysis by Mo et al. [19] indicated that the use of probiotics significantly lowers total cholesterol and low-density lipoprotein (LDL) cholesterol in hypercholesterolemic adults. Niamah et al. [20] also note that soy milk fermented (3 mL/day) by a probiotic starter (Log.11.1 cfu/mL) consisting of *S. thermophilis*, *L. acidophilus* LA-5 and *B. bifidum* BG-12 decreases the level of cholesterol and triglyceride compared with control.

Malik et al. [21] report that *L. plantarum* 299v (Lp299v) supplementation improves vascular endothelial function and reduces inflammatory biomarkers in men with stable coronary artery disease. In this experiment, twenty men with stable coronary artery disease consumed a drink containing 20 billion colony-forming units (cfu) of Lp299v per day for six weeks. Vascular endothelial function was measured by brachial artery flow-mediated dilation, and endothelial vasodilation was measured by video microscopy. It was also found that the administered probiotics can regulate the genes responsible for the intestinal transport of cholesterol (including *ABCG8*, *ABCG5* and *NPC1L1*), as well as some genes responsible for the homeostasis of cholesterol in the liver, including those controlling the production of 3-hydroxy-3-methylglutaryl-coenzyme A reductase (HMGCR) [21].

A recent study by Lew et al. [22] found *L. plantarum* DR7 to exert cholesterol-lowering properties via AMPK phosphorylation, resulting in the reduced expression of HMGCR. Nguyen et al. [23] also suggest that the probiotic *L. plantarum* PH40 may also possess cholesterol-lowering properties. Wang et al. [24]

reported that the four-week administration of *L. acidophilus* (10^9 cfu/mL) improves lipid-regulating activity in hypercholesterolemic rats, together with one of statin—rosuvastatin (10 mg/kg).

Systematic inflammation is commonly observed among CVDs, as are many risk factors, such as hypertension [25]. Oxidative stress is also known to play a role in the course of CVDs [24]. *Lactobacillus* and *Bifidobacterium* have been found to inhibit lipid peroxidation and ROS production, and hence may slow or even halt the development of CVDs and other oxidative stress-related diseases [26–28].

Yadav et al. [29] reported that the consumption of probiotic *L. fermentum* MTCC: 5898-fermented milk not only attenuated dyslipidemia, but also reduced oxidative stress and inflammation in male rats fed a cholesterol-enriched diet. Oxidative stress was measured by the activity of various anti-oxidative enzymes, such as catalase, superoxide dismutase and glutathione peroxidase, and the level of thiobarbituric acid reactive substances (TBARS) in the liver and kidney—a marker of lipid peroxidation. Inflammation, measured by the expression of inflammatory cytokines, including tumor necrosis factor-alpha (TNF-α) and interleukin-6 (IL-6), was also influenced at the genetic level. The study examined the effect of 90-day probiotic supplementation among male Wistar rats. The rats were divided into three groups: one was fed a standard diet (Group 1), another fed a cholesterol-enriched diet (Group 2), and another fed a cholesterol-enriched diet together with 2 mL MTCC: 5898-fermented milk (2×10^9 cfu) per day (Group 3). The probiotic-fermented milk was prepared by inoculating 1% of activated *L. fermentum* MTCC: 5898 (in skimmed milk) into fresh milk (2.5% fat), which was then incubated at 37 °C for 18 h before feeding.

Tenorio-Jimenez et al. [30] report that the 12-week administration of a daily dose of 5×10^9 cfu *L. reuteri* V3401 in capsules was associated with lower levels of inflammation biomarkers, such as TNF-α, IL-6, IL-8 and soluble intercellular adhesion molecule-1 (sICAM-1), in obese adults aged 18 to 65 years with metabolic syndrome, as well as with a reduced risk of CVD. Szulinska et al. [31] also observed that supplementation with the multispecies probiotic Ecologic® Barrier modified both the functional and biochemical parameters of vascular dysfunction in a group of 81 obese postmenopausal Caucasian women. The subjects were assigned to three groups: (1) placebo, (2) those receiving a low dose (2.5×10^9 cfu per day), and (3) those receiving a high dose (1×10^{10} cfu per day). The supplement was administered for 12 weeks. The authors note that the low and high doses decrease systolic blood pressure and serum vascular endothelial growth factor (VEGF), TNF-α and IL-6. Other clinical trials have also found probiotic use to be associated with a moderate or significant reduction in blood pressure among both healthy and obese participants [32–36]. The anti-hypertensive action of probiotics is believed to act via several mechanisms, including regulating the renin–angiotensin system [36].

The hyperactivation of blood platelets also plays a key role in thrombotic disorders. Although pharmacological strategies are available, such as those based on aspirin and its derivatives, these treatments are often accompanied by side-effects and complications that outweigh their benefits. In addition, blood platelet function is strongly influenced by diet, including the consumption of fruit and vegetables [37,38]. Although the precise roles played by probiotics in the modulation of hemostasis and its various elements, such as blood platelet function, are generally not well documented, a few in vitro and in vivo studies have nevertheless examined their effects on various elements of hemostasis, such as platelet activation. For example, Schreiber et al. reported that *L. reuteri* reduces P-selectin expression on the platelet surface and decreases blood platelet–endothelial cell interactions in rats treated with dextran sodium sulfate (DSS) [39]. In addition, Haro and Medina [40] also indicated that the oral administration of probiotic *L. casei* CRL431 may be a promising candidate for the prevention of thrombotic complications associated with pneumococcal pneumonia, especially in at-risk patients. It was found that the oral administration of CRL431 in a respiratory pneumococcal infection model in mice reduces blood platelet activation, measured by various parameters, including P-selectin expression, and modulates antithrombin levels within the normal range. These findings may indicate that *L. casei* may also influence the coagulation system [40]. In addition, in vitro experiments found no significant difference in the levels of blood platelet activation markers, such as ADP-induced platelet aggregation, between resting platelets and samples incubated with *L. rhamnosus* HN001 and *B. lactis*

HN019. The authors suggest that these probiotic strains do not appear to participate in the pathogenesis of thrombotic disorders [41].

It is likely that inflammatory processes play an important role in the pathogenesis and progression of atherosclerosis, as elevated levels of proinflammatory cytokines have been observed in patients with atherosclerosis [42]. However, although some studies have demonstrated that probiotics can decrease the production of pro-inflammatory cytokines, their underlying mechanism remains unclear [7].

A recent study by Majewska et al. [43] found probiotic supplementation (Ecologic® BARIER, containing 2.5×10^9 cfu/g; for 12 weeks) to inhibit the inflammation process, reduce oxidative stress, and decrease the concentration of homocysteine in obese women ($n = 50$; aged 45–70 years).

3. Prebiotics

Prebiotics contain no microorganisms—only substances which stimulate their growth. These do not undergo digestion; therefore, they reach the intestinal lumen unchanged, where they can then act. For food ingredients to be considered prebiotics, they must meet certain criteria: they must be resistant to the actions of stomach acids, bile salts and other hydrolyzing enzymes in the intestine, have a known chemical structure, provide a substrate for one or more strains of beneficial bacteria, stimulate the growth and activity of the desired groups of bacteria in the digestive tract, and possess proven health benefits [10,44].

Prebiotics can be obtained from various sources, including breast milk, soybeans and raw oats [10,45]. However, the most popular prebiotics are the oligosaccharides contained in plants, such as asparagus, artichokes, chicory and onions [10]. Oligosaccharides may benefit the gastrointestinal tract via fermentation and the proliferation of desirable bacterial species. For example, fructo-oligosaccharide promotes the growth of bifidobacteria in vivo. Oligofructose and inulin also increase the population of colonic bifidobacteria [46,47]. Hsu et al. [48] observed that xylo-oligosaccharides and fructo-oligosaccharides affect the intestinal microbiota and precancerous development of colonic lesions in rats. Nowadays, probiotics are often added as supplements to dairy products, meat products and beverages, such as health drinks. Recently, Cherry et al. [49] reported that seaweed may be a good source of polysaccharide components, which may act as prebiotics.

Prebiotics and CVDs

Parnell and Reiner [50] reported that probiotic supplementation lowers total serum cholesterol in a hypercholesterolemic rat model. In this experiment, rats were administered one of three diets supplemented with 0, 10 or 20% prebiotic fiber for 10 weeks. Both doses of prebiotic fiber reduced serum cholesterol concentrations by about 25%. In addition, this change was correlated with an increase in caeca digesta, as well as the up-regulation of genes involved in cholesterol biosynthesis and bile production. In addition, the obese rats with 10% prebiotic supplementation demonstrated an approximately 40% reduction in triacylglycerol accumulation in the liver (Table 1).

Obesity is often associated with the progression of CVDs. However, both probiotic and prebiotic supplementation have been reported to have anti-obesogenic effects in various clinical trials (Table 1) [51–55].

The role of prebiotics in preventing and treating hypertension is reviewed in greater detail by Ghaffari and Roshanravan [56].

4. Synbiotics

A synbiotic is a combination of probiotics and prebiotics, typically oligosaccharides or inulin, which demonstrate an additive action and are used to restore normal bacterial flora [10].

Synbiotics and CVDs

A number of studies have found synbiotics to demonstrate promising hypercholesterolemic properties [57–60]. For example, Mofid et al. [60] reported that the regular intake of synbiotic yoghurts reduces the risk of CVDs among hypercholesterolemic patients.

Haghighat et al. [59] noted that 12-week synbiotic supplementation reduces the concentration of intracellular adhesion molecule type 1 (ICAM-1), which is a risk factor for cardiovascular diseases in hemodialysis patients. The study included three groups of subjects: synbiotic, probiotic and placebo. Those in the synbiotic group received 15 g of prebiotic (three different fiber types: 5 g fructo-oligosaccharides, 5 g galacto-oligosaccharides and 5 g inulin) and 5 g probiotic powder (Bioflora®) containing *L. acidophilus* strain T16, *B. bifidum* strain BIA-6, *B. lactis* strain BIA-6, and *B. longum* strain LAF-5 (2.7×10^7 cfu/g each) in sachets. The probiotic group received 5 g probiotics, as in the synbiotic group, with 15 g of maltodextrin powder in sachets. The placebo group received 20 g of maltodextrin powder in sachets.

It has been found that a synbiotic containing *L. acidophilus* ATCC 4962 reduces total cholesterol, triacylglycerol, and LDL-cholesterol in hypercholesterolemic pigs, probably in the form of cholesterol esters, via the interrelated pathways of lipid transporters, including high-density lipoprotein (HDL), LDL and very low-density lipoprotein (VLDL). In this experiment, three commercially available prebiotics were used: mannitol, fructo-oligosacharides and inulin. The pigs on the symbiotic diet were supplemented with powdered *L. acidophilus* ATCC 4962 (1 g/pig per day), mannitol (1.56 g/pig per day), fructo-oligosacharides (1.25 g/pig per day) and inulin (2.2 g/pig per day). The animals were also given dietary fat (5 and 15%) (Table 1). In addition, it was found that the synbiotic reduces the deformation of erythrocytes via improved membrane permeability and fluidity [57,58].

5. The Effects of Probiotics, Prebiotics and Synbiotics on TMAO Levels

Trimethylamine-N-oxide ($(CH_3)_3NO$; TMAO) is an organic compound produced from choline, phosphatidylcholine, and carnitine precursors. These are converted into an intermediate compound, trimethylamine (TMA), by members of the gut microbiota, such as Acinetobacter; TMA is in turn oxidized into TMAO by the action of hepatic flavin monooxygenases (FMOs) [61]. As such, the consumption of carnitine-containing food products, such as some energy drinks and dietary supplements, results in increased TMAO levels in the blood [62].

However, the nature of the relationship between TMAO levels and CVDs remains unclear. Wilson et al. proposed that a high concentration of TMAO in the blood may be correlated with an increased risk of CVDs [63]. TMAO has also been indicated as a marker of cardiovascular events [64], and has been observed to influence the metabolism of cholesterol in the liver in the intestinal and artery walls. Hazen reported an increased deposition of cholesterol in peripheral cells, such as those in artery walls, in the presence of TMAO, together with the decreased removal of cholesterol [65]. In addition, carnitine intake and a high plasma concentration of TMAO have been found to correlate with low aortic lesions in ApoE -/- transgenic mice expressing cholesterol ester transfer protein (CETP) [66]. Ufnal et al. [67] and Tilg [68] suggest that TMAO may be involved in the etiology of hypertension and thrombosis, and in the regulation of arterial blood pressure. A review by Kanitsoraphan et al. [69] suggests that the concentration of TMAO could be incorporated into existing risk stratification tools, and could lead to novel prevention and treatment.

A recent study by Hardin et al. [70] described a possible mechanism connecting TMAO and the enhancement of atherosclerotic factors. They proposed that increased TMAO concentrations in plasma promoted the upregulation of macrophage scavenger receptors, which promote the recruitment of macrophages and associated inflammation. Being unable to properly metabolize the lipids inside them, the accumulated macrophages produce foamy cells. The resulting inflammation, foamy cell production and accumulation of macrophages promote the development of atherosclerosis and other CVDs. Leustean et al. [71] described other mechanisms of TMAO action in CVDs, including blood platelet aggregation and decreases in nitric oxide level (Figure 1).

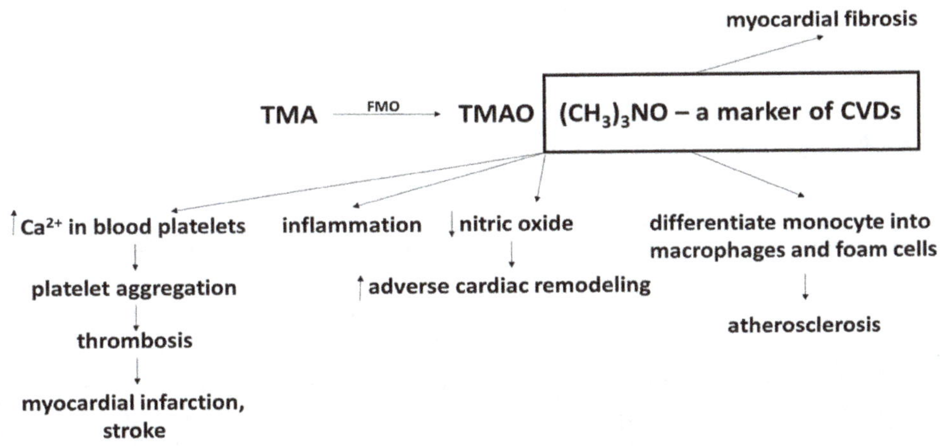

Figure 1. Effect of trimethylamine-N-oxide (TMAO) on cardiovascular diseases (CVDs) (modified) [70] More details in text.

Preliminary results suggest that antibiotic therapy may suppress TMAO levels, but the long-term stability of such therapy remains unknown [64]. It has been proposed that probiotic treatment may prevent the development of CVDs following TMAO accumulation (Figure 2). However, Malik et al. [21] noted that supplementation with a drink containing *L. plantarum* 299v (Lp299v), 20 billion cfu daily for six weeks, did not significantly change plasma TMAO concentrations in a group of 20 men aged 40–75 years with stable coronary artery disease. Tripolt et al. [72] also noted that supplementation with *L. casei* Shirota (6.5 × 109 cfu, daily) three times for 12 weeks does not change TMAO levels in subjects with metabolic syndrome. Similar results were observed by Boutagy et al. [73] in a study of nineteen non-obese subjects who consumed a mix of various probiotics (900 billion live bacteria) for four weeks.

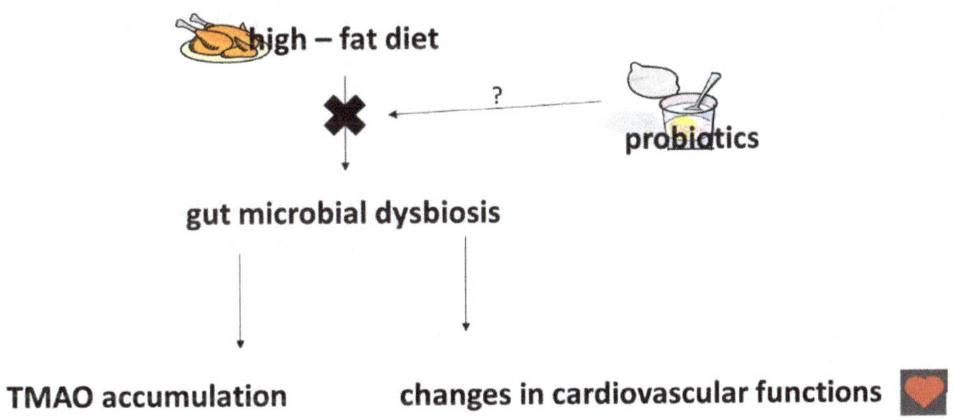

Figure 2. Effect of probiotics on trimethylamine-N-oxide (TMAO) accumulation and changes in cardiovascular functions. More details in text (modified) [69].

In contrast, Qui et al. [74] observed that *L. plantarum* ZDYO4 inhibits the development of TMAO-induced atherosclerosis in ApoE-/- 1.3% choline-fed mice, compared to controls. Tenore et al. [75] reported a decrease in TMAO level among a group of 90 individuals with CVD risk factors, including high total cholesterol and LDL levels, following the consumption of lactofermented annurca apple puree (125 g/day for 16 weeks). Each dose contained approximately 3×10^8 cfu *L. rhamnosus* LRH11 and *L. plantarum* SGL07.

Liu et al. reported that the consumption of probiotic-fermented purple sweet potato yoghurt may reverse congestive heart failure induced by hypertension; this was proposed to occur via the attenuation of cardiomyocyte apoptosis by the inhibition of Fas receptor-dependent apoptotic pathways [76]. It has also been indicated that the probiotic *B. animalis* subsp. *lactis* LKM512 may decrease TMA levels in healthy volunteers [77], and that probiotics may play an important role in atherosclerosis by modulating TMAO concentration [78].

Table 1. The effect of probiotics, prebiotics, and synbiotics on various risk factors of cardiovascular diseases (*in vivo* model).

Probiotic/Prebiotic/Synbiotic Consumption	Dose (Per Day)	Days/Weeks	Subjects	Risk Factors of Cardiovascular Diseases	Ref.
Probiotic					
L. plantarum 299v	20 billion cfu	6 weeks	Patients with stable coronary artery disease (people)	Reducing inflammatory biomarkers. No effect on trimethylamine-N-oxide (TMAO) level	[21]
L. plantarum PH04	10^7 cfu	14 days	Male mice fed a high-cholesterol diet containing 10% *w/v* skim milk and 10% *w/v* cream	Lowering total cholesterol and triglycerides	[23]
L. reuteri V3401	5×10^9 cfu	12 weeks	Obese adults (people) with metabolic syndrome	Reducing inflammation	[30]
Multispecies probiotic Ecologic® Barrier	2.5×10^9 cfu; 1×10^{10} cfu	12 weeks	Obese postmenopausal Caucasian women	Decreasing systolic blood pressure and inflammation	[31]
Multispecies probiotic Ecologic® Barrier	2.5×10^9 cfu	12 weeks	Obese women	Decreasing homocysteine	[43]
L. acidophilus	10^9 cfu/mL	4 weeks	Hypercholesterolemic rats	Lowering total cholesterol and low-density lipoprotein (LDL)	[24]
L. fermentum MTCC:5898-fermented milk	2×10^9 cfu	90 days		Reducing dyslipidemia, oxidative stress and inflammation	[29]
L. rhamnosus LRH11 and *L. plantarum* SGL07	3×10^8 cfu	16 weeks	People with CVDs risks	Reducing plasma trimethylamine-N-oxide (TMAO) level	[75]
B. animalis subsp. *lactis* LKM512	No described	12 weeks	Healthy people	Reducing plasma trimethylamine-N-oxide (TMAO) level	[77]
L. casei Shirota	6.5×10^9 cfu	12 weeks	Subjects with metabolic syndrome	No effect on trimethylamine-N-oxide (TMAO) level	[72]
S. thermophilis, *L. acidophilus* LA-5 and *B. bifidum* BG-12	No described (3 mL/day)	4 weeks	Healthy animals	Lowering cholesterol and triglyceride	[20]
Prebiotic					
Prebiotic fiber	10 or 20%	10 weeks	Obese hyperlipidemic rats	Lowering total serum cholesterol and triacylglycerol	[50]
Oligofructose	8 g/day	16 weeks	Overweight and obese children aged 7–12 years	Decreasing body weight	[53]
Oligofructose	21 g/day	12 weeks	Overweight and obese adults	Decreasing body weight	[51]
Synbiotic					
Prebiotic (three different fiber types: 5 g fructooligosaccharides, 5 g galactooligosaccharides and 5 g inulin) and probiotic powder (Bioflora®) containing *L. acidophilus* strain T16, *B. bifidum* strain BIA-6, *B. lactis* strain BIA-6, and *B. longum* strain LAF-5	15 g of prebiotic and 5 g probiotic in sachet	12 weeks	Hemodialysis patients	Reducing the concentration of intracellular adhesion molecule type 1	[59]
Synbiotic containing *L. acidophilus* ATCC 4962, and three commercially available prebiotics (mannitol, fructooligosacharides and inulin)	*L. acidophilus* ATCC 4962 (1 g/pig per day), mannitol (1.56 g/pig per day), fructooligosacharides (1.25 g/pig per day) and inulin (2.2 g/pig per day)	8 weeks	Hypercholesterolemic pigs	Reducing total cholesterol, triacylglycerol, low-density lipoprotein (LDL)-cholesterol	[57,58]

A recent study by Montrucchio et al. [79] found serum TMAO concentrations in people living with HIV (PLWH) to be correlated with higher cardiovascular risk and atherosclerosis, and to not be affected by high-dose probiotic supplementation—no change in TMAO concentration was observed after six months of probiotic supplementation. The study included 175 participants, with TMAO concentrations of about 165 ng/mL (Table 1). More information about the reduction of TMAO level by probiotics has been described in a review by Din et al. [58].

6. The Effects of Probiotics, Prebiotics and Synbiotics on Uric Acid Levels

Valdivielso et al. reported the existence of a correlation between the occurrence of chronic kidney disease (CKD) and CVDs, including atherosclerosis; they also noted that the progression of atherosclerosis appeared to be related to CKD progression, as well as to a higher uric acid level [80]. An increased level of uric acid in serum has been associated with the presence of CKD and CVDs due to various molecular mechanisms, such as oxidative stress and inflammation. Conversely, certain antioxidants, such as phenolic compounds, may decrease uric acid level [81]. It has been suggested that probiotics, prebiotic and synbiotics, i.e., a combination of probiotics and prebiotics, may also change the level of uric acid. For example, Rossi et al. [82] reported that a synbiotic intervention based on the administration of 15 g of prebiotics (including a combination of three different types of fibers), and 90 billion cfu from nine different strains of *Lactobacillus*, *Streptococcus* and *Bifidobacteria*, daily for three weeks, may influence the outcome of CVDs and CKDs. The authors also suggested that this mixture of pre- and probiotics may reduce the levels of various toxins, including indoxyl sulphate (IS) and p-cresyl sulphate (PCS) [80]. Like TMAO, IS and PCS have been identified as proatherogenic risk factors [83].

Al-Okbi et al. [84] also noted that a combination of encapsulated probiotic (*B. bifidum*, *L. delbrueckii*, and *S. thremophilus*) and green tea alcohol extract reduces the level of uric acid in rats with hepatorenal syndrome. Wang et al. [85] reported that supplementation with *Lactobacillus* DM9218 decreases serum uric acid in fructose-fed mice; the authors suggested that it may protect against high-fructose-induced liver damage and retinol uric acid accumulation by degrading inosine. The uric acid level was also significantly reduced in non-dialysis patients with CKD who received probiotics [86]. Moreover, the eight-week consumption of *L. gasseri* PA-3 yoghurt was found to decrease the level of serum uric acid in 25 patients [87].

However, Haghighat et al. reported that daily synbiotic supplementation for 12 weeks with sachets containing 15 g of prebiotics and 5 g of probiotic (2.7×10^7 cfu) did not appear to influence uric acid level in a group of 75 hemodialysis patients [58]. Garcia-Arrayo et al. [88] found that five-week probiotic supplementation with *L. acidophilus* KB27 (5 billion cfu/daily) and *L. rhamnosus* KB79 (5 billion cfu/daily) elevates uric acid extraction in rats; it was also found to increase oxonic acid- induced intrarenal accumulation, which is known to stimulate hyperuricemia and renal damage. Firouzi and Haghighatdoost [89] reported elevated uric acid levels in healthy people (n = 437) who consumed probiotics, prebiotics and synbiotics, compared with a placebo group.

7. Conclusions

Although it has been proposed that probiotic consumption may bestow anti-hypertensive properties and be associated with improved serum lipid profiles [57,58,90,91], these postulated benefits were based on an in vitro model. More recent in vivo trials indicate that the consumption of probiotics, prebiotics or a combination of the two, i.e., synbiotics, may assist in the prevention and treatment of cardiovascular diseases; however, few studies have examined the role of probiotics in this regard, and their precise medicinal and prophylactic doses for humans remain unknown (Table 1). It is also very difficult to demonstrate the specific correlation, relationship and synergic relationships between probiotics, prebiotics and synbiotics in the prevention and treatment of CVD. However, Liong et al. [57,59] and Haghighat et al. [59] indicated that probiotics, prebiotics and synbiotics may offer promise in the prevention and treatment of CVD; for example, a synbiotic containing *L. acidophilus*

ATCC 4962 and three commercially available prebiotics (mannitol, fructooligosacharides and inulin) has been found to reduce total cholesterol, triacylglycerol and LDL-cholesterol levels (Table 1). Moreover, other authors [21] describe the role of probiotics in patients with stable coronary artery disease. On the other hand, their role in patients with other CVDs, including stroke, cardiomyopathy, and carditis, is not known.

In addition, the mechanisms of action of probiotics, prebiotics and synbiotics remain poorly defined. Probiotics are believed to modulate various factors which may play an important role in CVDs (Figure 3). Similarly to prebiotics and synbiotics, they may lower cholesterol levels by increasing bile salt synthesis and bile acid deconjugation, and may offer protection from cardiovascular diseases. Moreover, probiotics have been found to have anti-oxidative, anti-platelet and anti-inflammatory properties (Figure 3). However, further experimental research, particularly well-designed clinical studies, are needed before these substances can effectively be used in the prevention and treatment of CVD. Finally, no studies have yet evaluated the effect of their use on CVDs in combination with classical therapy, for example aspirin; therefore, although no side-effects have been reported in clinical studies to date, it cannot be unequivocally stated whether probiotic, prebiotic and synbiotic use represents an effective strategy for the prevention and treatment of CVDs.

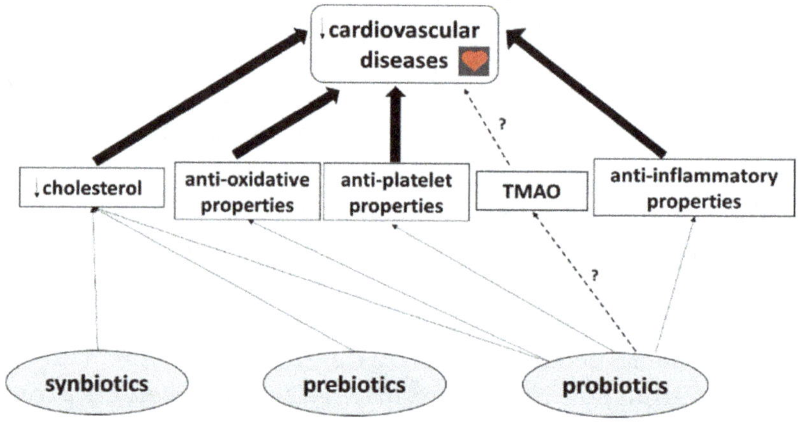

Figure 3. The effect of probiotics, prebiotics and synbiotics on cardiovascular disease. Probiotics lower the level of cholesterol by increasing bile salt synthesis and bile acid deconjugation. Probiotics also have anti-oxidative, anti-platelet and anti-inflammatory properties, and hence may offer protection from cardiovascular diseases. One proposed model of preventing the CVD-induced accumulation of TMAO may be probiotic supplementation. However, prebiotics and synbiotics may also decrease the level of total cholesterol and offer similar protection from cardiovascular disease. More details in text.

Abbreviations

cfu—colony-forming units; CKD—chronic kidney disease; FDA—Food and Drug Administration; FMO—flavin monooxygenases; HDL—high-density lipoprotein; IS—indoxyl sulphate; LDL—low-density lipoprotein; PCS—p-cresyl sulphate; TMA—trimethylamine; TMAO—trimethylamine-N-oxide; WHO—World Health Organization; VLDL—very low-density lipoprotein.

References

1. Shanthi, M.; Pekka, P.; Bo, N. *Global Atlas on Cardiovascular Diseases Prevention and Control*; World Health Organization in collaboration with the World Heart Federation and the World Stroke Organization: Geneva, Switzerland, 2011; pp. 3–18.
2. GBD. Mortality and Causes of Death Collaborators. 2013. Available online: https://doi.org/10.1016/S0140-6736(14)61682-2 (accessed on 17 December 2014).

3. Katsi, V.; Didagelos, M.; Skevofilax, S.; Armenis, I.; Kartalis, A.; Vlachopoulos, C.; Karvounis, H.; Tousoulis, D. Gut microbiota—Gut dysbiosis—Arterial hypertension: New horizons. *Curr. Hyperten. Rev.* **2018**, *12*, 1–14.
4. Pimenta, F.S.; Luaces-Regueira, M.; Ton, A.M.M.; Campagnaro, B.P.; Campos-Toimil, M.; Pereira, T.M.C.; Vasquez, E.C. Mechanisms of action of kefir in chronic cardiovascular and metabolic diseases. *Cell. Physiol. Biochem.* **2018**, *48*, 1901–1914. [CrossRef] [PubMed]
5. Rezac, S.; Kok, C.R.; Herrmann, M.; Hutkins, R. Fermented foods as a dietary source of live organisms. *Front. Microbiol.* **2018**, *9*, 1–29. [CrossRef] [PubMed]
6. Weis, M. Impact of the gut microbiome in cardiovascular and autoimmune diseases. *Clin. Sci.* **2018**, *132*, 2387–2389. [CrossRef]
7. O'Morain, V.L.; Ramji, D.P. The potential of probiotics in the prevention and treatment of atherosclerosis. *Mol. Nutr. Food Res.* **2020**, *64*, 1–15. [CrossRef]
8. Deng, X.; Ma, J.; Song, M.; Jin, Y.; Ge, W.; Guo, C. Effects of products designed to modulate the gut microbiota on hyperlipidaemia. *Eur. J. Nutr.* **2018**, *1*, 1–15. [CrossRef]
9. Vasquez, E.C.; Pereira, T.M.C.; Peotta, V.A.; Baldo, M.P.; Campos-Toimil, M. Probiotics as beneficial dietary supplements to prevent and treat cardiovascular diseases: Uncovering their impact on oxidative stress. *Oxid. Med. Cell. Longev.* **2019**, *7*, 1–12. [CrossRef]
10. Pandey, K.R.; Naik, S.R.; Vakil, B.V. Probiotics, prebiotics and synbiotics—A review. *J. Food Sci. Technol.* **2010**, *52*, 7577–7587. [CrossRef]
11. *Guildelines for the Evaluation of Probiotics in Food*; Joint FAO/WHO Working Group on Drafting Guidelines for the Evaluation of Probiotics in Food: London, ON, Canada, 2002.
12. Metchnikoff, E. Sur la lute des cellules de l'organisme centre l'invasion des microbes. *Ann. Inst. Pasteur.* **1887**, *1*, 321.
13. Khalesi, S.; Bellissimo, N.; Vandelanotte, C.; Williview, S.; Stanley, D.; Irwin, C. A review of probiotic supplementation in healthy adults: Helpful or hype? *Eur. J. Clin. Nutr.* **2018**, *26*, 1–16. [CrossRef]
14. Oberreuther-Moschner, D.L.; Jahreis, G.; Rechkemmer, G.; Pool-Zobel, B.L. Dietary intervention with the probiotics *Lactobacillus acidophilus* 145 and *Bifidobacterium longum* 913 modulates the potential of human faecal water to induce damage in HT29clone19A cells. *Br. J. Nutr.* **2004**, *91*, 925–932. [CrossRef] [PubMed]
15. Nowak, A.; Paliwoda, A.; Blasiak, J. Anti-proliferative, pro-apoptotic and anti-oxidative activity of *Lactobacillus* and *Bifidobacterium* strains: A review of mechanism and therapeutic perspectives. *Crit. Rev. Food. Sci. Nutr.* **2018**, *1*, 1–12. [CrossRef] [PubMed]
16. Sudha, M.R.; Chauhan, P.; Dixit, K.; Babu, S.; Jamil, K. Probiotics as complementary therapy for hypercholesterolemia. *Biol. Med.* **2009**, *1*, 1–13.
17. Bronzato, S.; Durante, A. Dietary supplements and cardiovascular diseases. *Inter. J. Cardiovas. Dis.* **2018**, *9*, 1–10.
18. Gadelha, C.J.M.U.; Bezerra, A.N. Effects of probiotics on the lipid profile: Systematic review. *J. Vasc. Bras.* **2019**, *9*, 1–18.
19. Mo, R.; Zhang, X.; Yang, Y. Effect of probiotics on lipid profiles in hypercholesterolaemic adults: A meta-analysis of randomized controlled trials. *Med. Clin.* **2018**, *19*, 1–12.
20. Niamah, A.K.; Sahi, A.A.; Al-Sharifi, A.S.N. Effect of feeding soy milk fermented by probiotic bacteria on some blood criteria and weight of experimental animals. *Prob. Antimicrob. Proteins* **2017**, *9*, 284–291. [CrossRef]
21. Malik, M.; Suboc, T.M.; Tyagi, S.; Salzman, N.; Wang, J.; Ying, R.; Tanner, M.J.; Kakarla, M.; Baker, J.E.; Widlansky, M.E. *Lactobacillus plantarum* 299v supplementation improves vascular endothelial function and reduces inflammatory biomarkers in med with stable coronary artery disease. *Circ. Res.* **2018**, *123*, 1091–1102. [CrossRef]
22. Lew, L.C.; Choi, S.B.; Khoo, B.Y.; Sreenivasan, S.; Ong, K.L.; Liong, M.T. *Lactobacillus plantarum* DR7 reduces cholesterol via phosphorylation of AMPK that down-regulated the mRNA expression of HMG-CoA reductase. *Kor. J. Food Sci. Animal Res.* **2018**, *38*, 350–361.
23. Nguyen, T.D.T.; Kang, J.H.; Lee, M.S. Characterization of *Lactobacillus plantarum* PH04, a potential probiotic bacterium with cholesterol-lowering effects. *Inter. J. Food Microbiol.* **2007**, *113*, 358–361. [CrossRef]
24. Wang, L.; Zhou, B.; Zhou, X.; Wang, Y.; Wang, H.; Jia, S.; Zhang, Z.; Chu, C.; Mu, J. Combined lowering effects of rosuvastatin and *L. acidophilus* on cholesterol levels in rat. *J. Microbiol. Biotechnol.* **2019**, *29*, 473–481. [CrossRef] [PubMed]

25. Del Pinto, R.; Pietropaoli, D.; Monaco, A.; Desideri, G.; Ferri, C.; Grassi, D. Non-pharmacological strategies against systemic inflammation: Molecular basis and clinical evidence. *Curr. Pharm. Des.* **2020**, *3*, 1–20.
26. Lin, M.Y.; Chang, F.J. Antioxidative effect of intestinal bacteria *Bifidobacterium longum* ATCC 15708 and *Lactobacillus acidophilus* ATCC 4356. *Dig. Dis. Sci.* **2000**, *45*, 1617–1622. [CrossRef] [PubMed]
27. El-Adawi, H.I.; Khalil, M.A.; El-Sheekh, M.M.; El-Deeb, N.M.; Hussein, M.Z. Cytotoxicity assay and antioxidant activities of the lactic acid bacterial strains. *Afric. J. Microbiol. Res.* **2012**, *6*, 1700–1712.
28. Zhong, C.; Qu, C.; Wang, B.; Liang, B.S.; Zeng, B. Probiotics for preventing and treating intestinal bacterial overgrowth: A meta-analysis and systematic review of current evidence. *J. Clin. Gastroenterol.* **2017**, *51*, 300–311. [CrossRef]
29. Yadav, R.; Khan, S.H.; Mada, S.B.; Meena, S.; Kapila, R.; Kaila, S. Consumption of probiotic *Lactobacillus fermentum* MTCC: 5898-fermented milk attenuates dyslipidemia, oxidative stress, and inflammation in male rats fed on cholesterol-enriched diet. *Probiotics Antimicro. Protein* **2018**, *1*, 1–10. [CrossRef]
30. Tenorio-Jimenez, C.; Martinez-Rmirez, M.J.; Tercero-Lozano, M.; Arraiza-Irigoyen, C.; Del Castillo-Codes, I.; Olza, J.; Plaza-Diaz, J.; Fontana, L.; Migueles, J.H.; Olivares, M.; et al. Evaluation of the effect of *Lactobacillus reuteri* V3401 on biomarkers of inflammation, cardiovascular risk and liver steatosis in obese adults with metabolic syndrome: A randomized clinical trial (PROSIR). *BMC Compl. Alter. Med.* **2018**, *18*, 1–8. [CrossRef]
31. Szulinska, M.; Loniewski, I.; Skrypnik, K.; Sobieska, M.; Korybalska, K.; Suliburska, J.; Bogdanska, P. Multispecies probiotic supplementation favorably affects vascular function and reduces arterial stiffness in obese postmenopausal women- A 12-week placebo-controlled and randomized clinical study. *Nutrients* **2018**, *10*, 1672. [CrossRef]
32. Agerholm-Larsen, L.; Raben, A.; Haulvik, N.; Hansen, A.S.; Manders, M.; Astrup, A. Effect of 8 week intake of probiotic milk products on risk factors for cardiovascular diseases. *Eur. J. Clin. Nutr.* **2000**, *54*, 288–297. [CrossRef]
33. Mizushima, S.; Ohshige, K.; Watanabe, J.; Kimura, M.; Kodowski, T.; Nakamurs, Y.; Tochikubo, O.; Ueshima, H. Randomized controlled trial of sour milk on blood pressure in bordeline hypertensive men. *Am. J. Hypertens* **2004**, *17*, 701–706. [CrossRef]
34. Aoyagi, Y.; Park, S.; Matsubara, S.; Honda, Y.; Amamoto, R.; Kushiro, A.; Miyazaki, K.; Shephard, R.J. Habitual intake of fermented milk products containing *Lactobacillus casei* strain Shirota and a reduced risk of hypertension in older people. *Benef. Microbes* **2017**, *8*, 23–29. [CrossRef] [PubMed]
35. Naruszewicz, M.; Johansson, M.L.; Zapolska-Downar, D.; Bukowska, H. Effect of *Lactobacillus plantarum* 299v on cardiovascular disease risk factors in smokers. *Microbiome* **2017**, *5*, 14–20. [CrossRef] [PubMed]
36. Matsumoto, T. Potential benefits of garlic and other dietary supplements for the management of hypertension. Review. *Exp. Ther. Med.* **2020**, *19*, 1479–1484.
37. Olas, B. Dietary supplements with antiplatelet activity: A solution for everyone? *Adv. Nutr.* **2018**, *9*, 51–57. [CrossRef] [PubMed]
38. Olas, B. Anti-aggregatory potential of selected vegetables—Promising dietary components for the prevention and treatment of cardiovascular disease. *Adv. Nutr.* **2019**, *10*, 280–290. [CrossRef]
39. Schreiber, O.; Petersson, J.; Phillipson, M.; Perry, M.; Ross, S.; Holm, L. *Lactobacillus reuteri* prevents colitis by reducing P-selectin-associated leukocyte- and platelet-endothelial cell interactions. *Am. J. Physiol. Gastrointest. Liver Physiol.* **2009**, *296*, G534–G542. [CrossRef]
40. Haro, C.; Medina, M. *Lactobacillus casei* CRL 431 improves endothelial and platelet functionality in a pneumococcal infection model. *Benef. Microbes* **2019**, *10*, 533–541. [CrossRef]
41. Zhou, J.S.; Rutherfurd, K.J.; Gill, H.S. Inability of probiotic bacterial strains *Lactobacillus rhamnosus* HN001 and *Bifidobacterium lactis* HN019 to induce human platelet aggregation I vitro. *J. Food Protect.* **2005**, *68*, 2459–2464. [CrossRef]
42. Libby, P. History of discovery: Inflammation in atherosclerosis. *Arterioscler. Thromb. Vasc. Biol.* **2012**, *32*, 2045–2051. [CrossRef]
43. Majewska, K.; Kregielska-Narożna, M.; Jakubowski, K.; Szulinska, M.; Bogdanski, P. The multispecies probiotic effectively reduces homocysteine concentration in obese women: A randomized double-blind placebo-controlled study. *J. Clin. Med.* **2020**, *4*, 1–11.
44. Kuo, S.M. The interplay between fiber and the intestinal microbiome in the inflammatory response. *Adv. Nutr.* **2013**, *4*, 16–28. [CrossRef] [PubMed]

45. Pokusaeva, K.; Fitzgerald, G.F.; van Sinderen, D. Carbohydrate metabolism in Bifidobacteria. *Genes Nutr.* **2011**, *6*, 285–306. [CrossRef] [PubMed]
46. Hidaka, H.; Eida, T.; Takizawa, T.; Tokunage, T.; Tashiro, Y. Effects of fructooligosacharides on intestinal flora and human health. *Bifidobact. Microflora* **1986**, *5*, 37–50. [CrossRef]
47. Hidaka, H.; Tashiro, Y.; Eida, T. Proliferation of bifidobacteria by oligosaccharides and their useful effects on human health. *Bifidobact. Microflora* **1991**, *10*, 65–79. [CrossRef]
48. Hsu, C.K.; Liao, J.W.; Chung, Y.C.; Hsieh, C.P.M.; Chan, Y.C. Xylooligosaccharides and fructooligosaccharides affect the intestinal microbiota and precancerous colonic lesion development in rats. *J. Nutr.* **2004**, *134*, 1523–1528. [CrossRef]
49. Cherry, P.; Vadav, S.; Strain, C.R.; Allsopp, P.J.; McSorley, E.M.; Ross, R.P.; Stanton, C. Probiotics from seaweeeds: An ocean of opportunity? *Marine Drugs* **2019**, *17*, 327. [CrossRef] [PubMed]
50. Parnell, J.A.; Reimer, R.A. Effect of prebiotic fibre supplementation on hepatic gene expression and serum lipids: A dose-response study in JCR:LA-cp rats. *Br. J. Nutr.* **2010**, *103*, 1177–1184. [CrossRef]
51. Parnell, J.A.; Reamer, R.A. Weight loss during oligofructose supplementation is associated with decreased ghrelin and increased peptide YY in overweight and obese adults. *Am. J. Clin. Nutr.* **2009**, *89*, 1751–1759. [CrossRef]
52. Hume, M.P.; Nicolucci, A.C.; Reimer, R.A. Prebiotic supplementation improves appetite control in children with overweight and obesity: A randomized controlled trial. *Am. J. Clin. Nutr.* **2017**, *105*, 790–799. [CrossRef]
53. Nicolucci, A.C.; Hume, M.P.; Martinez, I.; Mayengbam, S.; Walter, J.; Reimer, R.A. Prebiotics reduce body fat and alter intestinal microbiota in children who are overweight or with obesity. *Gastroenterology* **2017**, *153*, 711–722. [CrossRef]
54. Reimer, R.A.; Willis, H.J.; Tunnicliffe, J.M.; Park, H.; Madsen, K.L.; Sot-Vaca, A. Inulin-type fructans and whey protein both modulate appetite but only fructans alter gut microbiota in adults with overweight/obesity: A randomized controlled trial. *Mol. Nutr. Food Res.* **2017**, *61*, 1–17. [CrossRef] [PubMed]
55. Kim, B.; Choi, H.N.; Yim, J.E. Effect of diet on the gut microbiota associated with obesity. *J. Obesity Metab. Synd.* **2019**, *28*, 216–224. [CrossRef] [PubMed]
56. Ghaffari, S.; Roshanravan, N. The role of nutraceuticals in prevention and treatment of hypertension: An updated review of the literature. *Food Res. Int.* **2020**, *128*, 1–12. [CrossRef] [PubMed]
57. Liong, M.T. Probiotics: A critical review of their potential role as antihypertenstives, immune modulators, hypocholesterolemics, and perimenopausal treatments. *Nutr. Rev.* **2007**, *65*, 316–328. [CrossRef] [PubMed]
58. Liong, M.T.; Dunshea, F.R.; Shah, N.P. Effects of a symbiotic containing *Lactobacillus acidophilus* ATCC 4962 on plasma lipid profiles and morphology of erythrocytes in hypercholesterolemic pigs on high- and low-fat diets. *Br. J. Nutr.* **2007**, *98*, 736–744. [CrossRef] [PubMed]
59. Haghighat, N.; Mohammadshahi, M.; Shayanpour, S.; Haghighizadeh, M.H. Effect of symbiotic and probiotic supplementation on serum levels of endothelial cell adhesion molecules in hemodialysis patients: A randomized control study. *Probiotics Antimicro. Proteins* **2018**, *1*, 1–9.
60. Mofid, V.; Izadi, A.; Majtehedi, S.Y.; Khemoat, L. Therapeutic and nutritional effects of synbiotic yogurts in children and adults: A clinical review. *Probiotics Antimicrob. Proteins* **2019**, *10*, 1–17. [CrossRef]
61. Din, A.U.; Hassan, A.; Zhu, Y.; Yin, T.; Gregersen, H.; Wang, G. Amelioration of TMAO through probiotics and its potential role in atherosclerosis. *Appl. Microbiol. Biotechnol.* **2019**, *103*, 9217–9228. [CrossRef]
62. Janeiro, M.H.; Ramirez, M.J.; Milago, F.I.; Martinez, J.A.; Solas, M. Implication of trimethylamine N-oxide (TMAO) in disease: Potential biomarker or new therapeutic target. *Nutrients* **2018**, *10*, 1398. [CrossRef]
63. Wilson, T.W.H.; Wang, Z.; Levison, B.S.; Koeth, R.A.; Britt, E.B.; Fu, X.; Wu, Y.; Hazen, S.L. Intestinal microbial metabolism of phosphatidylcholine and cardiovascular risk. *N. Eng. J. Med.* **2013**, *368*, 1575–1584.
64. Moludi, J.; Alizadeh, M.; Yagin, N.L.; Pasdar, Y.; Nachvak, S.M.; Abdollahzad, H.; Tabaei, A.S. New insights on atherosclerosis: Endcananabinoid systems with gut microbiota. *J. Cardiovasc. Thorac. Res.* **2018**, *10*, 129–137. [CrossRef] [PubMed]
65. Hazen, S. *New Research on Red Meat and Heart Disease*; The Diane Rehm Show (Transcript); WAMU 88.5 American University Radio: Washington, DC, USA, 2013.
66. Collins, H.L.; Drazul-Schrader, D.; Sulpizio, A.C.; Koster, P.D.; Williamson, Y.; Adelman, S.J.; Owen, K.; Sanli, T.; Bellamine, A. L-Carnitine intake and high trimethylamine N-oxide plasma levels correlate with low aortic lesions in ApoE−/− transgenic mice expressing CETP. *Atherosclerosis* **2006**, *244*, 29–37. [CrossRef] [PubMed]

67. Ufnal, M.; Jazwiec, R.; Dadlez, M.; Drapala, A.; Sikora, M.; Skrzypecki, J. Trimethylamine-N-oxide: A carnitine-derived metabolite that prolongs the hypertensive effect of angiotensin II in rats. *Canad. J. Cardiol.* **2014**, *30*, 1700–1705. [CrossRef] [PubMed]
68. Tilg, H. A gut feeling about thrombosis. *N. Eng. J. Med.* **2016**, *374*, 2494–2496. [CrossRef]
69. Kanitsoraphan, C.; Rattanawong, P.; Charensri, S.; Vichai, S. Trimethylamine N-oxide and risk of cardiovascular disease and mortality. *Curr. Nutr. Rep.* **2018**, *7*, 2017–2213. [CrossRef] [PubMed]
70. Hardin, S.J.; Homme, R.; George, A.K.; Tyagi, S.C. Diet-induced chronic syndrome, metabolically transformed trimethylamine-N-oxide, and the cardiovascular functions. *Rev. Cardiovasc. Med.* **2019**, *20*, 121–128. [PubMed]
71. Leustean, A.M.; Ciocoiu, M.; Sava, A.; Costea, C.F.; Floria, M.; Tarniceriu, C.C.; Tanase, D.M. Implication of the intestinal microbiota in dignosisng the progression of diabetes and the presence of cardiovascular disease. *J. Diab. Res.* **2018**, 1–9. [CrossRef]
72. Tripolt, N.J.; Leber, B.; Triebl, A.; Kofeler, H.; Stadlbauer, V.; Sourij, H. Effect of Lactobacillus casei Shirota supplementation on trimethylamine-N-oxide levels in patients with metabolic syndrome: An open-label, randomized study. *Atherosclerosis* **2015**, *242*, 141–144. [CrossRef]
73. Boutagy, N.E.; Neilson, A.P.; Ostergerg, K.L.; Smithson, A.T.; England, T.R.; Davy, B.M.; Hulver, M.W.; Davy, K.P. Probiotic supplementation and trimethylamine-N-oxide production following a high-fat diet. *Obesity* **2015**, *23*, 2357–2363. [CrossRef]
74. Qui, L.; Tao, X.; Xiong, H.; Yu, J.; Wei, H. Lactobacillus plantarum ZDY04 exhibits a strain-specific property of lowering TMAO via the modulation of gut microbiota in mice. *Food Funct.* **2018**, *9*, 4299–4309.
75. Tenore, G.C.; Caruso, D.; Buonamo, G.; D'Avino, M.; Ciampaglia, R.; Maisto, M.; Schsano, C.; Bochino, B.; Novellino, E. Lactofermented annurca apple puree as a functional food indicated for the control of plasma lipid an oxidative amine levels: Results from a randomized clinical trial. *Nutrients* **2019**, *11*, 122. [CrossRef] [PubMed]
76. Liu, W.C.; Yang, M.C.; Wu, Y.Y.; Chen, P.H.; Hsu, C.M.; Chen, L.W. Lactobacillus plantarum revers diabetes-induced Fmo3 and iCAM expression in mice through enteric dysbiosis-related c-Jun NH2-terminal kinase pathways. *PLoS ONE* **2018**, *13*, e0196511.
77. Matsumoto, M.; Kitada, Y.; Shimomura, Y.; Naito, Y. Bifidobacterium animalis subsp. lactis LKM512 reduces levels of intestinal trimethylamine produced by intestinal microbiota in healthy volunteers: A double-blind, placebo-controlled study. *J. Funct. Food* **2017**, *36*, 94–101. [CrossRef]
78. Bogiatzi, C.; Gloor, G.; Allen-Vercoe, E.; Reid, G.; Wong, R.G.; Urquhart, B.L.; Dinculescu, V.; Reutz, K.N.; Velenosi, T.J.; Pignanelli, M.; et al. Metabolic products of the intestinal microbiome and extremes of atherosclerosis. *Atherosclerosis* **2018**, *273*, 91–97. [CrossRef] [PubMed]
79. Montrucchio, C.; De Nicolo, A.; D'Ettorre, G.; D'Ascenzo, F.; Lazzaro, A.; Fettoni, M.; D'Avolio, A.; Bonora, S.; Celani, L.; Di Perri, G.; et al. Serum trimethylamine-N-oxide concentrations in people living with HIV and the effect of probiotic supplementation. *Int. J. Antimicrob. Agents* **2020**, *55*, 1–10. [CrossRef] [PubMed]
80. Vadivielso, J.M.; Rodriquez-Puyol, D.; Pascual, J.; Barrios, C.; Bermudez-Lopez, M.; Sanchez-Nino, M.D.; Perez-Fernandez, M.; Ortiz, A. Atherosclerosis in chronic kidney disease: More, less, or just different? *Arterioscler. Thromb. Vasc. Biol.* **2019**, *10*, 1938–1966. [CrossRef]
81. Roumeliotis, S.; Roumeliotis, A.; Dounousi, E.; Eleftheriadis, T.; Liakopoulos, V. Dietary antioxidant supplements and uric acid in chronic kidney disease: A review. *Nutrients* **2019**, *11*, 1911. [CrossRef]
82. Rossi, M.; Johnson, D.W.; Morrison, M.; Pascoe, E.; Coombes, J.S.; Forbes, J.M.; McWhinney, B.C.; Ungerer, J.P.J.; Dimeski, G.; Campbell, K.L. SYNbiotics easing renal failure by improving gut microbiology (SYNERGY): A protocol of placebo-controlled randomized cross-over trial. *BMC Neprol.* **2014**, *15*, 1–10. [CrossRef]
83. Brown, J.M.; Hazen, S.L. Metaorganismal nutrient metabolism as a basis of cardiovascular disease. *Curr. Opin. Lipidol.* **2014**, *25*, 48–53. [CrossRef]
84. Al-Okbi, S.Y.; Mohamed, D.A.; Hamed, T.E.S.; Khalek, A.B.A.E.; Mohammed, S.E. Role of probiotic mixture with and without green tea extract in prevention of hepatorenal syndrome in rat model. *Pak. J. Biol. Sci.* **2019**, *22*, 21–27.
85. Wang, H.; Mei, L.; Deng, Y.; Liu, Y.; Wei, X.; Liu, M.; Zhou, J.; Ma, H.; Zheng, P.; Yuan, J.; et al. *Lactobacillus brevis* DM9218 ameliorates fructose-induced hyperuricemia through inosine degradation and manipulation of intestinal dysbiosis. *Nutrition* **2019**, *62*, 63–73. [CrossRef] [PubMed]
86. Tao, S.; Tao, S.; Cheng, Y.; Liu, J.; Ma, L.; Fu, P. Effects of probiotic supplements on the progression of chronic kidney disease: A meta-analysis. *Nephrology* **2019**, *24*, 1122–1130. [CrossRef] [PubMed]

87. Yamanaka, H.; Taniguchi, A.; Tsubai, H.; Kano, H.; Asami, Y. Hypouricaemic effects of yoghurt containing *Lactobacillus gasseri* PA-3 in patients with hyperuricaemia and/or gout: A randomized, double-blind, placebo-controlled study. *Mod. Rhematol.* **2019**, *29*, 146–150. [CrossRef] [PubMed]
88. Garcia-Arrayo, F.E.; Ganzaga, G.; Munoz-Jimenez, I.; Blas-Marron, M.G.; Silverio, O.; Tapia, E.; Soto, V.; Ranganathan, N.; Ranganathan, P.; Vyas, U.; et al. Probiotic supplements prevented oxonic acid-induced hyperuricemia and renal damage. *PLoS ONE* **2018**, *24*, e0202901.
89. Firouzi, S.; Haghighatdoost, F. The effects of prebiotic, probiotic, and synbiotic supplementation on blood parameters of renal function: A systematic review and meta-analysis of clinical trials. *Nutrition* **2018**, *51*, 104–113. [CrossRef]
90. Chi, C.; Li, C.; Wu, D.; Buys, N.; Wang, W.; Fan, H.; Sun, J. Effects of probiotics on patients with hypertension: A systematic review and meta-analysis. *Curr. Hypertens Rep.* **2020**, *21*, 1–12. [CrossRef]
91. Shah, B.R.; Li, B.; Al Sabbah, H.; Xu, W.; Mraz, J. Effects of prebiotic dietary fibers and probiotics on human health: With special focus on recent advancement in their encapsulated formulations. *Trends Food Sci. Technol.* **2020**, *102*, 178–192. [CrossRef]

2

Xenogeneic and Stem Cell-Based Therapy for Cardiovascular Diseases: Genetic Engineering of Porcine Cells and Their Applications in Heart Regeneration

Anne-Marie Galow [1,*], Tom Goldammer [1,2] and Andreas Hoeflich [1]

1 Institute of Genome Biology, Leibniz Institute for Farm Animal Biology, 18196 Dummerstorf, Germany; tom.goldammer@uni-rostock.de (T.G.); hoeflich@fbn-dummerstorf.de (A.H.)

2 Molecular Biology and Fish Genetics Unit, Faculty of Agriculture and Environmental Sciences, University of Rostock, 18059 Rostock, Germany

* Correspondence: galow@fbn-dummerstorf.de

Abstract: Cardiovascular diseases represent a major health concern worldwide with few therapy options for ischemic injuries due to the limited regeneration potential of affected cardiomyocytes. Innovative cell replacement approaches could facilitate efficient regenerative therapy. However, despite extensive attempts to expand primary human cells in vitro, present technological limitations and the lack of human donors have so far prevented their broad clinical use. Cell xenotransplantation might provide an ethically acceptable unlimited source for cell replacement therapies and bridge the gap between waiting recipients and available donors. Pigs are considered the most suitable candidates as a source for xenogeneic cells and tissues due to their anatomical and physiological similarities with humans. The potential of porcine cells in the field of stem cell-based therapy and regenerative medicine is under intensive investigation. This review outlines the current progress and highlights the most promising approaches in xenogeneic cell therapy with a focus on the cardiovascular system.

Keywords: cell transplantation; myocardial infarction; mesenchymal stem cells; graft rejection; triple knockout pigs; genome editing; iPSCs; CRISPR/Cas

---

1. Cardiac Wound Healing and the Road to Xenogeneic Cell Therapy

There are two pathological events representing the clinically most relevant incidents in the cardiovascular system, namely rupture of an atherosclerotic plaque and myocardial infarction (MI). Both events are accompanied with severe tissue damage and loss of cardiomyocytes. The subsequent healing process is divided in two transitional phases. The early inflammatory phase is initiated by immigration of immune cells that secrete pro-inflammatory factors and clean out the tissue. An orchestra of neutrophils, monocytes, and lymphocytes acts for hours to days to remove necrotic tissue, phagocytize bacteria that may have settled, and release growth factors. The release of transforming growth factor beta (TGF-β), fibroblast growth factors (FGFs), and platelet-derived growth factor (PDGF) stimulates fibroblast proliferation, thereby inducing the following reparative phase. The reparative phase is characterized by enhanced matrix synthesis, proliferation of fibroblasts, and scar formation and usually lasts for days to weeks but may continue over years depending on the extent of the injury [1]. Dying cardiomyocytes secrete a variety of pro-inflammatory chemokines dedicated to evoke actions from bone marrow-derived cells and to attract immune cells. Understanding the role of stem cells in the modulation of these wound healing phases is of major relevance for the development of reparative therapeutics and stem cell-based therapies for cardiac repair.

The first early stage clinical trials on stem cell transplantation suggested beneficial effects on cardiac repair for both bone marrow [2,3] and cardiac-derived stem cells [4,5] although they were only modest. To avoid immunogenicity, these trials were mainly conducted with autologous cells. Due to the fact that autologous stem cells need to be expanded for up to three weeks before they can be applied in sufficient numbers for cell therapy [6], the respective cells were applied only after endogenous repair had begun. Hence, the beneficial effects might be attenuated after initialization of scar formation. It seems apparent that besides the current technological difficulties regarding proliferative capacity and phenotype maintenance, also the time requirements limit the clinical use of primary human cells. Together with the lack of human donors, this stimulated the search for alternative sources of cells. Pigs emerged as promising candidates for the production of donor tissues as they resemble many anatomical and physiological features of humans. For the cardiovascular system in particular, properties like an identical heart weight to body weight ratio, similar coronary circulation and hemodynamics, as well as comparable healing characteristics of the myocardium [7] rendered pigs not only as a suitable model organism but also as a potential donor for heart xenotransplantation.

Beginning in the 1990s, studies in diabetic animal models have demonstrated that porcine islet cell transplantation was sufficient to normalize blood glucose in the recipients, thus proving physiologic activity and metabolic regulation across the species barrier [8,9]. These findings raised hope for the implementation of xenogeneic cell replacement as potential therapy for a multitude of human diseases and disorders and inspired a number of research activities in the newly emerging field of xenogeneic cell therapy [10–12]. In fact, translation into clinical trials was achieved for the application of porcine islets of Langerhans with [13] and without Sertoli cells [14] to treat diabetic patients. Long-term follow-up studies documented decreased insulin requirements in a majority of patients [15] and the recent development of encapsulation strategies is supposed to overcome remaining immunological complications [16].

2. Overcoming the Immunological Barrier and Graft Rejection

In general, the transplantation of foreign tissue into a recipient with a functioning immune system will trigger an immunological reaction, which needs to be contained to prevent graft rejection. This is true for allografts, but it becomes even more considerable when the graft is of xenogeneic origin. There are several challenges introduced by the interspecies differences that will be discussed in the following.

2.1. Multilayered Immunological Challenges

The oligosaccharide galactose-α1,3-galactose (Gal) is present in all mammals except for humans and old world nonhuman primates [17]. Natural anti-pig antibodies to this carbohydrate antigen activate the complement-mediated immune response, resulting in the destruction of transplanted organs and tissues within minutes or hours by primarily targeting the vascular endothelial cells [18–20]. Causative factors of this hyperacute rejection were considered similar to ABO incompatibility in allograft rejection, thus similar measures were attempted to prevent rejection. Acceptance of ABO-incompatible renal allografts could be accomplished by extracorporeal immunoadsorption of anti-A or anti-B antibodies from recipient's blood prior to the transplantation [21]. Accordingly, Taniguchi et al. depleted anti-Gal antibodies from baboon blood by specific immunoaffinity columns, thereby reducing serum cytotoxicity to pig kidney cells [22]. Thrombotic microangiopathy and subsequent graft failure can also be induced by activation of vascular endothelial cells by low levels of anti-nonGal antibodies or abnormal coagulation due to incompatibilities in the coagulation/anticoagulation factors [23,24].

For cellular xenotransplantation, the absence of vasculature attenuates the hyperacute xenograft rejection. However, there are additional immune responses that can be triggered by the xenogeneic cells, such as the activation of T-cells through direct and indirect pathways.

Direct activation is provoked by binding of recipient T cell receptors to swine leukocyte antigen class I and class II on porcine donor antigen-presenting cells, such as dendritic cells or endothelial cells constitutively expressing CD80/86 [25,26]. Indirect activation is initiated by the recognition of porcine donor peptides presented on the recipients major histocompatibility complex (MHC) class II. The subsequent T cell stimulation results in B cell activation and antibody production, thereby mediating humoral xenograft rejection [27].

Strategies to suppress xenoreactive T cells involved agents, such as CTLA4Ig (abatacept) and anti-CD40 mAb as well as anti-CD154 mAb, to block the T cell costimulation [28,29]. The soluble recombinant fusion protein, CTLA4Ig, attenuates costimulation mediated via CD28 by competing with its natural ligand B7 [30]. The costimulatory interaction of CD40 and its T cell-bound ligand CD154 is additionally involved in T cell-dependent B cell activity. Repeated administration of anti-CD154 mAb by intravenous injection could prevent an elicited antibody response to pig antigens in baboons [31]. However, combinatorial therapies targeting the CD28/B7 as well as the CD40/CD154 interaction represented the most effective approach for xenotransplantation as demonstrated for porcine skin [32], pancreas [33], and heterotopic heart transplants [34]. In all studies, agents were administered repeatedly every two to four days to maintain the effectiveness. Although these treatments improved xenogeneic graft survival to some extent, genetic engineering of the graft donor proved to be a far more successful approach.

2.2. *Genetic Engineering to Overcome the Barriers*

Pigs were genetically modified to render their tissues more resilient to the human humoral and cellular immune responses and to diminish the discrepancies to the human coagulation system. The first attempt was to introduce human complement-regulatory proteins, such as decay accelerating factor [35] and membrane cofactor protein (CD 46) [36], in porcine cells to protect them from the complement-mediated immune response of the recipient.

However, the breakthrough came only in the early 2000s when the first α1,3-galactosyltransferase gene-knockout (GTKO) pigs were generated by cloning [37] or nuclear transfer of spontaneous null mutant cells [38]. Knocking out the gene coding for the enzyme α1,3-galactosyltransferase prevents the production of Gal antigen, the main trigger for hyperacute rejections. Organs and cells from these GTKO pigs demonstrated prolonged graft survival. For example, heterotopically transplanted hearts were functional for more than two months in nonhuman primates, and in one animal, heart contractions ceased only after half a year. [39] However, xenograft rejection still occurred in GTKO pigs and was associated with activation of the innate immune system and coagulation [40]. Hence, to further improve the outcomes, GTKO pig cells were engineered to express human complement-regulatory proteins as investigated in vitro [41] and in vivo [42]. Whereas porcine endothelial cells transgenic for human complement regulatory protein CD46 were resistant to lysis by human and baboon serum [41], hearts from GTKO pigs expressing another complement regulatory protein CD55 did not show further extended graft survival in heterotopic cardiac pig-to-baboon transplantation, although local complement activation was restricted [42]. The observation of chronic vascular antibody deposition and endothelial cell activation suggested that rejection was initiated by non-Gal antigens.

In 2011, another porcine antigen, namely N-glycolylneuraminic acid (NeuGc), was found to elicit natural antibodies in humans, thereby increasing the transplant rejection risk [43]. NeuGc is expressed by most nonhuman mammals, which renders in vivo studies like in experimental pig-to-baboon organ transplantation problematic. However, the production of double knockout pigs by homozygous disruption of α1,3-galactosyltransferase (GGTA1), and cytidine monophosphate-N-acetylneuraminic acid hydroxylase (CMAH) prevents the adverse effects of these antibody–antigen interactions [44] and was a further step towards successful xenogeneic transplantation.

In 2015, the first triple knockout (TKO) pigs were created lacking the genes for GGTA1, CMAH, and additionally β4GalNT2, the gene coding for β1,4 *N*-acetylgalactosaminyltransferase (Sda), which was suggested to produce further xenoantigens for many humans [45]. Many humans display minimal or no natural antibodies to TKO pig cells, which leaves cellular rather than antibody-mediated rejection as the next hurdle for clinical application.

In order to address the T cell-mediated immune response, pigs overexpressing pCTLA4-Ig were produced both on a wild-type and GTKO background. However, these pigs exhibited reduced humoral immunity, which obliged the prophylactic use of antibiotics to promote their survival [46]. A promising alternative was proposed by the insertion of a mutant human MHC class II transactivator transgene in pigs that causes a downregulation of swine leukocyte class II expression and thereby reduces the human T cell response [47].

Another approach involves the overexpression of programmed cell death ligand 1 (PD-L1). In vitro studies with porcine PD-L1 expressing vascular endothelial cells and PD-L1 expressing B cells demonstrated a suppressed proliferation of human CD4 T cells and an enhanced expansion of regulatory T cells coupled with increased interleukin-10 production [48,49]. These results imply the potential of using human PD-L1-overexpressing porcine cells as a means to foster tolerance of other cell and tissue xenotransplants.

Human regulatory T cells can also be added directly in the context of xenotransplantation, where they have been shown to partly suppress the xenogeneic T cell response [50]. Besides regulatory T cells, mesenchymal stromal cells (MSCs) have unique anti-inflammatory and immunomodulatory properties and genetically modified porcine MSCs were shown to downregulate the human T cell response to porcine antigens in vitro, further implying considerable potential in xenotransplantation [51].

Complications with abnormal coagulation were tackled with additional genetic manipulations, such as the insertion of anticoagulant genes. Modification of GTKO pigs to express not only CD46 but also thrombomodulin resulted in prolonged graft survival [52]. Furthermore, porcine aortic endothelial cells transgenic for tissue factor pathway inhibitor were shown to exhibit a decreased expression of tissue factor, the primary initiator of blood coagulation [53].

In summary, the optimal xenogeneic donor might be a TKO pig that expresses minimally one human complement regulatory protein and another human coagulation regulatory protein. The introduction of further human transgenes, such as heme oxygenase 1 and CD47, might prove to be valuable for graft survival due to the general anti-inflammatory effects and the suppressive effect on monocyte and macrophage function, respectively [54]. Recent results with highly genetically engineered pigs were encouraging [55]; nevertheless, the study pointed at another pitfall, namely the influence of viruses [56].

3. Infection Risks in Xenogeneic Cell Therapy

The creation of TKO pigs constituted significant progress towards xenogeneic cell therapy. However, there are further risks and limitations associated with the transplantation of xenogeneic cells besides their immunological rejection. Complications during the engraftment, primary dysfunction of a graft, and potential transmission of infections are incidents to be considered attentively.

The infection risk associated with transplantation of porcine tissues into humans has been discussed already at the onset of research in this field [57,58] and is continuously curated today [59,60]. Hepatitis E virus (HEV), porcine cytomegalovirus (PCMV), porcine circovirus (PCV), and C-type porcine endogenous retroviruses (PERVs) are thought to pose a particular risk to possibly immunocompromised recipients. Detection systems for the respective viruses are discussed in a recent review [60].

HEV is a non-enveloped, single-stranded, positive-sense RNA virus that can induce hepatitis in humans. Besides two genotypes mainly found in humans, there are also two further genotypes (gt3 and gt4) that predominantly infect pigs [61]. However, HEV of the genotype 3 can be transmitted to humans by extensive contact with pigs or the consumption of undercooked pork [62]. Although the infections are asymptomatic in most cases and the rare symptomatic zoonotic diseases are usually mild, the virus might pose a risk in the setting of xenogeneic cell transplantations due to the potentially immunosuppressed status of the recipients. Therefore, different elimination strategies in herds generated for xenotransplantation are proposed.

The cytomegalovirus is an enveloped DNA virus belonging to the family *Herpesviridae*. For human cytomegalovirus, a negative impact on morbidity and mortality in allotransplantation is reported [63].

Thus, concern on the potential pathogenicity of porcine cytomegalovirus in xenotransplantation is deemed justified. The influence of PCMV on human transplant recipients is unclear. However, in baboons, PCMV transmission in orthotopic pig heart xenotransplantation was recently found to be associated with a shorter survival time of the transplant [64].

Circoviruses are non-enveloped spherical particles with a single-stranded circular small DNA genome belonging to the virus family *Circoviridae*. Porcine circovirus 3 (PCV3) is widespread among pigs and wild boars worldwide and was recently also detected in a herd of TKO pigs for xenotransplantation. After orthotopic heart transplantation, transmission of PCV3 to the recipient baboons was observed. A higher virus load in individuals with a longer survival time suggested an ongoing replication of the virus. However, in vitro experiments with 293T cells implicated that human cells could not be infected with PCV3 [65].

Of all the porcine viruses, PERVs are of particular concern due to the inherent characteristics of retroviruses. As endogenous viral elements in the genome, they cannot be eliminated by pathogen-free breeding. In contrast to human endogenous retroviruses that are in general inactive, PERVs have been shown to actively replicate in the pig [66]. Three closely related porcine endogenous retroviruses (PERV-A, -B, -C) were identified in pig [67], two of which are polytropic and can infect human cells [68,69]. Using clustered regularly interspaced short palindromic repeat-associated nuclease technology CRISPR/Cas, 62 PERVs could be inactivated in a porcine kidney cell line that normally releases high levels of infectious PERV in vitro [70]. Recently, the first PERV-inactivated pigs were successfully generated [71], suggesting that there might be completely PERV-free herds available for xenotransplantation in the future.

4. Stem Cells and Their Applications in Cardiovascular Regeneration

Stem cells can be subdivided in two categories, namely embryonic stem cells (ESCs) and adult stem cells. ESCs are derived from the inner cell mass of embryos in the blastocyst stage and can differentiate into any lineage. In contrast to adult stem cells, which demonstrate limited passage capacity, they can theoretically be maintained in culture indefinitely by continuous passaging. ESCs possess many further advantages, such as higher proliferation rate, stable morphology and telomerase activity under long-term cultivation, as well as pluripotency. Still, they turned out to be less favorable for cell-based therapies due to difficulties in efficient isolation, ethical concerns, and the widely reported tumorigenicity [72]. Therefore, research on clinical applications for cardiovascular diseases relies more heavily on adult stem cells nowadays.

A variety of adult stem cell types has been tested for their capacity for cardiac repair. A beneficial effect on cardiac function after injury was shown for cardiac progenitor cells [73,74], bone marrow-derived stem cells [75,76], induced pluripotent stem cells [77,78], as well as skeletal myoblasts [79,80]. These stem cell types display individual advantages, limitations, and practicability issues in clinical settings [81,82]. Progress in the application of different human stem populations as therapy for heart diseases in preclinical and clinical studies was recently evaluated [83].

Although stem cells derived from heart and bone marrow bear the capability to differentiate into the cardiac or mesenchymal lineage [84,85], it is now clear that they contribute minimally to newly formed cardiomyocytes [86–88]. Instead, stem cells induce neovascularization, stimulate endogenous stem cells, and modulate the post MI inflammatory response, thereby reducing scar formation [74,89,90].

4.1. Porcine Mesenchymal Stem Cells as a Promising Candidate in Cardiac Regeneration

Mesenchymal stem cells comprise a heterogeneous group of stromal cells holding postnatal capacity for self-renewal and multilineage differentiation [91]. They can be easily isolated from many tissues, such as bone marrow, adipose tissue, peripheral blood, and heart [92,93].

Due to their heterogeneity, a precise definition of MSCs remains problematic, but the International Society for Cellular Therapy defined minimal criteria to foster a more uniform characterization. Criteria are: (i) MSCs must be plastic adherent when maintained in standard culture conditions;

(ii) MSCs must express CD105, CD73, and CD90, while lacking expression of CD45, CD34, CD14 or CD11b, CD79alpha or CD19, and human leukocyte antigen (HLA)-DR surface molecules; and (iii) MSCs must differentiate into osteoblasts, adipocytes, and chondroblasts in vitro [94].

MSCs are attractive candidates for cell-based therapy not only for their secretion of bioactive molecules activating tissue repair processes but also for their lack of cell surface histocompatibility complex (HLA) class II molecules and T cell costimulatory molecules, rendering them immunoprivileged. These characteristics together with a paracrine-mediated immunomodulatory activity allowed for the usage of allogeneic MSCs without pharmacological immunosuppression in cardiomyopathy patients [95], thereby raising hope for a successful application of porcine MSCs in cardiovascular regeneration across the xenogeneic transplant barriers. In fact, several studies provided evidence that MSCs successfully engrafted and functioned across the species barrier without any immunosuppression as lined out in the literature search of Li et al. [96]. Although the majority of studies concerned the transplantation of human MSCs in other species, there is also evidence for the successful engraftments of porcine cells into rodent brain [97], bone marrow [98], and infarcted hearts [99].

A comprehensive review on the characteristics of porcine mesenchymal stem cells and their therapeutic potential towards various diseases was provided by Bharli et al. [100]. For cardiovascular regeneration in particular, the administration of MSCs to diseased hearts results in improved cardiac function and reduced scar size. The underlying mechanisms for these positive effects are manifold, including direct and indirect contribution to angio- and arteriogenesis, regulation of immune responses, activation of cytoprotective pathways in reversibly injured cardiomyocytes, and stimulation of resident cardiac cell proliferation [101,102]. However, the relative contribution of each mechanism to the regenerative effect is yet to be illuminated. Although transdifferentiation of MSCs into cardiomyocytes and vascular components was repeatedly described [103,104]; evidence consolidates that the contribution of MSCs to heart regeneration is mainly based on their release of numerous cytokines and paracrine factors, rather than direct cell replacement [89,105,106]. Allogeneic cell combination therapy utilizing not only mesenchymal stem cells but also cardiac stem cells was proven to elicit synergistic effects [107] and might also prove beneficial in prospective xenogeneic therapies. In fact, studies with human bone marrow-derived MSCs and c-kit-positive cardiac stem cells demonstrated that applications across the human–pig species barrier are feasible [108,109]. Table 1 presents a list of studies utilizing porcine mesenchymal stem cells in diverse disease models to explore their effect on cardiac regeneration. Notably, porcine mesenchymal stem cells were primarily applied in autologous or allogenic approaches, reflecting the significance of the pig as a preferential preclinical model for human cardiac pathologies but leaving open the question why there are no pig-to-baboon studies for stem cell transplantation. In fact, preclinical studies on stem cell therapy for cardiac diseases in non-human primates are scarce in general [110] and concentrated on human embryonic stem cell-derived cardiomyocytes [111,112] or iPSCs [113]. Thus, the lack of xenogeneic studies on porcine mesenchymal stem cells is most likely attributable to a combination of preference of the pig over the mouse as a preclinical model system and rareness of ethically more critically considered primate studies.

Table 1. Studies on the effect of porcine mesenchymal stem cells in heart regeneration. The table outlines the conditions and outcomes of mesenchymal stem cell-based therapies in several cardiovascular disease models published 2010–2020. ATMSCs: Adipose tissue-derived mesenchymal stem cells, ATSCs: adipose tissue-derived stem cell, CDCs: Cardiosphere-derived cells.

Cell Type and Cell Number	Delivery Method	Clinical Condition	Main Outcome	Study
Autologous MSC 3×10^7 cells	Direct left ventricular injection	Acute MI	Improved cardiac function Reduced oxidative stress and inflammatory response	[114]
Allogeneic ATMSCs 1×10^7 cells	Intracoronary infusion	Acute MI	Unaltered cardiac function Unaltered scar size Promoted revascularization	[115]

Table 1. *Cont.*

Cell Type and Cell Number	Delivery Method	Clinical Condition	Main Outcome	Study
Allogeneic ATMSCs 5×10^7 cells Overexpressing IGF-1 or HGF	Intramyocardial injection	Acute MI	Unaltered cardiac function Promoted revascularization Reduced inflammation Enhanced fibrosis	[116]
Allogeneic ATDPCs 1.75×10^6 cells	Recellularized myocardial scaffold	Acute MI	Improved cardiac function Reduced infarct size Promoted revascularization Attenuated fibrosis	[117]
Xenogeneic MSCs 1×10^6 cells	Intramyocardial injection	Acute MI	Improved cardiac function Unaltered infarct size Improved preservation of capillarity	[99]
Allogeneic MSCs 1.4×10^7 cells	Intramyocardial injection	Subacute MI	Unaltered cardiac function Reduced scar size	[118]
Autologous BMCs eNOS-transfected 1×10^7 cells	Intramyocardial injection	Subacute MI	Improved cardiac function Unaltered scar size Unaltered fibrosis	[119]
ATSCs 1×10^7 cells	Intramyocardial injection	Subacute MI	Improved cardiac function Reduced infarct size	[120]
Autologous MSC 6×10^7 cells	Intramyocardial injection	Chronic MI	Unaltered cardiac function Unaltered scar size Attenuation of LV wall thinning	[121]
Autologous BMCs 5×10^6	Left or right coronary artery infusion	Chronic MI	Improved cardiac function Promoted revascularization	[122]
Allogeneic MSC 2×10^8 cells	Intramyocardial injection	Chronic MI	Improved cardiac function Reduced scar size	[104]
Allogeneic MSC 1.5×10^7 cells	Recellularized collagen scaffold	Chronic MI	Improved cardiac function Reduced scar size Promoted revascularization	[123]
Allogeneic MSCs and CDCs 3.5×10^7 cells	Intracoronary infusion	Chronic ischemic cardiomyopathy (coronary stenosis)	Improved cardiac function Unaltered perfusion Improved remote wall thickening	[124]
Allogeneic MSCs and CSCs 2×10^8 cells	Transendocardial injection	Chronic ischemic cardiomyopathy	Improved cardiac function Reduced scar size Low-grade inflammatory infiltrates	[107]

4.2. Delivery and Final Fate

Cell dosing and the route of administration are crucial for the outcome of cell-based therapies. However, missing standards are still leading to inconsistent results in preclinical and clinical studies on stem cell-based therapy for cardiovascular disease [125]. Implementing efficient delivery methods and assuring long-term retention of grafted cells in the target area is challenging. There are a variety of methods for cell administration into a patient's myocardium, such as direct surgical intramyocardial injection, catheter-based intramyocardial administration, intravenous infusion, intracoronary artery administration, retrograde coronary venous delivery, and transplantation of engineered monolayer tissue [126], each with individual advantages and drawbacks.

Despite the availability of safe and technologically feasible delivery routes, benefits in cardiac function restoration observed in preclinical animal models could not be reproduced in humans so far. One underlying reason is that all delivery routes demonstrate rather low ratios of cell engraftment and survival in preclinical and clinical trials.

For example, early studies in an ischemic swine model demonstrated retention rates of peripheral blood mononuclear cells within the myocardium of only about 2.6%, 3.2%, and 11% after intracoronary, interstitial retrograde coronary venous, and intramyocardial delivery, respectively [127]. For these low retention rates, some of the delivery routes are controversially discussed regarding their actual impact on the recovery of cardiac function [126,128].

As a consequence, an increasing number of studies nowadays focuses on combining stem cells with synthetic or natural scaffolds. For cell delivery, both solid scaffolds used as biomimetic cardiac patches as well as soluble materials, such as injectable hydrogels, are commonly applied [129,130]. In general, these matrices are supposed to provide a suitable cellular microenvironment and ideally allow mechanical and electrical coupling with the host myocardium.

For preclinical trials, swine is commonly used as the translational model, for example, for the application of decellularized extracellular matrices (ECMs) of porcine as well as human origin as a scaffold for stem cells. Such bioactive constructs have been demonstrated to integrate well into cardiac tissues, where they support cardiac function and reduce myocardial scar formation [117,131,132]. However, decellularization of porcine heart tissue followed by efficient recellularization with patient-specific human induced pluripotent stem cells (iPSCs) to gain a fully functional cardiac patch poses a breakthrough that has yet to be achieved.

Interestingly, significant therapeutic effects in postischemic models were also observed when such constructs were used without cells. It is now understood that ECM can support cardiac regeneration by stimulating angiogenesis and cardiomyocyte proliferation via biochemical and biomechanical signaling [133–135]. Naturally occurring sources of suitable extracellular matrices include small intestinal submucosa, urinary bladder matrix, pericardium, as well as myocardial tissue itself [136].

4.3. Genetic Engineering to Improve Efficiency of Mesenchymal Stem Cells

Several mechanisms may account for the poor engraftment and survival rates of transplanted stem cells. During preparation of the cell suspensions, proapoptotic signaling might be triggered by compromised integrin-mediated survival and discontinuation of contacts and intercellular communication between cells and the extracellular matrix. After transplantation, apoptosis could be activated by several stressors present in the infarct and/or peri-infarct area, such as hypoxia, acidosis, nutrient deficiency, reactive oxygen species (ROS), inflammatory mediators, and cytotoxic agents [101]. The survival of transplanted MSCs is determined by the balance between these proapoptotic signals, mainly mediated through toll-like receptor 4 (TLR4) and G protein-coupled receptors, on the one hand and prosurvival pathways, such as the phosphoinositide 3-kinase (PI3K), protein kinase B (AKT), and extracellular signal-regulated kinase 1/2 (ERK1/2) pathways, on the other hand.

To increase the therapeutic effect of MSCs, several attempts have been made to render them more resistant to apoptosis. Targeted deletion of the proapoptotic TLR4 resulted in increased AKT activation and decreased hypoxia-induced apoptosis in murine MSCs [137] associated with improved myocardial recovery by elevated angiogenic factor production [138]. On the other side, porcine bone marrow-derived MSCs were transduced with AKT to strengthen prosurvival signals [139]. Indeed, AKT-MSCs showed reduced intracellular ROS levels and apoptosis induced by H_2O_2. Moreover, they demonstrated higher levels of vascular endothelial growth factor (VEGF) production and ERK1/2 activation, resulting in improved cardiac function after cellular transplantation.

Other genetic modifications for increased MSC survival target the heme oxygenase-1 gene; heat shock proteins; antiapoptotic proteins, such as Bcl-2, Bcl-xL, connexin 43, and survivin; or transcription factors, such as GATA-4 and HIF-1α, but are mainly conducted in rodent models and not yet translated to preclinical large animal models [101].

Retention could be improved by manipulation of the integrin signaling pathway. Porcine MSCs overexpressing integrin-linked kinase showed increased proliferation and reduced apoptosis, demonstrated by the TUNEL method (terminal deoxynucleotidyl transferase-mediated dUTP nick-end labeling). Upon transplantation, enhanced angiogenesis and cardiomyocyte proliferation was observed in pigs after MI while fibroses was reduced, resulting in improved ventricular remodeling and cardiac function [140].

Next to improving the retention and survival rates, there is another approach to improve the efficiency of stem cells, namely to increase their production of cardioprotective cytokines and growth factors. The most relevant factors for myocardial regeneration secreted by MSCs include VEGF, TGFβ, hepatocyte growth factor (HGF), platelet-derived growth factor (PDGF), stromal cell-derived factor 1 (SDF-1), fibroblast growth factor β (FGFβ), angiopoietin 1 (ANG-1), granulocyte colony-stimulating factor (G-CSF), and interleukin-8 (IL-8) [141].

The overexpression of both insulin-like growth factor 1 (IGF-1) and HGF in MSCs resulted in reduced inflammation and improved angiogenesis in a pig MI model. However, cardiac function parameters were not significantly improved [116]. In contrast, intramyocardial delivery of bone marrow mesenchymal stromal cells overexpressing mutant human HIF1-α reduced infarct size and improved LV systolic performance in another large animal model [142]. VEGF and ANGP-1 were significantly upregulated in the peri-infarct zone, supporting increased neovascularization and cardioprotective effects. Hypoxia-induced overexpression of VEGF facilitated its ischemia-responsive production and was sufficient to significantly increase myocardial neovascularization and attenuate left ventricular remodeling after myocardial infarction in a rat model [143].

The recent development and refinement of programmable nucleases, such as zinc-finger nucleases, transcription activator–like effector nucleases (TALENs), and clustered regularly interspaced short palindromic repeat (CRISPR)–Cas nucleases, may soon allow for a save application of gene editing in clinical practice. High nuclease activity and specificity was proven in various preclinical disease models and a number of clinical gene-editing trials are on the way [144].

However, despite the progress in DNA-based approaches, miRNA approaches might pose the more applicable method for future clinical translation as epigenetic modifications hold the possibility of transient action. There are three main strategies pursued with miRNAs: (i) improving the survival rates of transplanted cells, (ii) enhancing therapeutic efficacy by increased factor secretion, and (iii) supporting differentiation in cardiomyocytes.

The ability of miRNAs to protect MSCs during post-transplantation in the infarct heart has been demonstrated for miR-133 [145], miRNA-301a [146], and a cocktail of miR-21, miR-24, and miR-221 [147]. By employing miR-126 [148] or miR-146 [149], stem cells could be modified to enhance their paracrine release of angiogenic factors, such as VEGF, thereby improving ischemic angiogenesis and cell survival in the damaged heart. For the promotion of cardiomyocyte differentiation, overexpression of let-7 family members was shown to result in a matured morphology as well as increased force of contraction and respiratory capacity in human stem cell-derived cardiomyocytes [150]. Furthermore, overexpression of miR1-2 has been shown to promote cardiomyocyte differentiation in mouse MSCs via the activation of the Wnt/β-catenin signaling pathway [151]. Targeting the same pathway, also overexpression of miR-499 could induce mesenchymal stem cells toward cardiac differentiation [152]. Recently, first therapeutic miRNA-based applications inhibiting miR-132 (NCT04045405) or miR-92a (NCT03603431) were examined, marking the onset of translation of cardiac epigenetic modifications into the clinic.

The genetic engineering approaches in mesenchymal stem cell therapy as well as the other earlier mentioned xenogeneic approaches in heart regeneration therapy are illustrated in Figure 1.

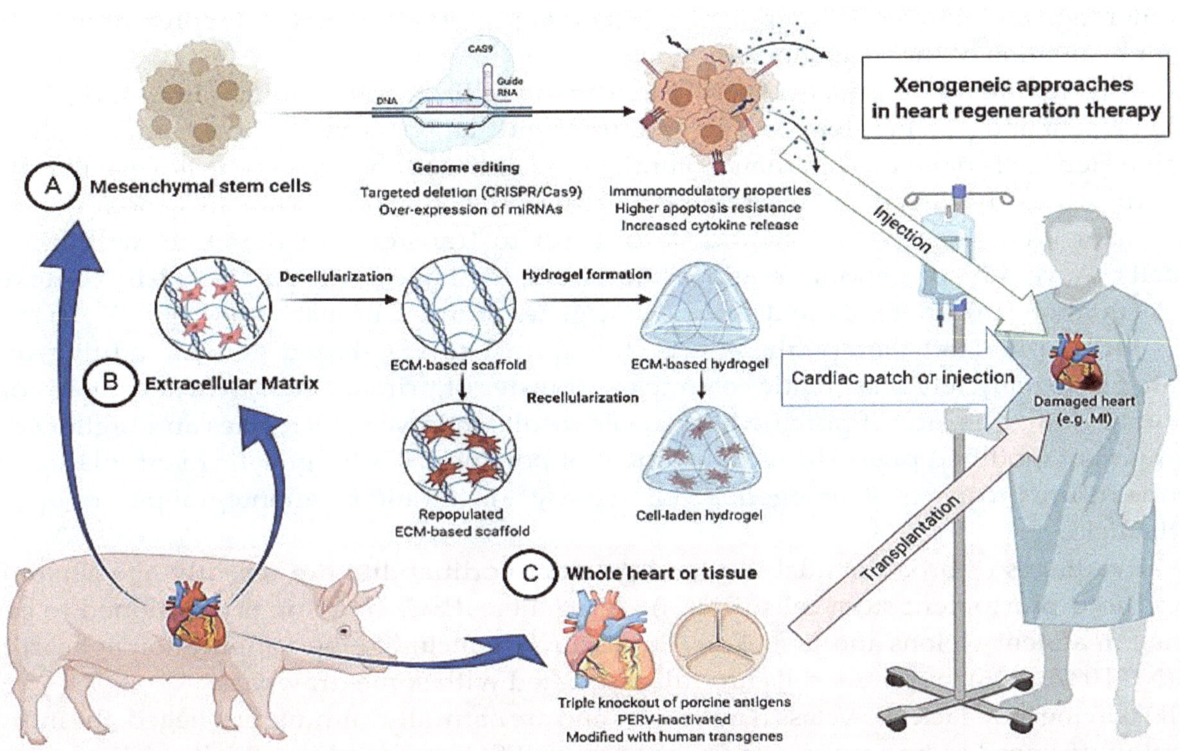

Figure 1. Summary of three conceivable xenogeneic approaches in heart regeneration therapy. Generally possible applications utilizing the pig as a donor include (**A**) transplantation of mesenchymal stem cells, (**B**) insertion of acellular or populated extracellular matrix, and (**C**) transplantation of the whole heart or heart valves of genetically engineered animals.

5. Future Prospects for Xenogeneic Cell Therapy

Allogenic cell transplantation as therapy to improve cardiac function was demonstrated to be feasible in pig [153] but also in human [154], where the administration of allogenic cells did not trigger immune-mediated events. Thus, one could question why xenogeneic cell therapy should be considered at all when allogeneic cell transplantation is possible, but there are major advantages coming with the pig as donor.

Even if one were to leave aside the lack of human donors, there is one basic and initiatory obstacle to the broad deployment of stem cell-based therapy. The low isolation rates of these primary cells cause the need for expansion before an application in the patient is appropriate. In clinical studies applying MSCs for the treatment of chronic and acute cardiovascular diseases, high cell numbers, ranging from 1×10^6 up to more than 1×10^9, are typically administered to compensate for the low survival and retention rates [155]. The time lapse between stem cell isolation and delivery renders early engraftment in acute MI impossible when relying on autologous cells or freshly isolated cells of allogenic donors.

Cryopreservation could bypass this bottleneck and allow for readily available cells, as it is the gold standard when cell storage and transportation is required. However, there are deviating observations regarding the impact of cryopreservation on various MSC features as discussed in detail in a recent review [156]. As opposed to physical damage, other aspects, such as gene expression alterations, stress responses, and epigenetic, changes after thawing are usually less assessed. The present data suggest that cryopreservation has no significant influence on proliferation, morphology, or differentiation of bone marrow-derived MSCs but does appear to influence viability, attachment, immunomodulation, and metabolism.

Since there is now general consent that the positive effect of transplanted MSCs in cardiac regeneration is mainly attributed to paracrine signaling instead of differentiation into cardiomyocytes, stable proliferation and differentiation potential after cryopreservation may not represent the adequate features for evaluation of their functional potency.

In contrast to human donors, genetically modified pig lines with minimal immunogenicity are constantly present and porcine stem cells of various origin can be harvested in advance at all times.

Porcine stem cells have proven their potential for cell-based therapy in cardiovascular diseases in many studies as discussed in this review. Furthermore, the possibility to genetically modify pigs is a major advantage, which would be difficult to transfer into the clinic with allogeneic human cells. A variety of genome engineering strategies have been employed in context with xenotransplantation [157], not only to delete porcine genes or insert human genes, but also to engineer stem cells with optimized therapeutic effects. In contrast to ESC-based genome editing in mice, these strategies usually rely on somatic cell nuclear transfer of primary cells, which is more complex and elaborate [158]. The lack of porcine ESC stocks results in lower efficiencies and higher costs for the generation of modified pigs. The establishment of porcine ESCs for genetic manipulation would advance the future prospects of xenogeneic cell therapy and should be an integral part of upcoming work in the field.

The advantages of broad availability and genetic modifiability are recently also shared with human-induced pluripotent stem cells (iPSCs). Allogeneic iPSCs banking is envisioned to provide off-the-shelf treatment options and first clinical trials already included their application in heart failure patients (NCT03763136), but these cells are still associated with some drawbacks.

While porcine MSC lack HLA class II molecules and are naturally immunoprivileged, the individual MHC haplotypes need to be considered for allogeneic iPSCs to avoid the T cell-mediated immune response and rejection of grafted cells. Interestingly, in murine models, even autologous iPSCs were shown to elicit an immune response when used in an undifferentiated state [159].

Generating one clinical-grade iPSC line is associated with financial expenses around 800,000USD [160]. Thus, instead of generating fully personalized iPSCs, HLA-haplotyped iPSC cell banks matching to the majority of recipients are discussed as an alternative approach [161]. The establishment of such cell banks is not free of barriers and the costs are still considerable [160,162], rendering the application of iPSCs for the production of cellular therapeutics commercially not necessarily superior to porcine MSCs. Furthermore, there is still some uncertainty on the actual impact of reported genetic aberrations in iPSCs in terms of functionality and the risk of teratoma formation [163].

On the other side, the size of adult pigs represents a husbandry challenge for standard laboratory facilities and costs for housing are substantial. For this reason, the generation of porcine MSCs might remain restricted to specialized laboratories, limiting the options for acute applications without employing potentially adverse cryopreservation for transportation. Both allogeneic and xenogeneic cell therapy approaches have their limitations. The future will show which strategy will be more feasible for applications in clinical settings.

Recently, genome editing by RNA-guided endonucleases (CRISPR/Cas9) in combination with iPSCs has paved the way for many exciting new opportunities, one of which is the creation of human cells and even organs from genetically modified chimeric pigs. In 2017, a pig blastocyst was successfully injected with human cells to create a chimeric pig for the first time [164]. Although chimeric pigs might provide an unrestricted resource of cells and organs that would be completely tolerated by the recipient's immune system, there are also fundamental ethical concerns [165].

An ethically uncontroversial approach is the application of decellularized tissues and matrices for cardiac regeneration therapy [166] as mentioned earlier. For this, decellularized extracellular matrix derived from porcine myocardium turned out to be the ideal scaffold for cardiac patches [167] or as a source for injectable matrix hydrogels [168], both shown to improve cardiac repair after myocardial infarction. Due to the limited access to healthy human hearts as a source for ECM, age-dependent shifts in ECM composition and significant patient-to-patient variability, human decellularized myocardium is not a well scalable option for the clinic. Thus, the pig remains as an optimal donor and xenogeneic therapy as a prospective clinical approach for heart regeneration. In 2019, a clinical trial on the application of a hydrogel derived from decellularized porcine myocardium proved its safety and feasibility and suggested improvements in 15 early and late myocardial infarction patients, warranting validation of efficacy in larger trials [169].

As research on cell therapies focuses more and more on iPSCs, the future of xenogeneic therapy approaches could shift towards acellular products. Either way, there will be special regulations to meet. Cell-based medicinal products, which apply also to xenogeneic products, are subject to specific regulations and directives guided by agencies, such as the US Food and Drug Administration or the European Medicines Agency [170]. Continuous monitoring for infectious pathogens in designated pathogen-free source animals must be accompanied by a standardized storage of samples and archiving of records from the donor animal. Acellular products like heart valves and other decellularized matrices are not classified as cell therapy products but are subject to their own regulations. Documents about safety and requirements for entering clinical trials are provided by the WHO and the International Xenotransplantation Association [144]. With appropriate regulatory frameworks in place, the way should be paved for xenogeneic cell therapy for cardiovascular diseases, in particular utilizing MSC and ECM products.

Acknowledgments: I would like to acknowledge BioRender (https://biorender.com/) who provided the publicly available illustrations that have been used to create Figure 1.

Abbreviations

ANG-1	angiopoietin 1
ATMSC	adipose tissue-derived mesenchymal stem cell
ATSC	adipose tissue-derived stem cell
CDC	cardiosphere-derived cells
CRISPR	clustered regularly interspaced short palindromic repeat
ECM	extracellular matrix
ERK1/2	extracellular signal-regulated kinase 1/2
ESC	embryonal stem cell
FGFβ	fibroblast growth factor β
G-CSF	granulocyte colony-stimulating factor
GTKO	galactosyltransferase knockout
HEV	hepatitis E virus
HGF	hepatocyte growth factor
HLA	human leukocyte antigen
IGF-1	Insulin-like growth factor 1
IL-8	interleukin-8
iPSCs	induced pluripotent stem cells
MHC	major histocompatibility complex
MI	myocardial infarction
MSC	mesenchymal stromal cells
PCMV	porcine cytomegalovirus
PCV	porcine circovirus
PDGF	platelet-derived growth factor
PD-L1	programmed cell death ligand 1
PERV	porcine endogenous retroviruses
PI3K	phosphoinositide 3-kinase
ROS	reactive oxygen species
SDF-1	stromal cell-derived factor 1
SLA	swine leukocyte antigen
TALEN	transcription activator-like effector nucleases

TGFβ	transforming growth factor β
TKO	triple knockout
TLR4	toll-like receptor 4
VEGF	vascular endothelial growth factor

References

1. Czubryt, M.P. Common threads in cardiac fibrosis, infarct scar formation, and wound healing. *Fibrogenesis Tissue Repair* **2012**, *5*, 19. [CrossRef] [PubMed]
2. Schächinger, V.; Erbs, S.; Elsässer, A.; Haberbosch, W.; Hambrecht, R.; Hölschermann, H.; Yu, J.; Corti, R.; Mathey, D.G.; Hamm, C.W.; et al. Intracoronary bone marrow–derived progenitor cells in acute myocardial infarction. *N. Engl. J. Med.* **2006**, *355*, 1210–1221. [CrossRef] [PubMed]
3. Chen, S.; Fang, W.; Ye, F.; Liu, Y.-H.; Qian, J.; Shan, S.; Zhang, J.; Chunhua, R.Z.; Liao, L.; Lin, S.; et al. Effect on left ventricular function of intracoronary transplantation of autologous bone marrow mesenchymal stem cell in patients with acute myocardial infarction. *Am. J. Cardiol.* **2004**, *94*, 92–95. [CrossRef] [PubMed]
4. Makkar, R.R.; Smith, R.R.; Cheng, K.; Malliaras, K.; Thomson, L.E.J.; Berman, D.; Czer, L.S.C.; Marbán, L.; Mendizabal, A.; Johnston, P.V.; et al. Intracoronary cardiosphere-derived cells for heart regeneration after myocardial infarction (CADUCEUS): A prospective, randomised phase 1 trial. *Lancet* **2012**, *379*, 895–904. [CrossRef]
5. Chugh, A.R.; Beache, G.; Loughran, J.H.; Mewton, N.; Elmore, J.B.; Kajstura, J.; Pappas, P.; Tatooles, A.; Stoddard, M.F.; Lima, J.A.C.; et al. Administration of cardiac stem cells in patients with ischemic cardiomyopathy (the SCIPIO Trial): Surgical aspects and interim analysis of myocardial function and viability by magnetic resonance. *Circulation* **2012**, *126*, S54–S64. [CrossRef]
6. Malik, N. *Allogeneic Versus Autologous Stem-Cell Therapy*; BioPharm International: San Mateo, CA, USA, 2012; Volume 25.
7. Lelovas, P.P.; Kostomitsopoulos, N.G.; Xanthos, T.T. A comparative anatomic and physiologic overview of the porcine heart. *J. Am. Assoc. Lab. Anim. Sci.* **2014**, *53*, 7.
8. Liu, X.; Federlin, K.F.; Bretzel, R.G.; Hering, B.J.; Brendel, M.D. Persistent reversal of diabetes by transplantation of fetal pig proislets into nude mice. *Diabetes* **1991**, *40*, 858–866. [CrossRef]
9. Tze, W.J.; Tai, J.; Cheung, S.S.; Bissada, N.; Tsang, A. A diabetic rabbit model for pig islet xenotransplantation. *Transplantation* **1993**, *56*, 1348–1352. [CrossRef]
10. Groth, C.G.; Korsgren, O.; Tibell, A.; Tollemar, J.; Möller, E.; Bolinder, J.; Ostman, J.; Reinholt, F.P.; Hellerström, C.; Andersson, A. Transplantation of porcine fetal pancreas to diabetic patients. *Lancet Lond. Engl.* **1994**, *344*, 1402–1404. [CrossRef]
11. Kordower, J.H.; Freeman, T.B.; Snow, B.J.; Vingerhoets, F.J.; Mufson, E.J.; Sanberg, P.R.; Hauser, R.A.; Smith, D.A.; Nauert, G.M.; Perl, D.P. Neuropathological evidence of graft survival and striatal reinnervation after the transplantation of fetal mesencephalic tissue in a patient with Parkinson's disease. *N. Engl. J. Med.* **1995**, *332*, 1118–1124. [CrossRef]
12. Isacson, O.; Deacon, T.W.; Pakzaban, P.; Galpern, W.R.; Dinsmore, J.; Burns, L.H. Transplanted xenogeneic neural cells in neurodegenerative disease models exhibit remarkable axonal target specificity and distinct growth patterns of glial and axonal fibres. *Nat. Med.* **1995**, *1*, 1189–1194. [CrossRef]
13. Valdés-González, R.A.; Dorantes, L.M.; Garibay, G.N.; Bracho-Blanchet, E.; Mendez, A.J.; Dávila-Pérez, R.; Elliott, R.B.; Terán, L.; White, D.J.G. Xenotransplantation of porcine neonatal islets of Langerhans and Sertoli cells: A 4-year study. *Eur. J. Endocrinol.* **2005**, *153*, 419–427. [CrossRef]
14. Wang, W.; Mo, Z.; Ye, B.; Hu, P.; Liu, S.; Yi, S. A clinical trial of xenotransplantation of neonatal pig islets for diabetic patients. *J. Cent. South Univ. Med Ed.* **2011**, *36*, 1134–1140. [CrossRef]
15. Valdes-Gonzalez, R.; Rodriguez-Ventura, A.L.; White, D.J.G.; Bracho-Blanchet, E.; Castillo, A.; Ramírez-González, B.; López-Santos, M.G.; León-Mancilla, B.H.; Dorantes, L.M. Long-term follow-up of patients with type 1 diabetes transplanted with neonatal pig islets. *Clin. Exp. Immunol.* **2010**, *162*, 537–542. [CrossRef]
16. Zhu, H.; Lu, L.; Liu, X.; Yu, L.; Lyu, Y.; Wang, B. Treatment of diabetes with encapsulated pig islets: An update on current developments. *J. Zhejiang Univ. Sci. B* **2015**, *16*, 329–343. [CrossRef]

17. Galili, U. Evolution of α1,3Galactosyltransferase and of the α-Gal Epitope. In *α-Gal and Anti-Gal: α1,3-Galactosyltransferase, α-Gal Epitopes, and the Natural Anti-Gal Antibody Subcellular Biochemistry*; Subcellular Biochemistry; Galili, U., Avila, J.L., Eds.; Springer: Boston, MA, USA, 1999; pp. 1–23. ISBN 978-1-4615-4771-6.
18. Galili, U. Interaction of the natural anti-Gal antibody with α-galactosyl epitopes: A major obstacle for xenotransplantation in humans. *Immunol. Today* **1993**, *14*, 480–482. [CrossRef]
19. Lexer, G.; Cooper, D.; Rose, A.G.; Wicomb, W.N.; Rees, J.; Keraan, M.; Du Toit, E. Hyperacute rejection in a discordant (pig to baboon) cardiac xenograft model. *J. Heart Transpl.* **1986**, *5*, 411–418.
20. Kobayashi, T.; Cooper, D.K. Anti-Gal, alpha-Gal epitopes, and xenotransplantation. *Subcell. Biochem.* **1999**, *32*, 229–257. [CrossRef]
21. Bannett, A.D.; McAlack, R.F.; Raja, R.; Baquero, A.; Morris, M. Experiences with known ABO-mismatched renal transplants. *Transpl. Proc.* **1987**, *19*, 4543–4546.
22. Taniguchi, S.; Neethling, F.A.; Korchagina, E.Y.; Bovin, N.; Ye, Y.; Kobayashi, T.; Niekrasz, M.; Li, S.; Koren, E.; Oriol, R.; et al. In vivo immunoadsorption of antipig antibodies in baboons using a specific Gal(alpha)1-3Gal column. *Transplantation* **1996**, *62*, 1379–1384. [CrossRef]
23. Houser, S.L.; Kuwaki, K.; Knosalla, C.; Dor, F.J.M.F.; Gollackner, B.; Cheng, J.; Shimizu, A.; Schuurman, H.-J.; Cooper, D.K.C. Thrombotic microangiopathy and graft arteriopathy in pig hearts following transplantation into baboons. *Xenotransplantation* **2004**, *11*, 416–425. [CrossRef]
24. Bühler, L.; Basker, M.; Alwayn, I.P.; Goepfert, C.; Kitamura, H.; Kawai, T.; Gojo, S.; Kozlowski, T.; Ierino, F.L.; Awwad, M.; et al. Coagulation and thrombotic disorders associated with pig organ and hematopoietic cell transplantation in nonhuman primates. *Transplantation* **2000**, *70*, 1323–1331. [CrossRef]
25. Yamada, K.; Sachs, D.H.; DerSimonian, H. Human anti-porcine xenogeneic T cell response. Evidence for allelic specificity of mixed leukocyte reaction and for both direct and indirect pathways of recognition. *J. Immunol.* **1995**, *155*, 5249–5256.
26. Murray, A.G.; Khodedoust, M.M.; Pober, J.S.; Bothwell, A.L.M. Porcine aortic endothelial cells activate human T cells: Direct presentation of MHC antigens and costimulation by ligands for human CD2 and CD28. *Immunity* **1994**, *1*, 57–63. [CrossRef]
27. Dorling, A.; Lombardi, G.; Binns, R.; Lechler, R.I. Detection of primary direct and indirect human anti-porcine T cell responses using a porcine dendritic cell population. *Eur. J. Immunol.* **1996**, *26*, 1378–1387. [CrossRef]
28. Kirk, A.D.; Harlan, D.M.; Armstrong, N.N.; Davis, T.A.; Dong, Y.; Gray, G.S.; Hong, X.; Thomas, D.; Fechner, J.H.; Knechtle, S.J. CTLA4-Ig and anti-CD40 ligand prevent renal allograft rejection in primates. *Proc. Natl. Acad. Sci. USA* **1997**, *94*, 8789–8794. [CrossRef]
29. Iwase, H.; Ekser, B.; Satyananda, V.; Bhama, J.; Hara, H.; Ezzelarab, M.; Klein, E.; Wagner, R.; Long, C.; Thacker, J.; et al. Pig-to-baboon heterotopic heart transplantation–exploratory preliminary experience with pigs transgenic for human thrombomodulin and comparison of three costimulation blockade-based regimens. *Xenotransplantation* **2015**, *22*, 211–220. [CrossRef]
30. Lin, H.; Bolling, S.F.; Linsley, P.S.; Wei, R.Q.; Gordon, D.; Thompson, C.B.; Turka, L.A. Long-term acceptance of major histocompatibility complex mismatched cardiac allografts induced by CTLA4Ig plus donor-specific transfusion. *J. Exp. Med.* **1993**, *178*, 1801–1806. [CrossRef]
31. Knosalla, C.; Ryan, D.J.J.; Moran, K.; Gollackner, B.; Schuler, W.; Sachs, D.H.; Awwad, M.; Schuurman, H.-J.; Cooper, D.K.C. Initial experience with the human anti-human CD154 monoclonal antibody, ABI793, in pig-to-baboon xenotransplantation. *Xenotransplantation* **2004**, *11*, 353–360. [CrossRef]
32. Elwood, E.T.; Larsen, C.P.; Cho, H.R.; Corbascio, M.; Ritchie, S.C.; Alexander, D.Z.; Tucker-Burden, C.; Linsley, P.S.; Aruffo, A.; Hollenbaugh, D.; et al. Prolonged acceptance of concordant and discordant xenografts with combined CD40 and C28 pathway blockade. *Transplantation* **1998**, *65*, 1422–1428. [CrossRef]
33. Lehnert, A.M.; Mottram, P.L.; Han, W.; Walters, S.N.; Patel, A.T.; Hawthorne, W.J.; Cowan, P.J.; d'Apice, A.J.F.; O'Connell, P.J. Blockade of the CD28 and CD40 pathways result in the acceptance of pig and rat islet xenografts but not rat cardiac grafts in mice. *Transpl. Immunol.* **2001**, *9*, 51–56. [CrossRef]
34. Wu, G.; Pfeiffer, S.; Schröder, C.; Zhang, T.; Nguyen, B.N.; Lea, W.; Kelishadi, S.; Atkinson, J.B.; Schuurman, H.-J.; White, D.J.G.; et al. Co-stimulation blockade targeting CD154 and CD28/B7 modulates the induced antibody response after a pig-to-baboon cardiac xenograft. *Xenotransplantation* **2005**, *12*, 197–208. [CrossRef] [PubMed]

35. Dalmasso, A.P.; Vercellotti, G.M.; Platt, J.L.; Bach, F.H. Inhibition of complement-mediated endothelial cell cytotoxicity by decay-accelerating factor. Potential for prevention of xenograft hyperacute rejection. *Transplantation* **1991**, *52*, 530–533. [CrossRef] [PubMed]
36. Adams, D.H.; Kadner, A.; Chen, R.H.; Farivar, R.S. Human membrane cofactor protein (MCP, CD 46) protects transgenic pig hearts from hyperacute rejection in primates. *Xenotransplantation* **2001**, *8*, 36–40. [CrossRef] [PubMed]
37. Phelps, C.J.; Koike, C.; Vaught, T.D.; Boone, J.; Wells, K.D.; Chen, S.-H.; Ball, S.; Specht, S.M.; Polejaeva, I.A.; Monahan, J.A.; et al. Production of alpha 1,3-galactosyltransferase-deficient pigs. *Science* **2003**, *299*, 411–414. [CrossRef] [PubMed]
38. Kolber-Simonds, D.; Lai, L.; Watt, S.R.; Denaro, M.; Arn, S.; Augenstein, M.L.; Betthauser, J.; Carter, D.B.; Greenstein, J.L.; Hao, Y.; et al. Production of -1,3-galactosyltransferase null pigs by means of nuclear transfer with fibroblasts bearing loss of heterozygosity mutations. *Proc. Natl. Acad. Sci. USA* **2004**, *101*, 7335–7340. [CrossRef] [PubMed]
39. Kuwaki, K.; Tseng, Y.-L.; Dor, F.J.M.F.; Shimizu, A.; Houser, S.L.; Sanderson, T.M.; Lancos, C.J.; Prabharasuth, D.D.; Cheng, J.; Moran, K.; et al. Heart transplantation in baboons using α1,3-galactosyltransferase gene-knockout pigs as donors: Initial experience. *Nat. Med.* **2005**, *11*, 29–31. [CrossRef]
40. Ezzelarab, M.; Garcia, B.; Azimzadeh, A.; Sun, H.; Lin, C.C.; Hara, H.; Kelishadi, S.; Zhang, T.; Lin, Y.J.; Tai, H.-C.; et al. The innate immune response and activation of coagulation in α1,3-galactosyltransferase gene-knockout xenograft recipients. *Transplantation* **2009**, *87*, 805–812. [CrossRef]
41. Hara, H.; Long, C.; Lin, Y.J.; Tai, H.-C.; Ezzelarab, M.; Ayares, D.; Cooper, D.K.C. In vitro investigation of pig cells for resistance to human antibody-mediated rejection. *Transpl. Int. Off. J. Eur. Soc. Organ Transpl.* **2008**, *21*, 1163–1174. [CrossRef]
42. McGregor, C.G.A.; Ricci, D.; Miyagi, N.; Stalboerger, P.G.; Du, Z.; Oehler, E.A.; Tazelaar, H.D.; Byrne, G.W. Human CD55 expression blocks hyperacute rejection and restricts complement activation in gal knockout cardiac xenografts. *Transplantation* **2012**, *93*, 686–692. [CrossRef]
43. Padler-Karavani, V.; Varki, A. Potential impact of the non-human sialic acid n-glycolylneuraminic acid on transplant rejection risk. *Xenotransplantation* **2011**, *18*, 1–5. [CrossRef] [PubMed]
44. Lutz, A.J.; Li, P.; Estrada, J.L.; Sidner, R.A.; Chihara, R.K.; Downey, S.M.; Burlak, C.; Wang, Z.-Y.; Reyes, L.M.; Ivary, B.; et al. Double knockout pigs deficient in N-glycolylneuraminic acid and galactose α-1,3-galactose reduce the humoral barrier to xenotransplantation. *Xenotransplantation* **2013**, *20*, 27–35. [CrossRef] [PubMed]
45. Estrada, J.; Martens, G.; Li, P.; Adams, A.; Newell, K.; Ford, M.; Butler, J.; Sidner, R.; Tector, M.; Tector, A. Evaluation of human and nonhuman primate antibody binding to pig cells lacking GGTA1/CMAH/β4GalNT2 genes. *Xenotransplantation* **2015**, *22*, 194–202. [CrossRef] [PubMed]
46. Phelps, C.J.; Ball, S.F.; Vaught, T.D.; Vance, A.M.; Mendicino, M.; Monahan, J.A.; Walters, A.H.; Wells, K.D.; Dandro, A.S.; Ramsoondar, J.J.; et al. Production and characterization of transgenic pigs expressing porcine CTLA4-Ig. *Xenotransplantation* **2009**. [CrossRef]
47. Hara, H.; Witt, W.; Crossley, T.; Long, C.; Isse, K.; Fan, L.; Phelps, C.J.; Ayares, D.; Cooper, D.K.C.; Dai, Y.; et al. Human dominant-negative class II transactivator transgenic pigs – effect on the human anti-pig T-cell immune response and immune status. *Immunology* **2013**, *140*, 39–46. [CrossRef]
48. Plege, A.; Borns, K.; Baars, W.; Schwinzer, R. Suppression of human T-cell activation and expansion of regulatory T cells by pig cells overexpressing PD-ligands. *Transplantation* **2009**, *87*, 975–982. [CrossRef]
49. Ding, Q.; Lu, L.; Zhou, X.; Zhou, Y.; Chou, K.-Y. Human PD-L1-overexpressing porcine vascular endothelial cells induce functionally suppressive human CD4+CD25hiFoxp3+ Treg cells. *J. Leukoc. Biol.* **2011**, *90*, 77–86. [CrossRef]
50. Lin, Y.J.; Hara, H.; Tai, H.-C.; Long, C.; Tokita, D.; Yeh, P.; Ayares, D.; Morelli, A.E.; Cooper, D.K.C. Suppresive efficacy and proliferative capacity of human regulatory t cells in allogeneic and xenogeneic responses. *Transplantation* **2008**, *86*, 1452–1462. [CrossRef]
51. Li, J.; Ezzelarab, M.B.; Ayares, D.; Cooper, D.K.C. The potential role of genetically-modified pig mesenchymal stromal cells in xenotransplantation. *Stem Cell Rev.* **2014**, *10*, 79–85. [CrossRef]
52. Mohiuddin, M.M.; Singh, A.K.; Corcoran, P.C.; Hoyt, R.F.; Thomas, M.L.; Ayares, D.; Horvath, K.A. Genetically engineered pigs and target-specific immunomodulation provide significant graft survival and hope for clinical cardiac xenotransplantation. *J. Thorac. Cardiovasc. Surg.* **2014**, *148*, 1106–1113. [CrossRef]

53. Lin, C.; Ezzelarab, M.; Hara, H.; Long, C.; Lin, C.; Dorling, A.; Cooper, D. Atorvastatin or transgenic expression of tfpi inhibits coagulation initiated by anti-nongal igg binding to porcine aortic endothelial cells. *J. Thromb. Haemost. JTH* **2010**, *8*, 2001–2010. [CrossRef] [PubMed]
54. Cooper, D.K.C.; Ezzelarab, M.; Iwase, H.; Hara, H. Perspectives on the optimal genetically-engineered pig in 2018 for initial clinical trials of kidney or heart xenotransplantation. *Transplantation* **2018**, *102*, 1974–1982. [CrossRef]
55. Längin, M.; Mayr, T.; Reichart, B.; Michel, S.; Buchholz, S.; Guethoff, S.; Dashkevich, A.; Baehr, A.; Egerer, S.; Bauer, A.; et al. Consistent success in life-supporting porcine cardiac xenotransplantation. *Nature* **2018**, *564*, 430–433. [CrossRef] [PubMed]
56. Reichart, B.; Längin, M.; Radan, J.; Mokelke, M.; Buttgereit, I.; Ying, J.; Fresch, A.K.; Mayr, T.; Issl, L.; Buchholz, S.; et al. Pig-to-non-human primate heart transplantation: The final step toward clinical xenotransplantation? *J. Heart Lung Transpl.* **2020**, *39*, 751–757. [CrossRef] [PubMed]
57. Bach, F.H.; Fishman, J.A.; Daniels, N.; Proimos, J.; Anderson, B.; Carpenter, C.B.; Forrow, L.; Robson, S.C.; Fineberg, H.V. Uncertainty in xenotransplantation: Individual benefit versus collective risk. *Nat. Med.* **1998**, *4*, 141–144. [CrossRef]
58. Weiss, R.A. Transgenic pigs and virus adaptation. *Nature* **1998**, *391*, 327–328. [CrossRef]
59. Fishman, J.A. Prevention of infection in xenotransplantation: Designated pathogen-free swine in the safety equation. *Xenotransplantation* **2020**, *27*, e12595. [CrossRef]
60. Denner, J. Sensitive detection systems for infectious agents in xenotransplantation. *Xenotransplantation* **2020**, e12594. [CrossRef]
61. Lu, L.; Li, C.; Hagedorn, C.H. Phylogenetic analysis of global hepatitis E virus sequences: Genetic diversity, subtypes and zoonosis. *Rev. Med. Virol.* **2006**, *16*, 5–36. [CrossRef]
62. Denner, J. Xenotransplantation and hepatitis E virus. *Xenotransplantation* **2015**, *22*, 167–173. [CrossRef]
63. Ramanan, P.; Razonable, R.R. Cytomegalovirus infections in solid organ transplantation: A review. *Infect. Chemother.* **2013**, *45*, 260–271. [CrossRef]
64. Denner, J.; Längin, M.; Reichart, B.; Krüger, L.; Fiebig, U.; Mokelke, M.; Radan, J.; Mayr, T.; Milusev, A.; Luther, F.; et al. Impact of porcine cytomegalovirus on long-term orthotopic cardiac xenotransplant survival. *bioRxiv* **2020**. [CrossRef]
65. Krüger, L.; Längin, M.; Reichart, B.; Fiebig, U.; Kristiansen, Y.; Prinz, C.; Kessler, B.; Egerer, S.; Wolf, E.; Abicht, J.-M.; et al. Transmission of porcine circovirus 3 (PCV3) by xenotransplantation of pig hearts into baboons. *Viruses* **2019**, *11*, 650. [CrossRef]
66. Denner, J. How active are porcine endogenous retroviruses (PERVs)? *Viruses* **2016**, *8*, 215. [CrossRef]
67. Takeuchi, Y.; Patience, C.; Magre, S.; Weiss, R.A.; Banerjee, P.T.; Le Tissier, P.; Stoye, J.P. Host range and interference studies of three classes of pig endogenous retrovirus. *J. Virol.* **1998**, *72*, 9986–9991. [CrossRef]
68. Le Tissier, P.; Stoye, J.P.; Takeuchi, Y.; Patience, C.; Weiss, R.A. Two sets of human-tropic pig retrovirus. *Nature* **1997**, *389*, 681–682. [CrossRef]
69. Martin, U.; Winkler, M.E.; Id, M.; Radeke, H.; Arseniev, L.; Takeuchi, Y.; Simon, A.R.; Patience, C.; Haverich, A.; Steinhoff, G. Productive infection of primary human endothelial cells by pig endogenous retrovirus (PERV). *Xenotransplantation* **2000**, *7*, 138–142. [CrossRef]
70. Yang, L.; Güell, M.; Niu, D.; George, H.; Lesha, E.; Grishin, D.; Aach, J.; Shrock, E.; Xu, W.; Poci, J.; et al. Genome-wide inactivation of porcine endogenous retroviruses (PERVs). *Science* **2015**, *350*, 1101–1104. [CrossRef]
71. Niu, D.; Wei, H.-J.; Lin, L.; George, H.; Wang, T.; Lee, I.-H.; Zhao, H.-Y.; Wang, Y.; Kan, Y.; Shrock, E.; et al. Inactivation of porcine endogenous retrovirus in pigs using CRISPR-Cas9. *Science* **2017**, *357*, 1303–1307. [CrossRef]
72. Blum, B.; Benvenisty, N. The tumorigenicity of human embryonic stem cells. *Adv. Cancer Res.* **2008**, *100*, 133–158. [CrossRef]
73. Beltrami, A.P.; Barlucchi, L.; Torella, D.; Baker, M.; Limana, F.; Chimenti, S.; Kasahara, H.; Rota, M.; Musso, E.; Urbanek, K.; et al. Adult cardiac stem cells are multipotent and support myocardial regeneration. *Cell* **2003**, *114*, 763–776. [CrossRef]
74. Marcello, R.; Padin-Iruegas, M.E.; Yu, M.; Antonella, D.A.; Silvia, M.; João, F.; Emanuela, F.; Raffaella, R.; Arcarese Michael, L.; Mitchell Thomas, S.; et al. Local activation or implantation of cardiac progenitor cells rescues scarred infarcted myocardium improving cardiac function. *Circ. Res.* **2008**, *103*, 107–116. [CrossRef]

75. Orlic, D.; Kajstura, J.; Chimenti, S.; Jakoniuk, I.; Anderson, S.M.; Li, B.; Pickel, J.; McKay, R.; Nadal-Ginard, B.; Bodine, D.M.; et al. Bone marrow cells regenerate infarcted myocardium. *Nature* **2001**, *410*, 701–705. [CrossRef] [PubMed]
76. Rota, M.; Kajstura, J.; Hosoda, T.; Bearzi, C.; Vitale, S.; Esposito, G.; Iaffaldano, G.; Padin-Iruegas, M.E.; Gonzalez, A.; Rizzi, R.; et al. Bone marrow cells adopt the cardiomyogenic fate in vivo. *Proc. Natl. Acad. Sci. USA* **2007**, *104*, 17783–17788. [CrossRef]
77. Jianhua, Z.; Wilson, G.F.; Soerens, A.G.; Koonce, C.H.; Junying, Y.; Palecek, S.P.; Thomson, J.A.; Kamp, T.J. Functional cardiomyocytes derived from human induced pluripotent stem cells. *Circ. Res.* **2009**, *104*, e30–e41. [CrossRef]
78. Zhu, W.; Zhao, M.; Mattapally, S.; Chen, S.; Zhang, J. CCND2 overexpression enhances the regenerative potency of human induced pluripotent stem cell–derived cardiomyocytes: remuscularization of injured ventricle. *Circ. Res.* **2018**, *122*, 88–96. [CrossRef]
79. Hoashi, T.; Matsumiya, G.; Miyagawa, S.; Ichikawa, H.; Ueno, T.; Ono, M.; Saito, A.; Shimizu, T.; Okano, T.; Kawaguchi, N.; et al. Skeletal myoblast sheet transplantation improves the diastolic function of a pressure-overloaded right heart. *J. Thorac. Cardiovasc. Surg.* **2009**, *138*, 460–467. [CrossRef]
80. Haider, H.K.; Tan, A.C.K.; Aziz, S.; Chachques, J.C.; Sim, E.K.W. Myoblast transplantation for cardiac repair: A clinical perspective. *Mol. J. Am. Soc. Gene* **2004**, *9*, 14–23. [CrossRef]
81. Wollert, K.C.; Helmut, D. Clinical applications of stem cells for the heart. *Circ. Res.* **2005**, *96*, 151–163. [CrossRef]
82. Duelen, R.; Sampaolesi, M. Stem cell technology in cardiac regeneration: A pluripotent stem cell promise. *EBioMedicine* **2017**, *16*, 30–40. [CrossRef]
83. Rikhtegar, R.; Pezeshkian, M.; Dolati, S.; Safaie, N.; Afrasiabi Rad, A.; Mahdipour, M.; Nouri, M.; Jodati, A.R.; Yousefi, M. Stem cells as therapy for heart disease: IPSCs, ESCs, CSCs, and skeletal myoblasts. *Biomed. Pharm.* **2019**, *109*, 304–313. [CrossRef]
84. Piero, A.; Jan, K.; Annarosa, L.; Roberto, B. Life and death of cardiac stem cells. *Circulation* **2006**, *113*, 1451–1463. [CrossRef]
85. Kucia, M.; Dawn, B.; Hunt, G.; Guo, Y.; Wysoczynski, M.; Majka, M.; Ratajczak, J.; Rezzoug, F.; Ildstad, S.T.; Bolli, R.; et al. Cells expressing early cardiac markers reside in the bone marrow and are mobilized into the peripheral blood after myocardial infarction. *Circ. Res.* **2004**, *95*, 1191–1199. [CrossRef]
86. Murry, C.E.; Soonpaa, M.H.; Reinecke, H.; Nakajima, H.; Nakajima, H.O.; Rubart, M.; Pasumarthi, K.B.S.; Ismail Virag, J.; Bartelmez, S.H.; Poppa, V.; et al. Haematopoietic stem cells do not transdifferentiate into cardiac myocytes in myocardial infarcts. *Nature* **2004**, *428*, 664–668. [CrossRef]
87. Van Berlo, J.H.; Kanisicak, O.; Maillet, M.; Vagnozzi, R.J.; Karch, J.; Lin, S.-C.J.; Middleton, R.C.; Marbán, E.; Molkentin, J.D. C-kit+ cells minimally contribute cardiomyocytes to the heart. *Nature* **2014**, *509*, 337–341. [CrossRef]
88. Nguyen, P.K.; Rhee, J.-W.; Wu, J.C. Adult stem cell therapy and heart failure, 2000 to 2016: A systematic review. *JAMA Cardiol.* **2016**, *1*, 831–841. [CrossRef] [PubMed]
89. Mirotsou, M.; Jayawardena, T.M.; Schmeckpeper, J.; Gnecchi, M.; Dzau, V.J. Paracrine mechanisms of stem cell reparative and regenerative actions in the heart. *J. Mol. Cell. Cardiol.* **2011**, *50*, 280–289. [CrossRef] [PubMed]
90. Li, T.-S.; Cheng, K.; Malliaras, K.; Smith, R.R.; Zhang, Y.; Sun, B.; Matsushita, N.; Blusztajn, A.; Terrovitis, J.; Kusuoka, H.; et al. Direct comparison of different stem cell types and subpopulations reveals superior paracrine potency and myocardial repair efficacy with cardiosphere-derived cells. *J. Am. Coll. Cardiol.* **2012**, *59*, 942–953. [CrossRef] [PubMed]
91. Pittenger, M.F.; Mackay, A.M.; Beck, S.C.; Jaiswal, R.K.; Douglas, R.; Mosca, J.D.; Moorman, M.A.; Simonetti, D.W.; Craig, S.; Marshak, D.R. Multilineage potential of adult human mesenchymal stem cells. *Science* **1999**, *284*, 143–147. [CrossRef] [PubMed]
92. Hass, R.; Kasper, C.; Böhm, S.; Jacobs, R. Different populations and sources of human mesenchymal stem cells (MSC): A comparison of adult and neonatal tissue-derived MSC. *Cell Commun. Signal.* **2011**, *9*, 12. [CrossRef] [PubMed]
93. Monsanto, M.M.; White, K.S.; Kim, T.; Wang, B.J.; Fisher, K.; Ilves, K.; Khalafalla, F.G.; Casillas, A.; Broughton, K.; Mohsin, S.; et al. Concurrent isolation of 3 distinct cardiac stem cell populations from a single human heart biopsy. *Circ. Res.* **2017**, *121*, 113–124. [CrossRef] [PubMed]

94. Dominici, M.; Le Blanc, K.; Mueller, I.; Slaper-Cortenbach, I.; Marini, F.; Krause, D.; Deans, R.; Keating, A.; Prockop, D.; Horwitz, E. Minimal criteria for defining multipotent mesenchymal stromal cells. The international society for cellular therapy position statement. *Cytotherapy* **2006**, *8*, 315–317. [CrossRef] [PubMed]
95. Hare, J.M.; Fishman, J.E.; Gerstenblith, G.; DiFede Velazquez, D.L.; Zambrano, J.P.; Suncion, V.Y.; Tracy, M.; Ghersin, E.; Johnston, P.V.; Brinker, J.A.; et al. Comparison of allogeneic vs autologous bone marrow–derived mesenchymal stem cells delivered by transendocardial injection in patients with ischemic cardiomyopathy. *JAMA* **2012**, *308*, 2369–2379. [CrossRef] [PubMed]
96. Li, J.; Ezzelarab, M.B.; Cooper, D.K.C. Do mesenchymal stem cells function across species barriers? Relevance for xenotransplantation. *Xenotransplantation* **2012**, *19*, 273–285. [CrossRef]
97. Medicetty, S.; Bledsoe, A.R.; Fahrenholtz, C.B.; Troyer, D.; Weiss, M.L. Transplantation of pig stem cells into rat brain: Proliferation during the first 8 weeks. *Exp. Neurol.* **2004**, *190*, 32–41. [CrossRef]
98. Eguchi, H.; Kuroiwa, Y.; Matsui, A.; Sada, M.; Nagaya, N.; Kawano, S. Intra-bone marrow cotransplantation of donor mesenchymal stem cells in pig-to-NOD/SCID mouse bone marrow transplantation facilitates short-term xenogeneic hematopoietic engraftment. *Transpl. Proc.* **2008**, *40*, 574–577. [CrossRef]
99. Nakamura, Y.; Wang, X.; Xu, C.; Asakura, A.; Yoshiyama, M.; From, A.H.L.; Zhang, J. Xenotransplantation of long-term-cultured swine bone marrow-derived mesenchymal stem cells. *Stem Cells Dayt. Ohio* **2007**, *25*, 612–620. [CrossRef]
100. Bharti, D.; Shivakumar, S.B.; Subbarao, R.B.; Rho, G.-J. Research advancements in porcine derived mesenchymal stem cells. *Curr. Stem Cell Res. Ther.* **2016**, *11*, 78–93. [CrossRef]
101. Karpov, A.A.; Udalova, D.V.; Pliss, M.G.; Galagudza, M.M. Can the outcomes of mesenchymal stem cell-based therapy for myocardial infarction be improved? Providing weapons and armour to cells. *Cell Prolif.* **2016**, *50*. [CrossRef]
102. Bagno, L.; Hatzistergos, K.E.; Balkan, W.; Hare, J.M. Mesenchymal stem cell-based therapy for cardiovascular disease: Progress and challenges. *Mol. Ther.* **2018**, *26*, 1610–1623. [CrossRef]
103. Moscoso, I.; Centeno, A.; López, E.; Rodriguez-Barbosa, J.I.; Santamarina, I.; Filgueira, P.; Sánchez, M.J.; Domínguez-Perles, R.; Peñuelas-Rivas, G.; Domenech, N. Differentiation "in vitro" of primary and immortalized porcine mesenchymal stem cells into cardiomyocytes for cell transplantation. *Transpl. Proc.* **2005**, *37*, 481–482. [CrossRef]
104. Quevedo, H.C.; Hatzistergos, K.E.; Oskouei, B.N.; Feigenbaum, G.S.; Rodriguez, J.E.; Valdes, D.; Pattany, P.M.; Zambrano, J.P.; Hu, Q.; McNiece, I.; et al. Allogeneic mesenchymal stem cells restore cardiac function in chronic ischemic cardiomyopathy via trilineage differentiating capacity. *Proc. Natl. Acad. Sci. USA* **2009**, *106*, 14022–14027. [CrossRef] [PubMed]
105. Gallina, C.; Turinetto, V.; Giachino, C. A new paradigm in cardiac regeneration: The mesenchymal stem cell secretome. *Stem Cells Int.* **2015**, *2015*, 765846. [CrossRef] [PubMed]
106. Cai, M.; Shen, R.; Song, L.; Lu, M.; Wang, J.; Zhao, S.; Tang, Y.; Meng, X.; Li, Z.; He, Z.-X. Bone marrow mesenchymal stem cells (BM-MSCs) improve heart function in swine myocardial infarction model through paracrine effects. *Sci. Rep.* **2016**, *6*, 28250. [CrossRef]
107. Natsumeda, M.; Florea, V.; Rieger, A.C.; Tompkins, B.A.; Banerjee, M.N.; Golpanian, S.; Fritsch, J.; Landin, A.M.; Kashikar, N.D.; Karantalis, V.; et al. A combination of allogeneic stem cells promotes cardiac regeneration. *J. Am. Coll. Cardiol.* **2017**, *70*, 2504–2515. [CrossRef] [PubMed]
108. Williams, A.R.; Hatzistergos, K.E.; Addicott, B.; McCall, F.; Carvalho, D.; Suncion, V.; Morales, A.R.; Silva, J.D.; Sussman, M.A.; Heldman, A.W.; et al. Enhanced effect of human cardiac stem cells and bone marrow mesenchymal stem cells to reduce infarct size and restore cardiac function after myocardial infarction. *Circulation* **2013**, *127*, 213–223. [CrossRef] [PubMed]
109. Karantalis, V.; Suncion-Loescher, V.Y.; Bagno, L.; Golpanian, S.; Wolf, A.; Sanina, C.; Premer, C.; Kanelidis, A.J.; McCall, F.; Wang, B.; et al. Synergistic effects of combined cell therapy for chronic ischemic cardiomyopathy. *J. Am. Coll. Cardiol.* **2015**, *66*, 1990–1999. [CrossRef] [PubMed]
110. Tompkins, B.A.; Wayne, B.; Johannes, W.; Mariann, G.; Georg, G.; Francisco, F.; Hare, J.M. Preclinical studies of stem cell therapy for heart disease. *Circ. Res.* **2018**, *122*, 1006–1020. [CrossRef] [PubMed]
111. Chong, J.J.H.; Yang, X.; Don, C.W.; Minami, E.; Liu, Y.-W.; Weyers, J.J.; Mahoney, W.M.; Van Biber, B.; Cook, S.M.; Palpant, N.J.; et al. Human embryonic-stem-cell-derived cardiomyocytes regenerate non-human primate hearts. *Nature* **2014**, *510*, 273–277. [CrossRef]

112. Keyang, Z.; Qiang, W.; Cheng, N.; Peng, Z.; Zhiwei, Z.; Yan, W.; Yingchao, W.; Yinchuan, X.; Minjian, K.; Haifeng, C.; et al. Lack of remuscularization following transplantation of human embryonic stem cell-derived cardiovascular progenitor cells in infarcted nonhuman primates. *Circ. Res.* **2018**, *122*, 958–969. [CrossRef]
113. Shiba, Y.; Gomibuchi, T.; Seto, T.; Wada, Y.; Ichimura, H.; Tanaka, Y.; Ogasawara, T.; Okada, K.; Shiba, N.; Sakamoto, K.; et al. Allogeneic transplantation of iPS cell-derived cardiomyocytes regenerates primate hearts. *Nature* **2016**, *538*, 388–391. [CrossRef] [PubMed]
114. Yue-Jin, Y.; Hai-Yan, Q.; Ji, H.; Jian-Jun, L.; Run-Lin, G.; Ke-Fei, D.; Guo-Sheng, Y.; Willerson, J.T.; Yong-Jian, G. Combined therapy with simvastatin and bone marrow–derived mesenchymal stem cells increases benefits in infarcted swine hearts. *Arter. Thromb. Vasc. Biol.* **2009**, *29*, 2076–2082. [CrossRef]
115. Bobi, J.; Solanes, N.; Fernández-Jiménez, R.; Galán-Arriola, C.; Dantas, A.P.; Fernández-Friera, L.; Gálvez-Montón, C.; Rigol-Monzó, E.; Agüero, J.; Ramírez, J.; et al. Intracoronary administration of allogeneic adipose tissue—Derived mesenchymal stem cells improves myocardial perfusion but not left ventricle function, in a translational model of acute myocardial infarction. *J. Am. Heart Assoc. Cardiovasc. Cereb. Dis.* **2017**, *6*. [CrossRef] [PubMed]
116. Gómez-Mauricio, G.; Moscoso, I.; Martín-Cancho, M.-F.; Crisóstomo, V.; Prat-Vidal, C.; Báez-Díaz, C.; Sánchez-Margallo, F.M.; Bernad, A. Combined administration of mesenchymal stem cells overexpressing IGF-1 and HGF enhances neovascularization but moderately improves cardiac regeneration in a porcine model. *Stem Cell Res. Ther.* **2016**, *7*, 94. [CrossRef] [PubMed]
117. Perea-Gil, I.; Prat-Vidal, C.; Gálvez-Montón, C.; Roura, S.; Llucià-Valldeperas, A.; Soler-Botija, C.; Iborra-Egea, O.; Díaz-Güemes, I.; Crisóstomo, V.; Sánchez-Margallo, F.M.; et al. A cell-enriched engineered myocardial graft limits infarct size and improves cardiac function: Pre-clinical study in the porcine myocardial infarction model. *JACC Basic Transl. Sci.* **2016**, *1*, 360–372. [CrossRef] [PubMed]
118. Amado, L.C.; Saliaris, A.P.; Schuleri, K.H.; John, S.M.; Xie, J.-S.; Cattaneo, S.; Durand, D.J.; Fitton, T.; Kuang, J.Q.; Stewart, G.; et al. Cardiac repair with intramyocardial injection of allogeneic mesenchymal stem cells after myocardial infarction. *Proc. Natl. Acad. Sci. USA* **2005**, *102*, 11474–11479. [CrossRef]
119. Ward, M.R.; Connelly, K.A.; Vijayaraghavan, R.; Vaags, A.K.; Graham, J.J.; Foltz, W.; Hough, M.R.; Stewart, D.J.; Dick, A. eNOS overexpressing bone marrow cells are safe and effective in a porcine model of myocardial regeneration following acute myocardial infarction. *Cardiovasc. Ther.* **2013**, *31*, e72–e78. [CrossRef]
120. Kim, M.C.; Kim, Y.S.; Kang, W.S.; Lee, K.H.; Cho, M.; Hong, M.H.; Lim, K.S.; Jeong, M.H.; Ahn, Y. Intramyocardial injection of stem cells in pig myocardial infarction model: The first trial in korea. *J. Korean Med. Sci.* **2017**, *32*, 1708–1712. [CrossRef]
121. Shake, J.G.; Gruber, P.J.; Baumgartner, W.A.; Senechal, G.; Meyers, J.; Redmond, J.M.; Pittenger, M.F.; Martin, B.J. Mesenchymal stem cell implantation in a swine myocardial infarct model: Engraftment and functional effects. *Ann. Thorac. Surg.* **2002**, *73*, 1919–1926. [CrossRef]
122. Yang, Z.; Ma, D.; Wang, W.; Xu, S.; Zhang, Y.; Chen, B.; Zhou, F.; Zhu, T.; Wang, L.; Jia, E.; et al. Neovascularization and cardiomyocytes regeneration in acute myocardial infarction after bone marrow stromal cell transplantation: Comparison of infarct-relative and noninfarct-relative arterial approaches in swine. *Clin. Chim. Acta* **2007**, *381*, 114–118. [CrossRef]
123. Pak, H.-N.; Qayyum, M.; Kim, D.T.; Hamabe, A.; Miyauchi, Y.; Lill, M.C.; Frantzen, M.; Takizawa, K.; Chen, L.S.; Fishbein, M.C.; et al. Mesenchymal stem cell injection induces cardiac nerve sprouting and increased tenascin expression in a swine model of myocardial infarction. *J. Cardiovasc. Electrophysiol.* **2003**, *14*, 841–848. [CrossRef] [PubMed]
124. Weil, B.R.; Suzuki, G.; Leiker, M.M.; Fallavollita, J.A.; Canty, J.M. Comparative efficacy of intracoronary allogeneic mesenchymal stem cells and cardiosphere-derived cells in swine with hibernating myocardium. *Circ. Res.* **2015**, *117*, 634–644. [CrossRef] [PubMed]
125. Golpanian, S.; Schulman, I.H.; Ebert, R.F.; Heldman, A.W.; DiFede, D.L.; Yang, P.C.; Wu, J.C.; Bolli, R.; Perin, E.C.; Moyé, L.; et al. Concise review: Review and perspective of cell dosage and routes of administration from preclinical and clinical studies of stem cell therapy for heart disease. *Stem Cells Transl. Med.* **2016**, *5*, 186–191. [CrossRef] [PubMed]
126. Sheng, C.C.; Zhou, L.; Hao, J. Current stem cell delivery methods for myocardial repair. *Biomed. Res. Int.* **2013**. [CrossRef]

127. Hou, D.; Youssef, E.A.-S.; Brinton, T.J.; Zhang, P.; Rogers, P.; Price, E.T.; Yeung, A.C.; Johnstone, B.H.; Yock, P.G.; March, K.L. Radiolabeled cell distribution after intramyocardial, intracoronary, and interstitial retrograde coronary venous delivery: Implications for current clinical trials. *Circulation* **2005**, *112*, I150–I156. [CrossRef]
128. Roura, S.; Gálvez-Montón, C.; Mirabel, C.; Vives, J.; Bayes-Genis, A. Mesenchymal stem cells for cardiac repair: Are the actors ready for the clinical scenario? *Stem Cell Res. Ther.* **2017**, *8*, 238. [CrossRef]
129. Perea-Gil, I.; Prat-Vidal, C.; Bayes-Genis, A. In vivo experience with natural scaffolds for myocardial infarction: The times they are a-changin'. *Stem Cell Res. Ther.* **2015**, 6. [CrossRef]
130. Nguyen, A.H.; Marsh, P.; Schmiess-Heine, L.; Burke, P.J.; Lee, A.; Lee, J.; Cao, H. Cardiac tissue engineering: State-of-the-art methods and outlook. *J. Biol. Eng.* **2019**, *13*, 57. [CrossRef]
131. Gálvez-Montón, C.; Bragós, R.; Soler-Botija, C.; Díaz-Güemes, I.; Prat-Vidal, C.; Crisóstomo, V.; Sánchez-Margallo, F.M.; Llucià-Valldeperas, A.; Bogónez-Franco, P.; Perea-Gil, I.; et al. Noninvasive assessment of an engineered bioactive graft in myocardial infarction: Impact on cardiac function and scar healing. *Stem Cells Transl. Med.* **2017**, *6*, 647–655. [CrossRef]
132. Shah, M.; Pawan, K.C.; Copeland, K.M.; Liao, J.; Zhang, G. A thin layer of decellularized porcine myocardium for cell delivery. *Sci. Rep.* **2018**, *8*, 16206. [CrossRef]
133. Wainwright, J.M.; Hashizume, R.; Fujimoto, K.L.; Remlinger, N.T.; Pesyna, C.; Wagner, W.R.; Tobita, K.; Gilbert, T.W.; Badylak, S.F. Right ventricular outflow tract repair with a cardiac biologic scaffold. *Cells Tissues Organs* **2012**, *195*, 159–170. [CrossRef] [PubMed]
134. Gálvez-Montón, C.; Fernandez-Figueras, M.T.; Martí, M.; Soler-Botija, C.; Roura, S.; Perea-Gil, I.; Prat-Vidal, C.; Llucià-Valldeperas, A.; Raya, Á.; Bayes-Genis, A. Neoinnervation and neovascularization of acellular pericardial-derived scaffolds in myocardial infarcts. *Stem Cell Res. Ther.* **2015**, 6. [CrossRef] [PubMed]
135. Mewhort, H.E.M.; Turnbull, J.D.; Satriano, A.; Chow, K.; Flewitt, J.A.; Andrei, A.-C.; Guzzardi, D.G.; Svystonyuk, D.A.; White, J.A.; Fedak, P.W.M. Epicardial infarct repair with bioinductive extracellular matrix promotes vasculogenesis and myocardial recovery. *J. Heart Lung Transpl.* **2016**, *35*, 661–670. [CrossRef] [PubMed]
136. Spinali, K.L.; Schmuck, E.G. Natural sources of extracellular matrix for cardiac repair. In *Cardiac Extracellular Matrix: Fundamental Science to Clinical Applications*; Advances in Experimental Medicine and Biology; Schmuck, E.G., Hematti, P., Raval, A.N., Eds.; Springer International Publishing: Cham, Switzerland, 2018; pp. 115–130. ISBN 978-3-319-97421-7.
137. Brewster, B.D.; Rouch, J.D.; Wang, M.; Meldrum, D.R. Toll-like receptor 4 ablation improves stem cell survival after hypoxic injury. *J. Surg. Res.* **2012**, *177*, 330–333. [CrossRef] [PubMed]
138. Wang, Y.; Abarbanell, A.M.; Herrmann, J.L.; Weil, B.R.; Manukyan, M.C.; Poynter, J.A.; Meldrum, D.R. TLR4 inhibits mesenchymal stem cell (MSC) STAT3 activation and thereby exerts deleterious effects on MSC–mediated cardioprotection. *PLoS ONE* **2010**, *5*, e14206. [CrossRef] [PubMed]
139. Lim, S.Y.; Kim, Y.S.; Ahn, Y.; Jeong, M.H.; Hong, M.H.; Joo, S.Y.; Nam, K.I.; Cho, J.G.; Kang, P.M.; Park, J.C. The effects of mesenchymal stem cells transduced with Akt in a porcine myocardial infarction model. *Cardiovasc. Res.* **2006**, *70*, 530–542. [CrossRef]
140. Mao, Q.; Lin, C.; Gao, J.; Liang, X.; Gao, W.; Shen, L.; Kang, L.; Xu, B. Mesenchymal stem cells overexpressing integrin-linked kinase attenuate left ventricular remodeling and improve cardiac function after myocardial infarction. *Mol. Cell. Biochem.* **2014**, *397*, 203–214. [CrossRef]
141. Hsiao, S.T.-F.; Asgari, A.; Lokmic, Z.; Sinclair, R.; Dusting, G.J.; Lim, S.Y.; Dilley, R.J. Comparative analysis of paracrine factor expression in human adult mesenchymal stem cells derived from bone marrow, adipose, and dermal tissue. *Stem Cells Dev.* **2012**, *21*, 2189–2203. [CrossRef]
142. Hnatiuk, A.P.; Ong, S.; Olea, F.D.; Locatelli, P.; Riegler, J.; Lee, W.H.; Jen, C.H.; De Lorenzi, A.; Giménez, C.S.; Laguens, R.; et al. Allogeneic mesenchymal stromal cells overexpressing mutant human hypoxia-inducible factor 1-α (HIF1-α) in an ovine model of acute myocardial infarction. *J. Am. Heart Assoc. Cardiovasc. Cereb. Dis.* **2016**, 5. [CrossRef]
143. Kim, S.H.; Moon, H.-H.; Kim, H.A.; Hwang, K.-C.; Lee, M.; Choi, D. Hypoxia-inducible vascular endothelial growth factor-engineered mesenchymal stem cells prevent myocardial ischemic injury. *Mol. Ther. J. Am. Soc. Gene* **2011**, *19*, 741–750. [CrossRef]
144. Cornu, T.I.; Mussolino, C.; Cathomen, T. Refining strategies to translate genome editing to the clinic. *Nat. Med.* **2017**, *23*, 415–423. [CrossRef] [PubMed]

145. Dakhlallah, D.; Zhang, J.; Yu, L.; Marsh, C.B.; Angelos, M.G.; Khan, M. MicroRNA-133a engineered mesenchymal stem cells augment cardiac function and cell survival in the infarct heart. *J. Cardiovasc. Pharm.* **2015**, *65*, 241–251. [CrossRef] [PubMed]
146. Lee, C.Y.; Shin, S.; Lee, J.; Seo, H.-H.; Lim, K.H.; Kim, H.; Choi, J.-W.; Kim, S.W.; Lee, S.; Lim, S.; et al. MicroRNA-mediated down-regulation of apoptosis signal-regulating kinase 1 (ASK1) attenuates the apoptosis of human mesenchymal stem cells (MSCs) transplanted into infarcted heart. *Int. J. Mol. Sci.* **2016**, *17*, 1752. [CrossRef] [PubMed]
147. Hu, S.; Huang, M.; Nguyen, P.K.; Gong, Y.; Li, Z.; Jia, F.; Lan, F.; Liu, J.; Nag, D.; Robbins, R.C.; et al. Novel microRNA pro-survival cocktail for improving engraftment and function of cardiac progenitor cell transplantation. *Circulation* **2011**, *124*, S27–S34. [CrossRef] [PubMed]
148. Huang, F.; Zhu, X.; Hu, X.-Q.; Fang, Z.-F.; Tang, L.; Lu, X.-L.; Zhou, S.-H. Mesenchymal stem cells modified with miR-126 release angiogenic factors and activate Notch ligand Delta-like-4, enhancing ischemic angiogenesis and cell survival. *Int. J. Mol. Med.* **2013**, *31*, 484–492. [CrossRef] [PubMed]
149. Seo, H.-H.; Lee, S.-Y.; Lee, C.Y.; Kim, R.; Kim, P.; Oh, S.; Lee, H.; Lee, M.Y.; Kim, J.; Kim, L.K.; et al. Exogenous miRNA-146a enhances the therapeutic efficacy of human mesenchymal stem cells by increasing vascular endothelial growth factor secretion in the ischemia/reperfusion-injured heart. *J. Vasc. Res.* **2017**, *54*, 100–108. [CrossRef] [PubMed]
150. Kuppusamy, K.T.; Jones, D.C.; Sperber, H.; Madan, A.; Fischer, K.A.; Rodriguez, M.L.; Pabon, L.; Zhu, W.-Z.; Tulloch, N.L.; Yang, X.; et al. Let-7 family of microRNA is required for maturation and adult-like metabolism in stem cell-derived cardiomyocytes. *Proc. Natl. Acad. Sci. USA* **2015**, *112*, E2785–E2794. [CrossRef]
151. Shen, X.; Pan, B.; Zhou, H.; Liu, L.; Lv, T.; Zhu, J.; Huang, X.; Tian, J. Differentiation of mesenchymal stem cells into cardiomyocytes is regulated by miRNA-1-2 via WNT signaling pathway. *J. Biomed. Sci.* **2017**, *24*, 29. [CrossRef]
152. Zhang, L.; Liu, J.; Liu, F.; Liu, W.; Wang, Y.; Zhu, B.; Yu, B. MiR-499 induces cardiac differentiation of rat mesenchymal stem cells through wnt/β-catenin signaling pathway. *Biochem. Biophys. Res. Commun.* **2012**, *420*, 875–881. [CrossRef]
153. Crisostomo, V.; Baez, C.; Abad, J.L.; Sanchez, B.; Alvarez, V.; Rosado, R.; Gómez-Mauricio, G.; Gheysens, O.; Blanco-Blazquez, V.; Blazquez, R.; et al. Dose-dependent improvement of cardiac function in a swine model of acute myocardial infarction after intracoronary administration of allogeneic heart-derived cells. *Stem Cell Res. Ther.* **2019**, *10*, 152. [CrossRef]
154. Fernández-Avilés, F.; Sanz-Ruiz, R.; Bogaert, J.; Casado Plasencia, A.; Gilaberte, I.; Belmans, A.; Fernández-Santos, M.E.; Charron, D.; Mulet, M.; Yotti, R.; et al. Safety and efficacy of intracoronary infusion of allogeneic human cardiac stem cells in patients with st-segment elevation myocardial infarction and left ventricular dysfunction. *Circ. Res.* **2018**, *123*, 579–589. [CrossRef] [PubMed]
155. Lemcke, H.; Voronina, N.; Steinhoff, G.; David, R. Recent progress in stem cell modification for cardiac regeneration. *Stem Cells Int.* **2018**, *2018*, 1909346. [CrossRef] [PubMed]
156. Bahsoun, S.; Coopman, K.; Akam, E.C. The impact of cryopreservation on bone marrow-derived mesenchymal stem cells: A systematic review. *J. Transl. Med.* **2019**, *17*, 397. [CrossRef] [PubMed]
157. Stevens, S. Genome engineering for xenotransplantation. *Genet. Eng. Glimpse Tech. Appl.* **2019**. [CrossRef]
158. Wilmut, I.; Beaujean, N.; de Sousa, P.A.; Dinnyes, A.; King, T.J.; Paterson, L.A.; Wells, D.N.; Young, L.E. Somatic cell nuclear transfer. *Nature* **2002**, *419*, 583–586. [CrossRef] [PubMed]
159. De Almeida, P.E.; Meyer, E.H.; Kooreman, N.G.; Diecke, S.; Dey, D.; Sanchez-Freire, V.; Hu, S.; Ebert, A.; Odegaard, J.; Mordwinkin, N.; et al. Transplanted terminally differentiated induced pluripotent stem cells are accepted by immune mechanisms similar to self-tolerance. *Nat. Commun.* **2014**, *5*, 3903. [CrossRef]
160. Bravery, C.A. Do human leukocyte antigen-typed cellular therapeutics based on induced pluripotent stem cells make commercial sense? *Stem Cells Dev.* **2014**, *24*, 1–10. [CrossRef]
161. Nakatsuji, N.; Nakajima, F.; Tokunaga, K. HLA-haplotype banking and iPS cells. *Nat. Biotechnol.* **2008**, *26*, 739–740. [CrossRef]
162. Huang, C.-Y.; Liu, C.-L.; Ting, C.-Y.; Chiu, Y.-T.; Cheng, Y.-C.; Nicholson, M.W.; Hsieh, P.C.H. Human iPSC banking: Barriers and opportunities. *J. Biomed. Sci.* **2019**, *26*, 87. [CrossRef]

163. Yoshihara, M.; Oguchi, A.; Murakawa, Y. Genomic instability of iPSCs and challenges in their clinical applications. In *Stem Cells: Therapeutic Applications*; Advances in Experimental Medicine and Biology; Ratajczak, M.Z., Ed.; Springer International Publishing: Cham, Switzerland, 2019; pp. 23–47. ISBN 978-3-030-31206-0.
164. Wu, J.; Platero-Luengo, A.; Sakurai, M.; Sugawara, A.; Gil, M.A.; Yamauchi, T.; Suzuki, K.; Bogliotti, Y.S.; Cuello, C.; Valencia, M.M.; et al. Interspecies chimerism with mammalian pluripotent stem cells. *Cell* **2017**, *168*, 473–486.e15. [CrossRef]
165. Koplin, J.; Wilkinson, D. Moral uncertainty and the farming of human-pig chimeras. *J. Med. Ethics* **2019**, *45*, 440–446. [CrossRef]
166. Pawan, K.C.; Hong, Y.; Zhang, G. Cardiac tissue-derived extracellular matrix scaffolds for myocardial repair: Advantages and challenges. *Regen. Biomater.* **2019**, *6*, 185–199. [CrossRef]
167. Huang, K.; Ozpinar, E.W.; Su, T.; Tang, J.; Shen, D.; Qiao, L.; Hu, S.; Li, Z.; Liang, H.; Mathews, K.; et al. An off-the-shelf artificial cardiac patch improves cardiac repair after myocardial infarction in rats and pigs. *Sci. Transl. Med.* **2020**, 12. [CrossRef] [PubMed]
168. Johnson, T.D.; Dequach, J.A.; Gaetani, R.; Ungerleider, J.; Elhag, D.; Nigam, V.; Behfar, A.; Christman, K.L. Human versus porcine tissue sourcing for an injectable myocardial matrix hydrogel. *Biomater. Sci.* **2014**, *2014*, 60283D. [CrossRef] [PubMed]
169. Traverse, J.H.; Henry, T.D.; Nabil, D.; Patel, A.N.; Carl, P.; Schaer, G.L.; DeQuach, J.A.; Kinsey, A.M.; Paul, C.; Christman, K.L. First-in-man study of a cardiac extracellular matrix hydrogel in early and late myocardial infarction patients. *JACC Basic Transl. Sci.* **2019**, *4*, 659–669. [CrossRef] [PubMed]
170. Schuurman, H.-J. Regulatory aspects of clinical xenotransplantation. *Int. J. Surg.* **2015**, *23*, 312–321. [CrossRef] [PubMed]

3

Interleukin-1β Mediates Arterial Thrombus Formation via NET-Associated Tissue Factor

Luca Liberale [1,2], Erik W. Holy [3], Alexander Akhmedov [1], Nicole R. Bonetti [1,4], Fabian Nietlispach [3], Christian M. Matter [1,3], François Mach [5], Fabrizio Montecucco [2,6], Jürg H. Beer [1,4], Francesco Paneni [1,3,7], Frank Ruschitzka [3], Peter Libby [8], Thomas F. Lüscher [1,9] and Giovanni G. Camici [1,3,7,*]

1 Center for Molecular Cardiology, Schlieren Campus, University of Zurich, 8952 Schlieren, Switzerland; luca.liberale@uzh.ch (L.L.); alexander.akhmedov@uzh.ch (A.A.); nicole.bonetti@uzh.ch (N.R.B.); christian.matter@uzh.ch (C.M.M.); juerg-hans.beer@ksb.ch (J.H.B.); francesco.paneni@uzh.ch (F.P.); thomas.luescher@zhh.ch (T.F.L.)
2 First Clinic of Internal Medicine, Department of Internal Medicine, University of Genoa, 16132 Genoa, Italy; fabrizio.montecucco@unige.it
3 Department of Cardiology, University Hospital Zurich, 8091 Zurich, Switzerland; erik.holy@usz.ch (E.W.H.); fabian.nietlispach@usz.ch (F.N.); frank.ruschitzka@usz.ch (F.R.)
4 Department of Internal Medicine, Cantonal Hospital of Baden, 5404 Baden, Switzerland
5 Department of Cardiology, Hopital Universitaire de Geneve, 1206 Geneve, Switzerland; francois.mach@unige.ch
6 IRCCS Ospedale Policlinico San Martino Genoa—Italian Cardiovascular Network, 16132 Genoa, Italy
7 Department of Research and Education, University Hospital Zurich, 8001 Zurich, Switzerland
8 Division of Cardiovascular Medicine, Department of Medicine, Brigham and Women's Hospital, Harvard Medical School, 02115 Boston, MA, USA; plibby@bwh.harvard.edu
9 Royal Brompton and Harefield Hospitals and Imperial College, London SW3 6NP, UK
* Correspondence: Giovanni.camici@uzh.ch

Abstract: CANTOS reported reduced secondary atherothrombotic events in patients with residual inflammatory risk treated with the inhibitory anti-IL-1β antibody, Canakinumab. Yet, mechanisms that underlie this benefit remain elusive. Recent work has implicated formation of neutrophil extracellular traps (NETosis) in arterial thrombosis. Hence, the present study explored the potential link between IL-1β, NETs, and tissue factor (TF)—the key trigger of the coagulation cascade—in atherothrombosis. To this end, ST-elevation myocardial infarction (STEMI) patients from the Swiss multicenter trial SPUM-ACS were retrospectively and randomly selected based on their CRP levels. In particular, 33 patients with STEMI and high C-reactive protein (CRP) levels (≥ 10 mg/L) and, 33 with STEMI and low CRP levels (≤ 4 mg/L) were investigated. High CRP patients displayed elevated circulating IL-1β, NETosis, and NET-associated TF plasma levels compared with low CRP ones. Additionally, analysis of patients stratified by circulating IL-1β levels yielded similar results. Moreover, NETosis and NET-associated TF plasma levels correlated positively in the whole population. In addition to the above, translational research experiments provided mechanistic confirmation for the clinical data identifying IL-1β as the initial trigger for the release of the pro-coagulant, NET-associated TF. In conclusion, blunted TF presentation by activated neutrophils undergoing NETosis may provide a mechanistic explanation to reduced secondary atherothrombotic events as observed in canakinumab-treated patients in CANTOS.

Keywords: IL-1β; Canakinumab; arterial thrombosis; tissue factor; neutrophil extracellular traps

1. Introduction

The Canakinumab Anti-inflammatory Thrombosis Outcomes Study (CANTOS) [1] affirmed in humans the inflammatory theory of atherosclerosis [2]. In CANTOS, over 10,000 post-myocardial infarction patients with residual inflammatory risk (defined as high-sensitivity C-reactive protein (hs-CRP) concentrations ≥ 2 mg/L) and treated with currently mandated concomitant cardiovascular (CV) therapy randomly received placebo or one of 3 doses of the interleukin (IL)-1β neutralizing antibody canakinumab. Canakinumab treatment reduced the primary composite endpoint (non-fatal myocardial infarction or stroke and cardiovascular death) by 15%, and blunted circulating levels of hsCRP and IL-6 by 35–40% without lowering atherogenic lipids [1]. Yet, the molecular mechanisms underlying this clinical benefit, particularly its thrombotic component, remain incompletely understood.

Occlusive arterial thrombus formation following plaque rupture or erosion causes most myocardial infarctions and many ischemic strokes [3]. Several experimental observations suggest a strong bidirectional link between inflammation, atherosclerosis and arterial thrombosis [4–8]. Indeed, inflammatory conditions favour atherothrombosis as reflected by increased plaque burden and CV event rates in patients with chronic inflammatory diseases [9]. Moreover, thrombosis itself can also induce and enhance inflammation thus setting the stage for a vicious cycle involving different pathways, and more prominently the tissue factor (TF)-thrombin axis [10]. Recent work has implicated neutrophil extracellular traps (NETs) in thrombosis by various mechanisms including presentation of tissue factor procoagulant activity [11–13]. Formation of NETs contributes to the host defence properties of neutrophils. Various infectious and non-infectious stimuli induce NETs which consist of extracellular strands of unwound DNA in complex with histones and proteins from neutrophil granules [13,14].

Hence, the present study explored the molecular mechanisms by which canakinumab reduces atherothrombotic events, as observed in CANTOS. To this end, we tested the hypothesis that IL-1β, NETosis, and TF-bearing NETs interrelate in a cohort of patients with ST-elevation myocardial infarction (STEMI) and different degree of systemic inflammation randomly selected from the Swiss SPUM-ACS trial (ClinicalTrials.gov number NCT01000701) [15]. To provide mechanistic explanations for these clinical findings, mouse experiments used a murine canakinumab-surrogate antibody (01BSUR) IL-1β to inhibit this cytokine in lipopolysaccharide (LPS)-treated mice before induction of arterial thrombosis by endothelial-specific photochemical injury.

2. Experimental Section

2.1. Patient Enrollment and Blood Sampling

The SPUM–ACS study (Special Program University Medicine–Acute Coronary Syndromes) is a prospective cohort study of consecutive acute coronary syndrome (ACS) patients hospitalized in different Swiss university hospitals registered in ClinicalTrials.gov (NCT01000701). Details of the study have been reported previously [15]. Briefly, patients with ACS undergoing coronary angiography were consecutively enrolled in four Swiss medical centres between December 2009 and October 2012. Exclusion criteria were severe physical disability, inability to give consent owing to dementia, and life expectancy of <1 year for non-cardiac reasons. Inclusion criteria were age ≥18 years, ST-segment elevation myocardial infarction (STEMI), non-ST-segment–elevation myocardial infarction, or unstable angina. The local ethics committees approved the study and all patients gave written informed consent in compliance with the Declaration of Helsinki as listed under ClinicalTrials.gov number NCT01000701.

STEMI patients were enrolled at the Andreas-Grüntzig-Catheterisation laboratory of the Department of Cardiology at the University Hospital Zurich, Switzerland, within 72 h after pain onset, and subdivided into two groups. Specifically, plasma samples of 33 STEMI patients with high circulating C-reactive protein (CRP) levels ≥ 10 mg/L and 33 STEMI patients with low CRP levels ≤ 4 mg/L and were analysed. Liver or kidney failure, active cancer, infections, or autoimmune disease were exclusion criteria. Blood was drawn from the arterial sheath into EDTA tubes at the time of diagnostic coronary angiography and centrifuged at 2700 g for 10 min at room temperature to obtain plasma, and frozen and stored in aliquots at −80 °C until serial measurement in the core laboratory (Department of Clinical Chemistry, University Hospital Zurich, Switzerland).

2.2. *IL-1β Quantification in Human Plasma*

Plasma levels of IL-1β were measured by high-sensitivity ELISA following the manufacturer's instructions (Quantikine® HSLB00D, R&D Systems, Minneapolis, MN). Plasma samples with an absorbance value below the lowest IL-1β concentration included in the standard curve (assessed in duplicates) were assigned an absorbance equal to that of the lowest point of the standard curve.

2.3. *NETosis Assessment in Human and Murine Plasma*

Quantification of circulating NET remnants such as myeloperoxidase (MPO)-DNA complexes by ELISA appears to be the current, most specific and objective assay to monitor NETosis in vivo [12,16,17]. As previously described [12,17], microtiter plates were coated with anti-MPO antibody (5 μg/mL, Cat No. 07-496, Merck, Darmstadt, Germany) overnight at 4 °C. After blocking with 1% BSA, the serum was added in combination with the peroxidase-conjugated anti-DNA monoclonal antibody (part of the commercial cell death detection kit; Roche, Basel, Switzerland) according to the manufacturer's instructions. After 2 h of incubation and accurate washing with PBS, the peroxidase substrate (ATBS) from the kit was added to each plate. The absorbance at 405 nm wavelength was measured after 40 min incubation in the dark, 490 nm was used as reference wavelength.

2.4. *Tissue Factor-DNA Complexes Quantification in Human and Murine Plasma*

To assess the NET contribution to circulating TF levels, we sought to quantify the fraction of TF associated with circulating DNA. This protocol adapted that used for MPO-DNA complex assessment to detect TF–DNA complexes. Briefly, microtiter plate was coated with either human or mouse TF capture antibody (parts of the commercial DuoSet® ELISA kits from R&D Systems, Cat No. DY2339 and DY3178-05, respectively) according to the manufacturer's instructions. After overnight incubation and blocking with 1% BSA, serum was added in combination with the peroxidase-conjugated anti-DNA monoclonal antibody (component No.2 of the commercial cell death detection kit from Roche, cat No. 11774425001) following the manufacturer's instructions. Validation experiments measured MPO-DNA and TF–DNA complexes in human plasma incubated with increasing concentration of LPS to stimulate NETosis (Supplemental Figure S1). Briefly, blood was collected in EDTA tubes (Vacutainer, BD Diagnostics) from a healthy donor and aliquoted in tubes containing increasing concentration of LPS dissolved in PBS (0–25 μg/mL) [18]. After 2 h, plasma was isolated by centrifugation at 2700 g for 15 min and MPO-DNA and TF–DNA complexes assessed as mentioned above (Supplemental Figure S1).

2.5. *Animals*

Experiments used 12-week-old male C57BL/6 wild-type mice (Charles-River Lab, Freiburg im Breisgau, Germany); all rodents were kept in a temperature-controlled animal facility under normal light/dark cycle with free access to food and water. All procedures were approved by the Committee for Animal Testing of the Canton of Zurich, Switzerland (ZH023/17). Animal experiments were performed conform to the Directive 2010/63/EU of the European Parliament and of the Council of 22 September 2010 on the protection of animals used for scientific purposes.

2.6. *Monoclonal anti IL-1β Antibody*

Dr. Hermann Gram (Novartis, Basel, Switzerland) kindly provided the highly specific canakinumab-surrogate anti-mouse IL-1β antibody 01BSUR. Since the human anti IL-1β antibody (i.e., canakinumab) does not neutralize the rodent antigen, experiments used this monoclonal anti-IL-1β antibody instead. Novartis used 01BSUR, a murine IgG2a/k isotype, in all parallel pre-clinical studies performed for the development of canakinumab [19,20].

2.7. Treatments and Arterial Thrombosis

As previously described [21], mice received 5 mg/kg lipopolysaccharide (LPS) (E. coli O111: B4, Sigma–Aldrich, St. Louis, MO, USA) by intraperitoneal (i.p.) injection 10 h before the laser-induced arterial thrombosis to trigger inflammation. Five hours after LPS administration and for the remaining 5 h before exposure to the thrombosis protocol, animals randomly received the murine canakinumab-surrogate antibody (01BSUR, 10 μg/g) or vehicle (i.e., NaCl 0.9%) via tail vein injection. The unique dose was chosen to reproduce the canakinumab concentration in sera from patients enrolled in the clinical trial CACZ885A2102 (NCT00487708), as previously described [20,22–25].

Ten hours after i.p. LPS injection and five hours after i.v. treatment with the canakinumab-surrogate antibody, mice underwent photochemical injury of the common carotid artery CCA as previously described (Figure 1A) [26–28]. Briefly, mice were anaesthetized using pentobarbital (87 mg/kg body weight); after midline neck incision, the right common carotid artery was exposed under an operating microscope. To induce photochemical injury of the endothelium, rose bengal (50 mg/kg body weight) was injected into the tail vein and the common carotid artery was exposed to a laser light beam (1.5 mW, 540 nm, Mellesgriot Inc., Carlsbad, CA, USA) at a distance of 6 cm for 60 min. Carotid blood flow and heart rate were monitored (Doppler flow probe carotid artery Transonic Systems Inc., 0.5 VB) until occlusion (flow ≤0.1 mL for 1 min) or for a maximum of 120 min, in case arterial thrombosis was not detected.

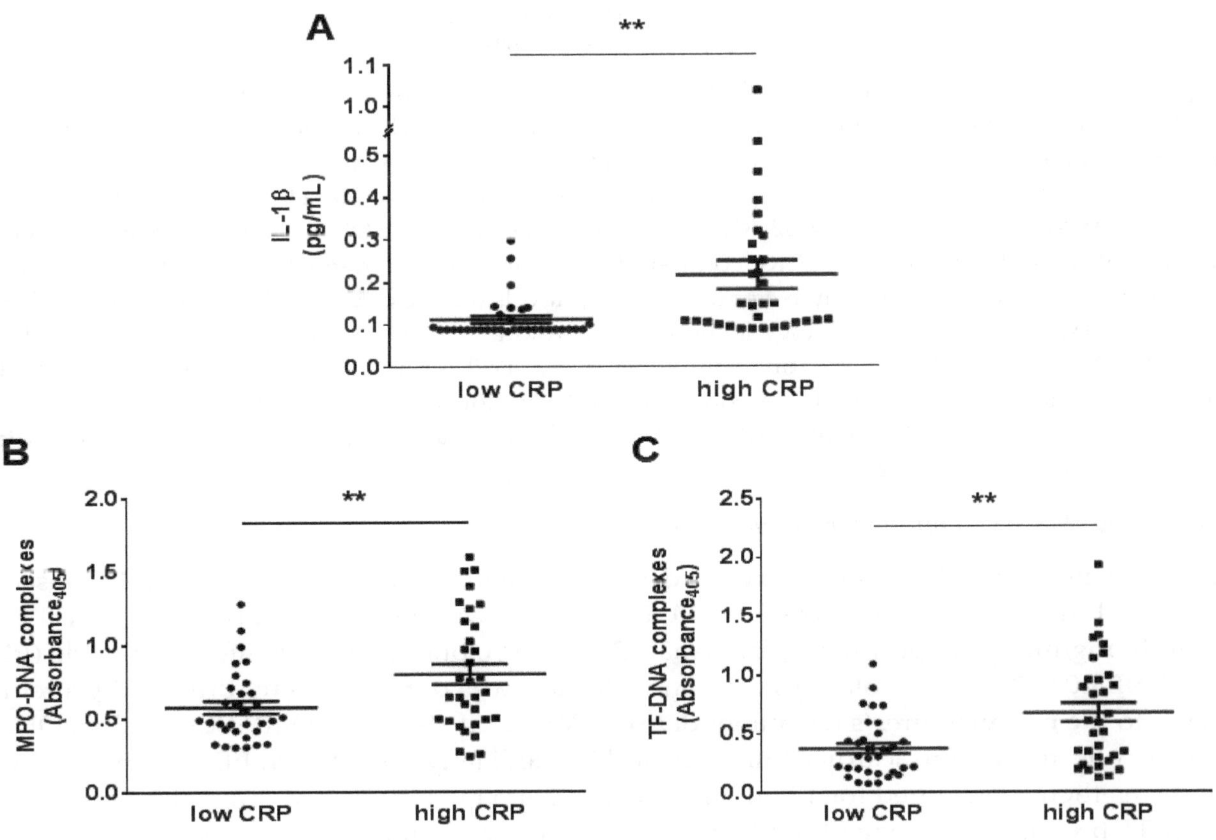

Figure 1. *Cont.*

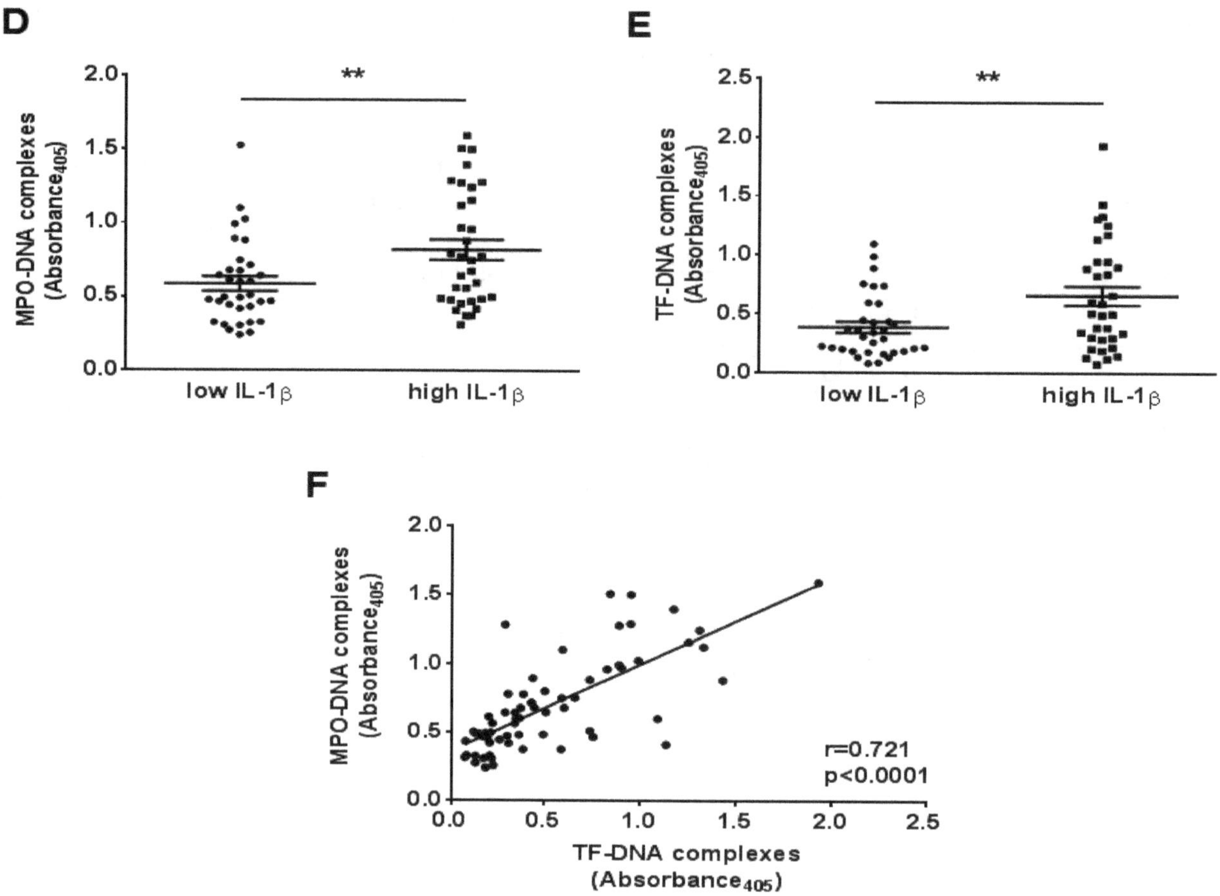

Figure 1. Levels of IL-1β, neutrophil extracellular traps (NETosis), NET-associated tissue factor and their relationships in patients with coronary disease. (**A**) STEMI patients with high systemic inflammation have higher IL-1β plasma levels than those with lower C-reactive protein (CRP) levels ($n = 33$). (**B**) Patients with STEMI and high CRP levels showed increased levels of NETosis assessed by plasma MPO-DNA complexes ($n = 32$–33) (**C**) Plasma tissue factor TF)-DNA complexes rose in patients with STEMI and high circulating CRP compared to less inflamed patients ($n = 33$). (**D–E**) Similarly, in patients categorized according to circulating IL-1β levels (above or below the median value of our cohort 0.1041 pg/mL), those with high levels of this cytokine also showed increased myeloperoxidase (MPO)-DNA and TF–DNA circulating complexes ($n = 33$) (**F**) A positive relationship was detectable among plasma IL-1β and MPO-DNA complexes in the whole cohort ($n = 66$). ** $p < 0.01$. CRP = C reactive protein, IL-1β = interleukin-1β, MPO = myeloperoxidase, STEMI = ST-elevated myocardial infarction, TF = tissue factor.

2.8. Artery and Plasma Sampling for Tissue Factor Assessment

Aortas were collected after euthanasia and snap frozen in liquid nitrogen. They were subsequently homogenized in the lysis buffer (Tris 50 mM, NaCl 150 mM, EDTA 1 mM, NaF 1 mM, DTT 1 mM, aprotinin 10 mg/mL, leupeptin 10 mg/mL, Na3VO4 0.1 mM, phenylmethylsulfonyl fluoride (PMSF) 1 mM, and NP-40 0.5%); next, total protein concentration was determined by Bradford protein assay according to the manufacturer's recommendations (VWR Life Science AMRESCO, Solon, OH, USA). Blood was collected via intracardiac puncture and immediately mixed with EDTA. The EDTA-blood solution was then centrifuged for 15 min at 3000 g. Plasma was collected and snap-frozen in liquid nitrogen. TF protein measurement used a colorimetric enzyme-linked immunosorbent assay (ELISA) specific for the mouse protein (DY3178-05; R&D systems, Minneapolis, MN, USA) following the manufacturer's instructions. For aortas, TF concentration measured by ELISA was normalized to the total protein content of the sample. TF content was expressed as pg/mg of total protein.

2.9. *Statistical Analysis*

Data are expressed as mean ± SEM. All statistical analyses used GraphPad Prism 6 software (GraphPad Software, Inc, La Jolla, CA, USA). Data were analysed by one-way analysis of variance (ANOVA) with Bonferroni *post hoc* test for multiple comparisons or unpaired two-tailed Student's *t*-test as appropriate. Fisher's exact test was used for comparison of categorical data between study subjects, and Pearson's correlation analysis was used to test the correlation between two quantitative variables. A probability p value below 0.05 was considered as statistically significant.

3. Results

3.1. *IL-1β levels, NETosis and TF–DNA Complexes Increase in STEMI Patients with High Systemic Inflammation*

To explore the relationship between IL-1β, NETosis, and TF-bearing NETs we have retrospectively and randomly selected patients with STEMI and different degree of systemic inflammation (CRP ≤ 4 mg/L or ≥ 10 mg/L) from the Swiss SPUM-ACS trial. Then, IL-1β levels as well as circulating MPO-DNA and TF–DNA complexes were measured by ELISA and compared between the high CRP and low CRP groups.

66 STEMI patients (33 for each degree of inflammation group) with a median age of 66 years were enrolled. Table 1 reports a complete assessments of demographic and clinic characteristics of the whole cohort. As expected, patients were at high cardiovascular risk with 65.2% of them being active smokers, 50.0% suffering from hypertension and another 50% showing dyslipidaemia. Ongoing medical therapy at the time of angiography (i.e., anti-platelets, diuretic, anti-hypertensive or lipid-lowering drugs) is detailed in Table 1. Of importance, the two groups did not differ in blood pressure, BMI, smoking habits, comorbidities (i.e., dyslipidaemia and diabetes mellitus) or medications.

Table 1. Demographic and clinical characteristics of the study cohort.

	Whole Cohort (n = 66)	Low CRP * (n = 33)	High CRP (n = 33)	p
Demographic				
Age, years	66 ± 12	66 ± 12	65 ± 12	NS
Gender, m/f	46/20	23/10	23/10	NS
Clinical and biochemical				
Systolic BP †, mmHg	130 ± 23	130 ± 26	123 ± 20	NS
Diastolic BP, mmHg	78±15	81±16	75±12	NS
BMI ‡, Kg/m^2	25.5±3.6	25.2±3.6	25.8±3.6	NS
Hypertension	33 (50.0%)	17 (51.5%)	16 (48.5%)	NS
Diabetes	9 (13.6%)	5 (15.2%)	4 (12.1%)	NS
Active smokers	43 (65.2%)	10 (30.0%)	18 (54.5%)	NS
Total-c §, mmol/L	4.93±1.12	5.15±1.26	4.70±0.93	NS
HDL-c ‖, mmol/L	1.22±0.31	1.24±0.27	1.21±0.34	NS
LDL-c #, mmol/L	3.31±1.13	3.57±1.23	3.07±0.97	NS
Dyslipidaemia	33 (50.0%)	17 (51.5%)	16 (48.5%)	NS
Medications				
Aspirin	17 (25.8%)	9 (27.3%)	8 (24.2%)	NS
Clopidogrel	2 (3.0%)	1 (3.0%)	1 (3.0%)	NS
ACE-I ** or ARBs ††	17 (26.2%)	11 (33.3%)	6 (18.8%)	NS
β-blockers	10 (15.2%)	7 (21.2%)	3 (9.1%)	NS
Diuretics	6 (9.1%)	4 (12.1%)	2 (6.1%)	NS
Statins	12 (18.2%)	4 (12.1%)	8 (24.2%)	NS

* CRP: C reactive protein; † BP: blood pressure; ‡ BMI: body mass index; § Total-c: total cholesterol; ‖ HDL-c: high density lipoprotein cholesterol; # LDL-c: low density lipoprotein cholesterol; ** ACE-I: angiotensin converting enzyme inhibitors; †† ARBs: angiotensin receptor blockers.

Circulating IL-1β levels increased significantly in STEMI patients with high CRP concentrations as compared to those with lower CRP (0.215 ± 0.034 vs. 0.111 ± 0.009 pg/mL; $p < 0.01$; Figure 1A).

Circulating plasma MPO-DNA complexes were also higher in the high CRP group compared to patients with low CRP (0.80 ± 0.07 vs. 0.58 ± 0.04; $p < 0.01$; Figure 1B). Furthermore, patients with STEMI and elevated CRP had statistical significantly higher levels of circulating TF–DNA complexes than those with low CRP levels as compared the less inflamed subjects (0.67 ± 0.08 vs. 0.37 ± 0.04; $p < 0.01$; Figure 1C). Categorization of patients according to circulating IL-1β levels (above or below its median value in the cohort: 0.1041 pg/mL) yielded similar results to those observed with lower and higher CRP cut-off points as defined above (0.821 ± 0.07 vs. 0.586 ± 0.05 for MPO-DNA and 0.66 ± 0.08 vs. 0.39 ± 0.05 for TF–DNA; $p < 0.01$ for both; Figure 1D–E). Moreover, a strong positive correlation was observed in the entire STEMI cohort between the NETosis marker MPO-DNA and NET-associated TF in plasma (r = 0.721; $p < 0.001$; Figure 1F).

3.2. IL-1β Neutralization Delays Arterial Thrombotic Occlusion In Vivo in LPS-Treated Mice

Murine thrombosis experiments sought to mimic an underlying inflammatory condition by administering LPS, as done previously [21]. Next, animals received the canakinumab-surrogate antibody (01BSUR, 10 μg/g) and underwent the thrombosis protocol (Figure 2A). This pre-treatment resembles the situation of recurrent events in CANTOS participants, who were stable at time of enrollment (≥ 30 d post qualifying event.). Compared to controls, inflamed mice treated with anti-IL-1β antibody showed a 50% increase in time to occlusion (24.9 ± 2.2 vs. 39.2 ± 2.3 min, $p < 0.001$, Figure 2B,C). The two study groups had comparable initial mean flow and heart rates (0.66 ± 0.05 vs. 0.67 ± 0.04 mL/min and 333 ± 15 vs. 354 ± 16 beats/min, respectively; Figure 2D,E).

3.3. Treatment with Canakinumab-Surrogate Anti-Mouse IL-1β Antibody Reduces Plasma Levels of Tissue Factor

To investigate the mechanisms that underlie the decreased thrombotic potential observed in canakinumab-surrogate treated mice, plasma and aortic lysates were analysed for TF levels, the key trigger of the extrinsic coagulation cascade. TF plasma levels decreased in mice treated with the anti-IL-1β antibody (37.07 ± 4.14 vs. 49.49 ± 3.17 pg/mL; Figure 3A) as compared to controls. On the other hand, TF levels in aortic extracts from the two treatment arms did not differ (1413 ± 101.8 vs. 1623 ± 130.8 pg/mg of protein; Figure 3B).

3.4. Anti-IL-1β Treatment Reduces NETosis and NET-Associated Tissue Factor Levels

Since arterial TF levels did not differ between treated and untreated animals, the current study focused on circulating protein as a possible mediator of the retarded thrombosis post IL-1β inhibition. Several cell types contribute to the circulating TF pool during arterial thrombosis. Indeed, NETs can promote thrombus formation by presenting active TF in the setting of myocardial infarction.[12] Animals treated with anti-IL-1β antibody have reduced levels of circulating MPO-DNA complexes (a marker of in vivo NETosis) after thrombus formation, as compared to vehicle-treated animals (0.082 ± 0.010 vs. 0.152 ± 0.024; $p < 0.05$; Figure 4A). To determine whether the reduced circulating TF levels observed in the treatment group related directly to the reduced NETosis, TF–DNA complexes were assessed in plasma from the two treatment arms. IL-1β inhibition significantly reduced levels of TF–DNA complexes after thrombus formation, as compared to control treatment (0.048 ± 0.012 vs. 0.099 ± 0.018; $p < 0.05$; Figure 4B). Blood cell counts did not differ in the two study subgroups (Table 2).

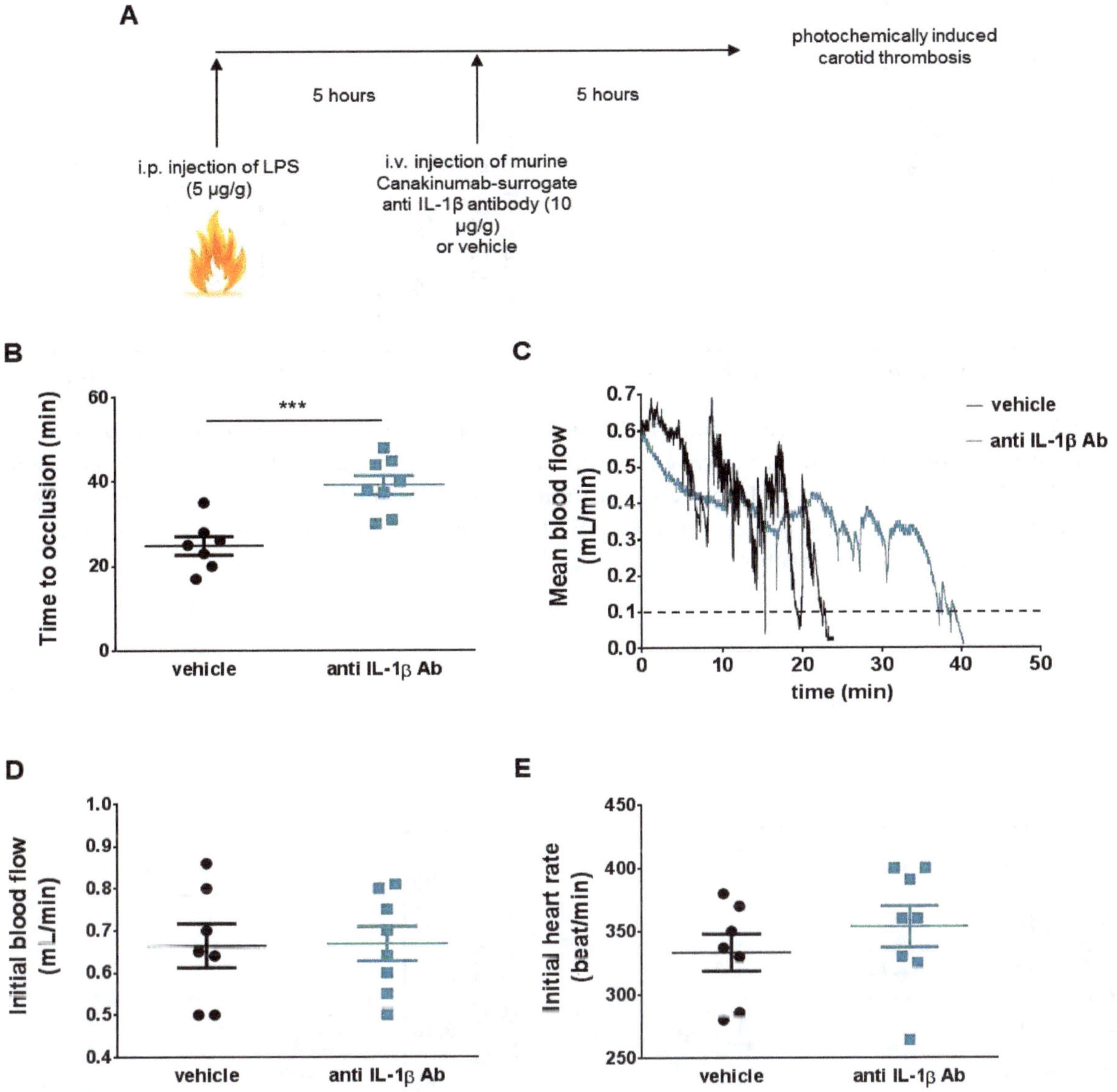

Figure 2. Anti-IL-1β antibody retards arterial thrombosis. (**A**) In an attempt to simulate the design of Canakinumab Anti-inflammatory Thrombosis Outcomes Study (CANTOS), which enrolled patients with residual inflammatory risk, animals received lipopolysaccharide (LPS) (5 μg/g, i.p) 10 h before undergoing photochemically induced carotid thrombosis. The anti-mouse IL-1β monoclonal antibody was administered to the animal intravenously via tail vein injection 5 h before thrombosis at a single dose of 10 μg/g, vehicle (i.e., NaCl 0.9%) was used as negative control. (**B**) Animals treated with monoclonal antibody against IL-1β (anti IL-1β Ab) showed increased time to occlusion as compared to vehicle-treated ones (n = 7–8). (**C**) Representative trace of mean blood flow until occlusion (mean flow ≤ 0.1 mL for 1 min) in the two study groups. (**D**,**E**) Baseline blood flow and heart rate did not differ among treated and untreated animals (n = 7–8). ***$p < 0.001$. IL-1β = interleukin-1β, LPS = lipopolysaccharide.

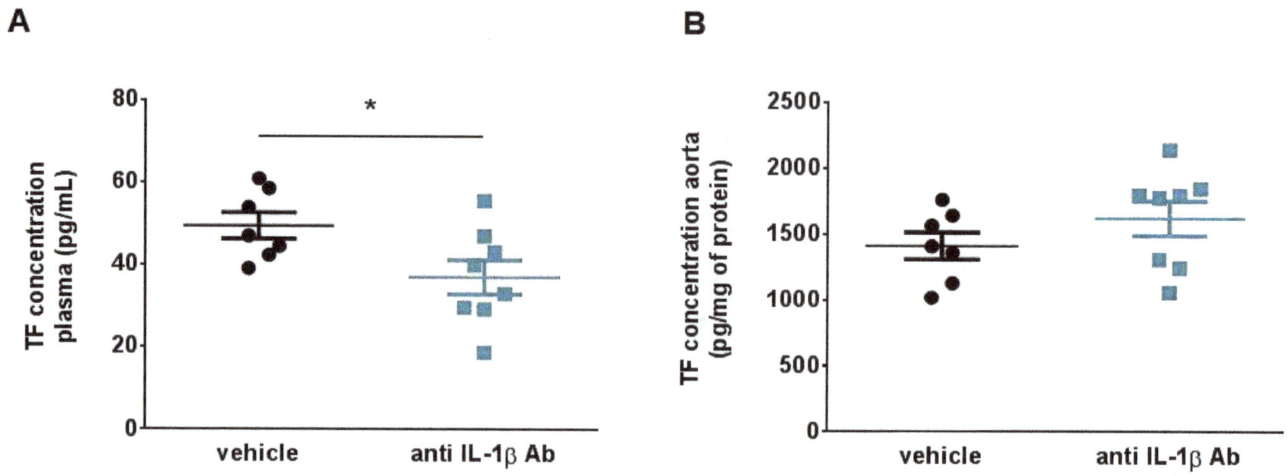

Figure 3. IL-1β blockade reduces different tissue factor pools in mice with arterial thrombosis. (**A**) Treatment with the canakinumab-surrogate antibody (anti IL-1β Ab) reduced plasma TF levels as assessed by ELISA ($n = 7$–8). (**B**) Treated and untreated animals showed no difference in terms of TF concentration in aorta lysates ($n = 7$). * $p < 0.05$. ELISA = enzyme-linked immunosorbent assay, IL-1β = interleukin-1β, TF = tissue factor.

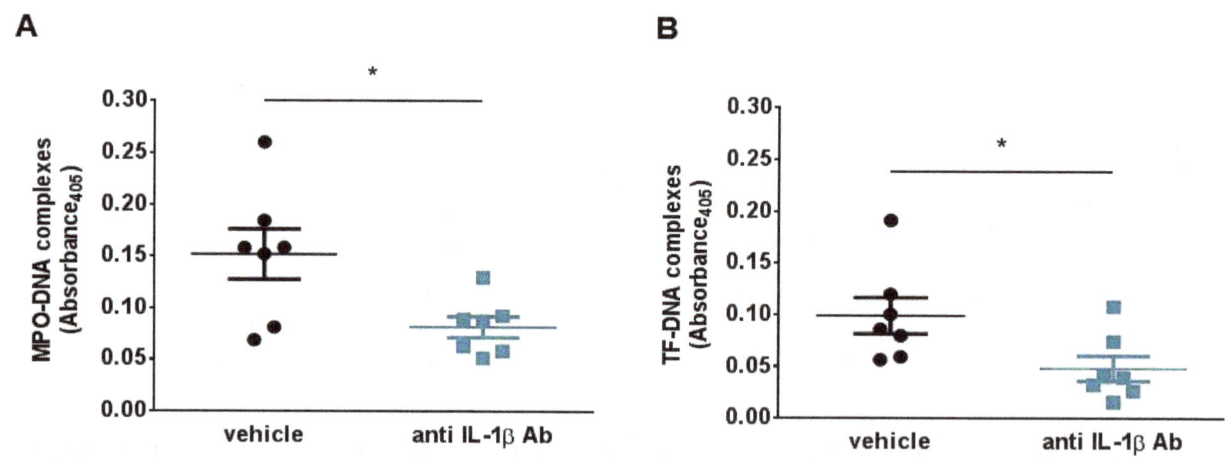

Figure 4. IL-1β blockade limits NETosis and NET-associate tissue factor levels. (**A**) Animal treated with the murine anti IL-1β antibody showed a significant reduction in the level of NETosis plasma marker MPO-DNA complexes ($n = 7$) (**B**) Levels of NET-associated TF fell after thrombosis in animals treated with the anti-IL-1β antibody as assessed by plasma TF–DNA complexes ($n = 7$). * $p < 0.05$. IL-1β = interleukin-1β, MPO = myeloperoxidase, NET = neutrophil extracellular trap, TF = tissue factor.

Table 2. Peripheral blood cell count.

	Vehicle	Anti IL *-1β	p
Total WBC ‡ ($10^3/mm^3$)	1.37 ± 0.13	1.38 ± 0.18	NS
Lymphocytes (%)	43.1 ± 5.2	32.3 ± 4.2	NS
Neutrophils (%)	51.4 ± 5.0	62.7 ± 4.2	NS
Monocytes (%)	5.5 ± 0.6	5.0 ± 0.7	NS
NLR †	1.5 ± 0.3	2.7 ± 0.7	NS
Platelets ($10^3/mm^3$)	297.6 ± 44.2	312.8 ± 28.8	NS

* IL: interleukin; † NLR: neutrophil to lymphocyte ratio; ‡ WBC: white blood cells.

4. Discussion

Ischaemic heart disease and stroke caused by atherothrombotic complications lead global causes of morbidity and mortality triggered by inflammatory bursts [29–31]. Recently, CANTOS established a causal role of inflammation in humans with previous ACS and residual inflammatory risk by showing reduced recurrent cardiovascular events after treatment with canakinumab (an anti-IL-1β antibody) [1]. The present study probed the potential mechanisms by which canakinumab may reduce thrombotic events.

This study tested the hypothesis that IL-1β influences NET formation and NETs' association with tissue factor (TF) the key trigger of the coagulation cascade in atherothrombosis. To assess the role of inflammation, ACS patients with different degree of systemic inflammation—so as to simulate the conditions observed in patients enrolled in CANTOS—were selected. In particular, 33 patients with STEMI and high C-reactive protein (CRP) levels ($\geq$ 10 mg/L) and, 33 with STEMI and low CRP levels ($\leq$ 4 mg/L), were investigated.

Patients were retrospectively and randomly selected from the Swiss multi-center trial SPUM-ACS (n = 1639, NCT01000701). The SPUM–ACS study (Special Program University Medicine–Acute Coronary Syndromes) is a prospective cohort study of consecutive acute coronary syndrome (ACS) patients hospitalized in different Swiss university hospitals. Details of the study have been reported previously [15]. Previous investigations have implicated NETs in coronary artery disease [14,32], and the present report correlates systemic inflammation and IL-1β with MPO-DNA complexes, currently considered an established assay for NETosis in vivo [16]. We further assessed circulating NETs-associated TF by measuring plasma TF–DNA complexes and documented their significant elevation in STEMI patients with high CRP plasma levels compared to those with lower CRP. Additionally, categorization of patients according to circulating IL-1β levels showed higher NETosis rate and levels of TF–DNA complexes in patients with higher levels of this cytokine. Moreover, the levels of NET-associated TF correlated with MPO-DNA circulating levels, a novel finding that indicates their strong interdependency. Stakos et al. recently reported NET-associated TF isolated from the culprit coronary artery of ACS patients [12]. Furthermore, these authors found that TF required the intact NET scaffold to be biologically active [12]. The relationship reported here between levels of systemic inflammation, IL-1β, NETosis and NET-associated TF production indicates a common regulating pathway and supports the hypothesis of TF arising from neutrophil undergoing NETosis, as a possible mediator of the benefits of canakinumab treatment.

Experimental data have long suggested a role for IL-1β in atherothrombosis [33,34]; indeed, IL-1β causes vascular smooth muscle cell dysfunction, activates endothelial cells and induces pro-coagulant and adhesion protein expression [35,36]. Furthermore, experimental and human atherosclerotic plaques contain IL-1β and its loss of function limits experimental atherosclerosis [37,38]. Similarly, CANTOS demonstrated that IL-1β blockade reduces recurrent myocardial infarction in human after ACS [1]. The current study sought to experimentally investigate the mechanisms of this effect and showed blunted thrombosis in inflamed mice treated with canakinumab surrogate to resemble the IL-1β-mediated inflammatory risk of patients enrolled in CANTOS.

Arterial thrombosis mediated by activation of platelets and TF causes most ACS [39]. Patients with CV risk factors as well as those with ACS have increased levels of TF [40–42]. Various cell types produce TF including endothelial cells, monocytes/macrophages and smooth muscle cells in response to different pro-inflammatory cytokines, among which IL-1β is one of the best-characterized [43–45]. In light of the above, we hypothesized that treatment with IL-1β antibody could reduce thrombus formation by targeting TF in vascular and/or circulating cells. IL-1β neutralization in mice reduced TF levels in plasma but not in arterial tissue, suggesting that in our experimental setting IL-1β inhibition primarily targets circulating TF.

As recently reported, activated neutrophils can contribute to blood-borne TF and thrombus formation by binding the injured endothelium [10,46]. Although neutrophils contain TF, either endogenous or acquired via microparticle internalization, questions remained on how these cells release it [10]. In 2012, Kambas et al [47]. reported that neutrophils can release large amounts of TF in the form of NETs. They further showed that NET-associated TF indeed derives from neutrophils, and that the thrombin eventually formed can activate platelets. The same authors reported a requirement for neutrophil priming with pro-inflammatory cytokines (i.e., IL-1β and TNF-α) for TF mRNA translation [47]. In line with the above, the current study found blunted NETosis (MPO-DNA complexes) in IL-1β-blocked animals after thrombus formation, thus underscoring the important role of IL-1β in priming neutrophils for NETosis during inflammatory conditions [48]. Next, we assessed whether blunted NETosis could account for the reduction in TF levels as seen in anti-IL-1β-treated animals by measuring TF–DNA complex in the plasma. Affirming our hypothesis, animals pretreated with IL-1β antibody showed significantly reduced NET-associated TF levels compared to controls. A possible role for IL-1β in NETosis induction has long been hypothesized [49] and recently confirmed in a publication by Meher et al [50]. Here, the authors report that IL-1β localizes within NETs in mice with experimental abdominal aortic aneurysms and that IL-1β blockade inhibits NETosis in isolated neutrophils [50]. They proposed a mechanism by which IL-1β–induced ceramide synthesis triggers the release of NETs by inducing nuclear Cer 16:0 synthesis, which permeabilizes the nuclear membrane and triggers NETosis. Accordingly, attenuation of NETosis can result from either inhibition of IL-1β signaling (IL-1 receptor antagonist treatment) or inhibition of ceramide synthases (fumonisin B1 treatment) [50]. Furthermore, we recently investigated IL-1 isoform association with NETs [51]. Curiously, we found that NET-associated cathepsin G degrades IL-1β to inactive fragments, but actually cleaves IL-1α to a more active form. The IL-1α isoform rather than IL-1β isoform accounts for activation of tissue factor expression and activity on human endothelial cells by NETs [51]. Thus, canakinumab might reduce thrombosis rate by blunting IL-1β-mediated NETosis synergistically with the reduction of other known IL-1β pro-thrombotic features such as its agonist role on platelets [52].

The current study has some limitations which merit consideration. First, patients enrolled in this clinical cohort had less use of CV medications at baseline than in CANTOS, as would be expected in a group that included individuals with a first MI, in contrast to the secondary prevention population in CANTOS. Animal experiments permit in-depth investigation of molecular mechanisms but do not necessarily faithfully replicate the clinical setting. CANTOS enrolled patients with a previous ACS with comorbidities and treated with many medications, conditions that do not apply to the rodents used in this study. Also, while CANTOS reported a reduction of secondary CV events, we here show a reduction of the thrombotic potential in the non-atherosclerotic mouse carotid arteries. Lastly, to mirror the pro-inflammatory state of the CANTOS cohort, we challenged mice with LPS to induce an inflammatory response. This intervention does not fully reproduce the low-grade inflammation observed in patients enrolled in CANTOS. Yet, low-dose LPS treatment is a well-established and reproducible method for experimental induction of inflammation that does not rely on altered metabolic conditions or genetic manipulations, unlike many other models (e.g., dyslipidaemia and obesity models, cytokine overexpressing animals), and thus avoids numerous variables in the experimental conditions. Furthermore, hsCRP—the inclusion criteria for the CANTOS trial—is not a reliable marker of inflammation in mice [53].

5. Conclusions

In conclusion, this study proposes reduced TF production by neutrophils undergoing NETosis as a novel mechanistic contributor to the reduction in CV events achieved by treatment with canakinumab in the CANTOS trial. The results affirm the tight interrelationship of inflammation with thrombosis, and point to processes and biomarkers that merit monitoring in further attempts to address residual cardiovascular risk with anti-inflammatory interventions.

Author Contributions: L.L., P.L., F.P., T.F.L. and G.G.C. conceived the project and the experimental set-up; L.L., A.A. and N.R.B. performed experiments; C.M.M., F.Ma. and T.F.L. coordinated the enrollment of the patients

(SPUM-ACS study); L.L. and G.G.C. wrote the manuscript; E.W.H., F.N., J.H.B., F.Mo. and F.R. provided critical input for the set-up and analysis for the clinical part of the study; all authors critically reviewed the manuscript and contributed to discussion and interpretation of results.

Acknowledgments: We thank Hermann Gram from the Novartis Institutes for BioMedical Research for kindly supplying the anti-mouse IL-1β monoclonal antibody. We are grateful to the principal investigators of the SPUM-ACS study: Stephan Windecker, University of Bern, Peter Jüni, University of Bern, Nicholas Rodondi, MD, University of Lausanne, Switzerland. Furthermore, we acknowledge the diligent work of the independent clinical events committee for SPUM-ACS: Matthias Pfisterer, University of Basel (chair), Tiziano Moccetti, CardioCentro Lugano, Lukas Kappenberger, University of Lausanne, Switzerland. We also thank the local study nurses (Anika Adam and Christine Hager), the lab technicians, the central data monitors, the electronic data capturing system (2mt GmbH Ulm, Germany) and the members of the local catheter teams for their invaluable work.

References

1. Ridker, P.M.; Everett, B.M.; Thuren, T.; MacFadyen, J.G.; Chang, W.H.; Ballantyne, C.; Fonseca, F.; Nicolau, J.; Koenig, W.; Anker, S.D.; et al. Antiinflammatory Therapy with Canakinumab for Atherosclerotic Disease. *N. Engl. J. Med.* **2017**, *377*, 1119–1131. [CrossRef] [PubMed]
2. Libby, P. Inflammation in atherosclerosis. *Nature* **2002**, *420*, 868–874. [CrossRef] [PubMed]
3. Lippi, G.; Franchini, M.; Targher, G. Arterial thrombus formation in cardiovascular disease. *Nat. Rev. Cardiol.* **2011**, *8*, 502–512. [CrossRef] [PubMed]
4. Montecucco, F.; Liberale, L.; Bonaventura, A.; Vecchie, A.; Dallegri, F.; Carbone, F. The Role of Inflammation in Cardiovascular Outcome. *Curr. Atheroscler. Rep.* **2017**, *19*, 11. [CrossRef]
5. Hansson, G.K.; Libby, P.; Tabas, I. Inflammation and plaque vulnerability. *J. Intern. Med.* **2015**, *278*, 483–493. [CrossRef]
6. Libby, P.; Simon, D.I. Inflammation and thrombosis: The clot thickens. *Circulation* **2001**, *103*, 1718–1720. [CrossRef]
7. Jackson, S.P.; Darbousset, R.; Schoenwaelder, S.M. Thromboinflammation: Challenges of therapeutically targeting coagulation and other host defense mechanisms. *Blood* **2019**, *133*, 906–918. [CrossRef]
8. Casula, M.; Montecucco, F.; Bonaventura, A.; Liberale, L.; Vecchié, A.; Dallegri, F.; Carbone, F. Update on the role of Pentraxin 3 in atherosclerosis and cardiovascular diseases. *Vascul. Pharmacol.* **2017**, *99*, 1–12. [CrossRef]
9. Carbone, F.; Bonaventura, A.; Liberale, L.; Paolino, S.; Torre, F.; Dallegri, F.; Montecucco, F.; Cutolo, M. Atherosclerosis in Rheumatoid Arthritis: Promoters and Opponents. *Clin. Rev. Allergy Immunol.* **2018**, 1–14. [CrossRef]
10. Kambas, K.; Mitroulis, I.; Ritis, K. The emerging role of neutrophils in thrombosis-the journey of TF through NETs. *Front. Immunol.* **2012**, *3*, 385. [CrossRef]
11. Martinod, K.; Wagner, D.D. Thrombosis: Tangled up in NETs. *Blood* **2014**, *123*, 2768–2776. [CrossRef] [PubMed]
12. Stakos, D.A.; Kambas, K.; Konstantinidis, T.; Mitroulis, I.; Apostolidou, E.; Arelaki, S.; Tsironidou, V.; Giatromanolaki, A.; Skendros, P.; Konstantinides, S.; et al. Expression of functional tissue factor by neutrophil extracellular traps in culprit artery of acute myocardial infarction. *Eur. Heart. J.* **2015**, *36*, 1405–1414. [CrossRef] [PubMed]
13. Bonaventura, A.; Montecucco, F.; Dallegri, F.; Carbone, F.; Lüscher, T.F.; Camici, G.G.; Liberale, L. Novel findings in neutrophil biology and their impact on cardiovascular disease. *Cardiovasc. Res.* **2019**, *115*, 1266–1285. [CrossRef] [PubMed]
14. Bonaventura, A.; Liberale, L.; Carbone, F.; Vecchié, A.; Díaz-Cañestro, C.; Camici, G.; Montecucco, F.; Dallegri, F. The Pathophysiological Role of Neutrophil Extracellular Traps in Inflammatory Diseases. *Thromb. Haemost.* **2018**, *118*, 6–27. [CrossRef]
15. Weidmann, L.; Obeid, S.; Mach, F.; Shahin, M.; Yousif, N.; Denegri, A.; Muller, O.; Räber, L.; Matter, C.M.; Lüscher, T.F. Pre-existing treatment with aspirin or statins influences clinical presentation, infarct size and inflammation in patients with de novo acute coronary syndromes. *Int. J. Cardiol.* **2019**, *275*, 171–178. [CrossRef]

16. Masuda, S.; Nakazawa, D.; Shida, H.; Miyoshi, A.; Kusunoki, Y.; Tomaru, U.; Ishizu, A. NETosis markers: Quest for specific, objective, and quantitative markers. *Clin. Chim. Acta* **2016**, *459*, 89–93. [CrossRef]
17. Kessenbrock, K.; Krumbholz, M.; Schönermarck, U.; Back, W.; Gross, W.L.; Werb, Z.; Gröne, H.-J.; Brinkmann, V.E.; Jenne, D. Netting neutrophils in autoimmune small-vessel vasculitis. *Nat. Med.* **2009**, *15*, 623–625. [CrossRef]
18. Khan, M.A.; Farahvash, A.; Douda, D.N.; Licht, J.-C.; Grasemann, H.; Sweezey, N.; Palaniyar, N. JNK Activation Turns on LPS- and Gram-Negative Bacteria-Induced NADPH Oxidase-Dependent Suicidal NETosis. *Sci. Rep.* **2017**, *7*, 3409. [CrossRef]
19. European Medicines Evaluation Agency (EMEA). CHMP Assessment Report for Ilaris. Available online: http://www.ema.europa.eu/docs/en_GB/document_library/EPAR_-_Public_assessment_report/human/001109/WC500031679.pdf (accessed on 5 March 2019).
20. Osborn, O.; Brownell, S.E.; Sanchez-Alavez, M.; Salomon, D.; Gram, H.; Bartfai, T. Treatment with an Interleukin 1 beta antibody improves glycemic control in diet-induced obesity. *Cytokine* **2008**, *44*, 141–148. [CrossRef]
21. Gaul, D.S.; Weber, J.; Van Tits, L.J.; Sluka, S.; Pasterk, L.; Reiner, M.F.; Calatayud, N.; Lohmann, C.; Klingenberg, R.; Pahla, J.; et al. Loss of Sirt3 accelerates arterial thrombosis by increasing formation of neutrophil extracellular traps and plasma tissue factor activity. *Cardiovasc. Res.* **2018**, *114*, 1178–1188. [CrossRef]
22. Awan, Z.; Denis, M.; Roubtsova, A.; Essalmani, R.; Marcinkiewicz, J.; Awan, A.; Gram, H.; Seidah, N.G.; Genest, J. Reducing Vascular Calcification by Anti-IL-1beta Monoclonal Antibody in a Mouse Model of Familial Hypercholesterolemia. *Angiology* **2016**, *67*, 157–167. [CrossRef]
23. Liberale, L.; Diaz-Cañestro, C.; Bonetti, N.R.; Paneni, F.; Akhmedov, A.; Beer, J.H.; Montecucco, F.; Lüscher, T.F.; Camici, G.G. Post-ischaemic administration of the murine Canakinumab-surrogate antibody improves outcome in experimental stroke. *Eur. Heart J.* **2018**, *39*, 3511–3517. [CrossRef]
24. Chakraborty, A.; Tannenbaum, S.; Rordorf, C.; Lowe, P.J.; Floch, D.; Gram, H.; Roy, S. Pharmacokinetic and pharmacodynamic properties of canakinumab, a human anti-interleukin-1beta monoclonal antibody. *Clin. Pharmacokinet.* **2012**, *51*, e1–e18. [CrossRef]
25. Diaz-Canestro, C.; Reiner, M.F.; Bonetti, N.R.; Liberale, L.; Merlini, M.; Wüst, P.; Amstalden, H.; Briand-Schumacher, S.; Semerano, A.; Sessa, M.; et al. AP-1 (Activated Protein-1) Transcription Factor JunD Regulates Ischemia/Reperfusion Brain Damage via IL-1beta (Interleukin-1beta). *Stroke* **2019**, *50*, 469–477. [CrossRef]
26. Holy, E.W.; Akhmedov, A.; Speer, T.; Camici, G.G.; Zewinger, S.; Bonetti, N.; Tanner, F.C.; Beer, J.H.; Lüscher, T.F. Carbamylated Low-Density Lipoproteins Induce a Prothrombotic State Via LOX-1: Impact on Arterial Thrombus Formation In Vivo. *J. Am. Coll. Cardiol.* **2016**, *68*, 1664–1676. [CrossRef]
27. Breitenstein, A.; Stämpfli, S.F.; Reiner, M.F.; Shi, Y.; Keller, S.; Akhmedov, A.; Clerigué, A.S.; Spescha, R.D.; Beer, H.-J.; Lüscher, T.F.; et al. The MAP kinase JNK2 mediates cigarette smoke-induced arterial thrombosis. *Thromb. Haemost.* **2017**, *117*, 83–89.
28. Stampfli, S.F.; Akhmedov, A.; Gebhard, C.; Lohmann, C.; Holy, E.W.; Rozenberg, I.; Spescha, R.; Shi, Y.; Luscher, T.F.; Tanner, F.C.; et al. Aging induces endothelial dysfunction while sparing arterial thrombosis. *Arterioscler. Thromb. Vasc. Biol.* **2010**, *30*, 1960–1967. [CrossRef]
29. Organization, W.H. The Top 10 Causes of Death. Available online: http://www.who.int/news-room/fact-sheets/detail/the-top-10-causes-of-death (accessed on 5 March 2019).
30. Liberale, L.; Camici, G.G. The Role of Vascular Aging in Atherosclerotic Plaque Development and Vulnerability. *Curr. Pharm. Des.* **2019**, *25*, 3098–3111. [CrossRef]
31. Carbone, F.; Liberale, L.; Bonaventura, A.; Cea, M.; Montecucco, F. Targeting Inflammation in Primary Cardiovascular Prevention. *Curr. Pharm. Des.* **2016**, *22*, 5662–5675. [CrossRef]
32. Borissoff, J.I.; Joosen, I.A.; Versteylen, M.O.; Brill, A.; Fuchs, T.A.; Savchenko, A.S.; Gallant, M.; Martinod, K.; Cate, H.T.; Hofstra, L.; et al. Elevated levels of circulating DNA and chromatin are independently associated with severe coronary atherosclerosis and a prothrombotic state. *Arterioscler. Thromb. Vasc. Biol.* **2013**, *33*, 2032–2040. [CrossRef]
33. Libby, P. Interleukin-1 Beta as a Target for Atherosclerosis Therapy: Biological Basis of CANTOS and Beyond. *J. Am. Coll. Cardiol.* **2017**, *70*, 2278–2289. [CrossRef] [PubMed]

34. Fearon, W.F.; Fearon, D.T. Inflammation and cardiovascular disease: Role of the interleukin-1 receptor antagonist. *Circulation* **2008**, *117*, 2577–2579. [CrossRef] [PubMed]
35. Bevilacqua, M.P.; Pober, J.S.; Majeau, G.R.; Cotran, R.S.; Gimbrone, M.A., Jr. Interleukin 1 (IL-1) induces biosynthesis and cell surface expression of procoagulant activity in human vascular endothelial cells. *J. Exp. Med.* **1984**, *160*, 618–623. [CrossRef] [PubMed]
36. Bevilacqua, M.P.; Pober, J.S.; Wheeler, M.E.; Cotran, R.S.; Gimbrone, M.A., Jr. Interleukin 1 acts on cultured human vascular endothelium to increase the adhesion of polymorphonuclear leukocytes, monocytes, and related leukocyte cell lines. *J. Clin. Investig.* **1985**, *76*, 2003–2011. [CrossRef]
37. Galea, J.; Armstrong, J.; Gadsdon, P.; Holden, H.; Francis, S.E.; Holt, C.M. Interleukin-1 beta in coronary arteries of patients with ischemic heart disease. *Arterioscler. Thromb. Vasc. Biol.* **1996**, *16*, 1000–1006. [CrossRef]
38. Kirii, H.; Niwa, T.; Yamada, Y.; Wada, H.; Saito, K.; Iwakura, Y.; Asano, M.; Moriwaki, H.; Seishima, M. Lack of interleukin-1beta decreases the severity of atherosclerosis in ApoE-deficient mice. *Arterioscler. Thromb. Vasc. Biol.* **2003**, *23*, 656–660. [CrossRef]
39. Breitenstein, A.; Tanner, F.C.; Luscher, T.F. Tissue factor and cardiovascular disease: Quo vadis? *Circ. J.* **2010**, *74*, 3–12. [CrossRef]
40. Lim, H.S.; Blann, A.D.; Lip, G.Y. Soluble CD40 ligand, soluble P-selectin, interleukin-6, and tissue factor in diabetes mellitus: Relationships to cardiovascular disease and risk factor intervention. *Circulation* **2004**, *109*, 2524–2528. [CrossRef]
41. Sambola, A.; Osende, J.; Hathcock, J.; Degen, M.; Nemerson, Y.; Fuster, V.; Crandall, J.; Badimon, J.J. Role of risk factors in the modulation of tissue factor activity and blood thrombogenicity. *Circulation* **2003**, *107*, 973–977. [CrossRef]
42. Suefuji, H.; Ogawa, H.; Yasue, H.; Kaikita, K.; Soejima, H.; Motoyama, T.; Mizuno, Y.; Oshima, S.; Saito, T.; Tsuji, I.; et al. Increased plasma tissue factor levels in acute myocardial infarction. *Am. Heart J.* **1997**, *134*, 253–259. [CrossRef]
43. Puhlmann, M.; Weinreich, D.M.; Farma, J.M.; Carroll, N.M.; Turner, E.M.; Alexander, H.R., Jr. Interleukin-1beta induced vascular permeability is dependent on induction of endothelial tissue factor (TF) activity. *J. Transl. Med.* **2005**, *3*, 37. [CrossRef] [PubMed]
44. Osnes, L.T.; Westvik, A.B.; Joo, G.B.; Okkenhaug, C.; Kierulf, P. Inhibition of IL-1 induced tissue factor (TF) synthesis and procoagulant activity (PCA) in purified human monocytes by IL-4, IL-10 and IL-13. *Cytokine* **1996**, *8*, 822–827. [CrossRef] [PubMed]
45. Schecter, A.D.; Spirn, B.; Rossikhina, M.; Giesen, P.L.A.; Bogdanov, V.; Fallon, J.T.; Fisher, E.A.; Schnapp, L.M.; Nemerson, Y.; Taubman, M.B. Release of active tissue factor by human arterial smooth muscle cells. *Circ. Res.* **2000**, *87*, 126–132. [CrossRef] [PubMed]
46. Darbousset, R.; Thomas, G.M.; Mezouar, S.; Frere, C.; Bonier, R.; Mackman, N.; Renné, T.; Dignat-George, F.; Dubois, C.; Panicot-Dubois, L. Tissue factor-positive neutrophils bind to injured endothelial wall and initiate thrombus formation. *Blood* **2012**, *120*, 2133–2143. [CrossRef]
47. Kambas, K.; Mitroulis, I.; Apostolidou, E.; Girod, A.; Chrysanthopoulou, A.; Pneumatikos, I.; Skendros, P.; Kourtzelis, I.; Koffa, M.; Kotsianidis, I.; et al. Autophagy mediates the delivery of thrombogenic tissue factor to neutrophil extracellular traps in human sepsis. *PLoS ONE* **2012**, *7*, e45427. [CrossRef]
48. Keshari, R.S.; Jyoti, A.; Dubey, M.; Kothari, N.; Kohli, M.; Bogra, J.; Barthwal, M.K.; Dikshit, M. Cytokines induced neutrophil extracellular traps formation: Implication for the inflammatory disease condition. *PLoS ONE* **2012**, *7*, e48111. [CrossRef]
49. Mitroulis, I.; Kambas, K.; Chrysanthopoulou, A.; Skendros, P.; Apostolidou, E.; Kourtzelis, I.; Drosos, G.I.; Boumpas, D.T.; Ritis, K. Neutrophil extracellular trap formation is associated with IL-1beta and autophagy-related signaling in gout. *PLoS ONE* **2011**, *6*, e29318. [CrossRef]
50. Meher, A.K.; Spinosa, M.; Davis, J.P.; Pope, N.; Laubach, V.E.; Su, G.; Serbulea, V.; Leitinger, M.; Ailawadi, N.; Upchurch, G.R., Jr. Novel Role of IL (Interleukin)-1beta in Neutrophil Extracellular Trap Formation and Abdominal Aortic Aneurysms. *Arterioscler. Thromb. Vasc. Biol.* **2018**, *38*, 843–853. [CrossRef]
51. Folco, E.J.; Mawson, T.L.; Vromman, A.; Bernardes-Souza, B.; Franck, G.; Persson, O.; Nakamura, M.; Newton, G.; Luscinskas, F.W.; Libby, P. Neutrophil Extracellular Traps Induce Endothelial Cell Activation and Tissue Factor Production through Interleukin-1α and Cathepsin G. *Arterioscler. Thromb. Vasc. Biol.* **2018**, *38*, 1901–1912. [CrossRef]

4

The Circulating GRP78/BiP is a Marker of Metabolic Diseases and Atherosclerosis: Bringing Endoplasmic Reticulum Stress into the Clinical Scenario

Josefa Girona [1,2], Cèlia Rodríguez-Borjabad [1,2], Daiana Ibarretxe [1,2], Joan-Carles Vallvé [1,2], Raimon Ferré [1,2], Mercedes Heras [1,2], Ricardo Rodríguez-Calvo [1,2], Sandra Guaita-Esteruelas [1], Neus Martínez-Micaelo [1,2], Núria Plana [1,2] and Lluís Masana [1,2,*]

[1] Vascular Medicine and Metabolism Unit, Research Unit on Lipids and Atherosclerosis, Sant Joan University Hospital, Universitat Rovira i Virgili, IISPV, 43201 Reus, Spain; josefa.girona@urv.cat (J.G.); celia.nutricio@gmail.com (C.R.-B.); daiana.ibarretxe@urv.cat (D.I.); jc.vallve@urv.cat (J.-C.V.); rferre@grupsagessa.cat (R.F.); mercedes.heras@urv.cat (M.H.); ricardo.rodriguez@ciberdem.com (R.R.-C.); sandra.guaita@urv.cat (S.G.-E.); neus.martinez@urv.cat (N.M.-M.); nplana@grupsagessa.cat (N.P.)

[2] Spanish Biomedical Research Centre in Diabetes and Associated Metabolic Disorders (CIBERDEM), 28029 Madrid, Spain

* Correspondence: luis.masana@urv.cat

Abstract: Background: Glucose-regulated protein 78/Binding immunoglobulin protein (GRP78/BiP) is a protein associated with endoplasmic reticulum stress and is upregulated by metabolic alterations at the tissue-level, such as hypoxia or glucose deprivation, and it is hyper-expressed in fat tissue of obese individuals. Objective: To investigate the role of the GRP78/BiP level as a metabolic and vascular disease biomarker in patients with type 2 diabetes (DM), obesity and metabolic syndrome (MS). Methods: Four hundred and five patients were recruited, of whom 52.5% were obese, 72.8% had DM, and 78.6% had MS. The intimae media thickness (cIMT) was assessed by ultrasonography. The plasma GRP78/BiP concentration was determined, and its association with metabolic and vascular parameters was assessed. Circulating GRP78/BiP was also prospectively measured in 30 DM patients before and after fenofibrate/niacin treatment and 30 healthy controls. Results: In the cross-sectional study, the GRP78/BiP level was significantly higher in the patients with obesity, DM, and MS. Age-, gender- and BMI-adjusted GRP78/BiP was directly associated with LDL-cholesterol, non-HDL-cholesterol, triglycerides, apoB, and cIMT. GRP78/BiP was positively associated to carotid plaque presence in the adjusted model, irrespective of obesity, DM and MS. In the prospective study, nicotinic acid treatment produced a significant reduction in the GRP78/BiP levels that was not observed with fenofibrate. Conclusions: GRP78/BiP plasma concentrations are increased in patients with both metabolic derangements and subclinical atherosclerosis. GRP78/BiP could be a useful marker of metabolic and cardiovascular risk.

Keywords: GRP78/BiP; endoplasmic reticulum stress; atherosclerosis; carotid intima–media thickness; obesity; type 2 diabetes; metabolic syndrome; cardiovascular risk; fenofibrate/niacin treatment

1. Introduction

Glucose-regulated protein 78/Binding immunoglobulin protein (GRP78/BiP) is an endoplasmic reticulum stress (ERS) protein that belongs to the Hsp70 multigene family and is located in the inner membrane of the endoplasmic reticulum. Its main function is associated with the unfolded protein response (UPR) in ERS situations. GRP78/BiP chaperons newly synthesized proteins until full maturation. In ERS situations, the proteins are titrated away, which frees ERS proteins that function to reduce protein synthesis and increase misfolded protein degradation and the protein-folding capacity [1]. GRP78/BiP is overexpressed in several tissues under ERS. The GRP78/BiP mRNA levels are elevated in the livers of obese mice, and high glucose levels result in reduced GRP78/BiP expression [2]. Additionally, the GRP78/BiP levels are increased in the adipose tissue of patients with diabetes and obesity [3,4]. Hypoxia and glucose deprivation account for the induction of GRP78/BiP [5,6]. Interestingly, this protein has also been detected in cell membranes, where it acts as a multireceptor and signal receptor transducer and mediates other functions [7,8]. These aspects are particularly relevant in some neoplastic tissues [9]. GRP78/BiP is released into culture medium from challenged cells to induce ERS. A soluble part of the protein can be detected in circulation, probably due to active secretion rather than simply a result of cell necrosis or apoptosis [10–12].

Alterations in ER homeostasis have been observed in obese and diabetic subjects [13]. The pathophysiological role of the UPR in obesity, insulin resistance and diabetes has been demonstrated in several studies in animal models [14] and humans [15,16]. One of the main findings was the demonstration that both genetically and diet-induced obese mice exhibited chronic activation of the UPR [2]. Consistent with these findings, treatment of obese and diabetic mice with chemical chaperones alleviated ERS and restored glucose homeostasis in the liver, muscle, and adipose tissues [17]. Furthermore, mice heterozygous for Grp78/BiP ($Grp78^{+/-}$) were protected from the metabolic disorders linked to a high-fat diet [18]. A decrease in the BMI resulting from bariatric surgery reduced ERS in insulin-resistant, obese, human patients [19]. In this regard, physical exercise alleviates ERS in obese individuals through reduction of GRP78/BiP expression and release [4].

Atherosclerosis is the major cause of cardiovascular disease, and UPR activation occurs at all stages of atherosclerotic lesion development. GRP78/BiP has been found to be highly expressed in macrophages, smooth muscle cells, and endothelial cells of atherosclerotic lesions [20]. Increased ERS occurs in unstable plaques, suggesting that ERS-induced apoptosis of smooth muscle cells and macrophages may contribute to plaque vulnerability. Moreover, unstable atherosclerotic plaques present abnormal numbers of apoptotic cells, which is related to ERS [21] mainly via robust CHOP expression. ERS markers, such as GRP78/BiP, are strongly associated with atherosclerotic plaques in human coronary artery lesions [22]. Hemodynamic shear stress in atherosclerotic regions regulates GRP78/BiP expression in vivo and in vitro, and GRP78/BiP upregulation in the endothelium has been hypothesized to provide a protective compensatory effect in response to ERS within early or developing atherosclerotic lesions [23].

ERS is a pathophysiological process that is involved in many metabolic derangements. Therefore, an ERS biomarker should be highly informative at the clinical level.

To the best of our knowledge, no studies have addressed the relationship between GRP78/BiP, diabetes, metabolic alterations, and subclinical atherosclerosis. In the present study, we have studied the associations between GRP78/BiP and metabolic indexes and atherosclerosis in patients with obesity, type 2 diabetes mellitus (DM), and/or metabolic syndrome (MS). We have also investigated the effect of lipid-modifying drugs on GRP78/BiP in patients with DM.

2. Research Design and Methods

2.1. Design and Study Subjects

Cross-Sectional Study: For the cross-sectional study, we recruited 405 consecutive individuals attending the vascular medicine and metabolism unit of our university hospital due to lipid metabolism disturbances and associated disorders (obesity, DM, and MS) who were willing to participate. DM, MS, and obesity were diagnosed according to standard clinical criteria. Prediabetes was diagnosed according to the fasting glucose level (>100 mg/dL and <126 mg/dL). Subjects with chronic lung, renal, or liver disease, cancer, or any other serious disease were excluded. Patients on lipid-lowering drugs underwent a 6-week wash-out period (8 weeks if they were on fibrates). Anamnesis, anthropometric, and physical examination data were recorded.

Prospective Study: GRP78/BiP was analyzed in deep-frozen stored sera from 29 patients with DM and 30 gender- and age-matched, apparently healthy, individuals (control group) who participated in an open randomized control trial to evaluate the impact of fenofibrate and niacin on HDL quality in DM patients. The details of this study including the flow chart scheme have been published [24] (ClinicalTrials.gov Identifier: NCT02153879). Briefly, after a 6-week lipid-lowering drug wash-out period, the patients with DM were randomly distributed into two groups. One group received 20 mg of simvastatin plus 145 mg of fenofibrate, and the other group received 20 mg of simvastatin plus 2 g of niacin plus laropiprant for a 12-week period. After a new 6-week lipid-lowering drug wash-out period, they were shifted to the other lipid-lowering drug in a crossover design for a 12-week period.

The Hospital Ethics Committee approved the study, and all patients provided their written consent to participate in the study.

2.2. Clinical and Laboratory Determinations

A blood sample was obtained from each patient in the study cohort after overnight fasting. Aliquots were prepared for immediate storage at −80 °C in the BioBanc at our center prior to use. Biochemical parameters, lipids, and apolipoproteins were measured using colorimetric, enzymatic and immunoturbidimetric assays, respectively (Spinreact, SA, Spain; Wako Chemicals GmbH, Germany; and Polymedco, New York, NY, USA; CV < 4%), which were adapted to the Cobas Mira Plus Autoanalyser (Roche Diagnostics, Spain). The lipid profile was analyzed according to the Spintrol "H" CAL (Spinreact, SA, Spain) GC–MS reference methods. Spintrol "H" Normal was used as a quality control. The circulating PCSK9 levels were measured by an enzyme-linked immunosorbent assay (ELISA) kit (R&D Systems, Minneapolis, MN, USA). The FABP5, FABP4 and HMW-adiponectin levels were assessed using commercial ELISA kits (BioVendor Laboratory Medicine Inc., Brno, Czech Republic; RayBiotech, Inc., Georgia, GA, USA; CV, 5%). The serum GRP78/BiP levels were measured with an ELISA kit (Enzo Life Sciences, Inc., New York, NY, USA) following the reagent manufacturer's instructions. The optical density (OD) of the well was measured at a wavelength of 450 nm ± 2 nm (Synergy, BioTek Instruments, Inc., Winooski, VT, USA). Each sample was analyzed in duplicate. The serum GRP78/BiP levels were measured using a standard curve constructed with the kit's standards. The homeostasis model assessment–insulin resistance (HOMA–IR) index was calculated from the fasting glucose and insulin concentrations, as previously reported [25].

2.3. Carotid Ultrasound Imaging

A total of 316 subjects from the entire cohort underwent a vascular study with the Mylab 50 X-Vision ultrasound (Esaote, Italy). A 7.5 MHz linear array and semiautomated software were used to measure the carotid intima–media thickness (cIMT) in the far wall of both common carotid arteries. The cIMT mean was the average of 2 territories. Bifurcations and internal carotids were also measured using a manual method. A plaque was defined as a focal structure that either encroached into the arterial lumen by at least 0.5 mm or 50% of the surrounding cIMT value or demonstrated a thickness >1.5 mm, as measured from the media–adventitia interface to the intima-lumen interface, according to the Mannheim carotid intima–media thickness consensus [26].

2.4. Statistical Analyses

Data are presented as medians and 25th and 75th percentiles or percentages, unless otherwise indicated. The normality of continuous variables was determined by the Kolmogorov–Smirnov test. GRP78/BiP was log-transformed to reduce skewness. Unadjusted associations between GRP78/BiP and continuous variables were assessed by Spearman's correlation test. Differences in GRP78/BiP between patients with obesity, DM, and MS were analyzed by the Mann–Whitney test, and differences between MS components were analyzed using the Kruskal–Wallis test. Group differences between treatments in the validation cohort were analyzed with the paired Wilcoxon test. Adjusted differences were investigated using analysis of covariance (ANCOVA). Multivariate linear regression models were constructed to search for independent relationships between GRP78/BiP (dependent variable) and clinical and biochemical variables in the whole study group and in the obese, type 2 diabetic, and MS subjects. Logistic binary regression models were also performed for dichotomous variables to assess the risk of obesity, DM, MS, or atherosclerotic plaques based on the serum GRP78/BiP levels. All statistical analyses were conducted with SPSS 25 (IBM, Armonk, NY, USA). A p value < 0.05 was considered statistically significant.

3. Results

3.1. Subjects' Characterisctics

The clinical, anthropometric, and biochemical characteristics of the patients participating in the cross-sectional study are shown in Table 1. The median (25th percentile–75th percentile) age of the study subjects was 60 (50–67) years, and 50.9% were women. Obesity was present in 52.5%, DM in 72.8%, and MS in 78.6% of the patients. Carotid atherosclerotic plaques were present in 33.2% of the patients. The median GRP/BiP level was 7.43 (4.42–13.49) µg/mL. Analysis of our full cohort revealed no differences in GRP78/BiP between genders, and the level was unrelated to age.

Table 1. Clinical and biochemical characteristics of the study subjects.

	$N = 405$
Women (%)	50.9
Age (years)	60 (50–67)
BMI (kg/m^2)	27.53 (27.33–34.75)
Waist circumference (cm)	103.0 (95.0–112.0)
Systolic BP (mmHg)	133 (124–146)
Diastolic BP (mmHg)	80 (71–85)
Glucose (mg/dL)	126.7 (101.0–163.0)
Insulin (%) *	10.43 (6.95–16.48)
HbA1c (%) †	6.40 (5.70–7.50)
HOMA-IR *	3.13 (1.75–6.19)
Lipids and Apolipoproteins	
Total cholesterol (mmol/L)	5.20 (4.50–6.19)
LDL-C (mmol/L)	3.18 (2.55–3.97)
HDL-C (mmol/L)	1.38 (1.19–1.59)
Non-HDL-C (mmol/L)	3.80 (3.14–4.73)
Total triglycerides (mmol/L)	1.65 (1.04–2.58)
ApoB100 (mg/dL)	103 (85–120)
ApoA1 (mg/dL)	136 (128–146)
Lp(a) (mg/dL)	8.10 (2.70–22.00)
Protein Biomarkers	
GRP78/BiP (µg/mL)	7.43 (4.42–13.49)
PCSK9 (ng/mL)	320.2 (254.4–404.7)
hsCRP (mg/L)	2.09 (1.12–3.75)
FABP4 (ng/mL)	26.06 (16.84–37.24)
FABP5 (ng/mL)	7.74 (6.13–9.92)
HMW-Adiponectin (µg/mL)	5.44 (2.96–8.98)
Disease	
Obesity (%)	52.5
Type 2 diabetes (%)	72.8
Metabolic syndrome (%)	78.6
Subclinical Atherosclerosis	
cIMT (mm) ‡	0.685 (0.619–0.776)
Carotid atherosclerotic plaque (%) §	33.2

Data are shown as n (percentage) or median (25th percentile–75th percentile). BMI = body mass index; BP = blood pressure; LDL-C = LDL cholesterol; HDL-C = HDL cholesterol; Non-HDL-C = non-HDL cholesterol; ApoB100 = apolipoprotein B100; ApoA1 = apolipoprotein A1, Lp(a) = lipoprotein a; GRP78/BiP = 78 kDa glucose-regulated protein/binding immunoglobulin protein; PCSK9 = proprotein convertase subtilisin/kexin type 9; hsCRP = high-sensitivity C-reactive protein; FABP4 = fatty acid binding protein 4; FABP5 = fatty acid binding protein 5; HMW-adiponectin = high-molecular-weight adiponectin; cIMT = carotid intima–media thickness. Measurements were available in a subpopulation of: * $n = 168$; † $n = 314$; ‡ $n = 312$; § $n = 316$.

3.2. *Association of GRP78/BiP with the Metabolic Status*

The GRP78/BiP serum concentrations were higher in patients with obesity, DM, and MS compared with patients without metabolic disturbances (5.67 (3.74–11.62) μg/mL vs. 9.15 (5.74–16.38) μg/mL, $p < 0.001$; 4.72 (3.63–9.94) μg/mL vs. 8.57 (5.27–16.73) μg/mL, $p < 0.001$ and 4.15 (2.91–5.76) μg/mL vs. 9.15 (5.85–16.73) μg/mL, $p < 0.001$, respectively) (Figure 1A,B,C). A direct and positive association was found with the number of MS components ($p < 0.001$) (Figure 1D). The differences were independent of covariates ($p < 0.001$ for obesity, DM, and MS) (Figure 1).

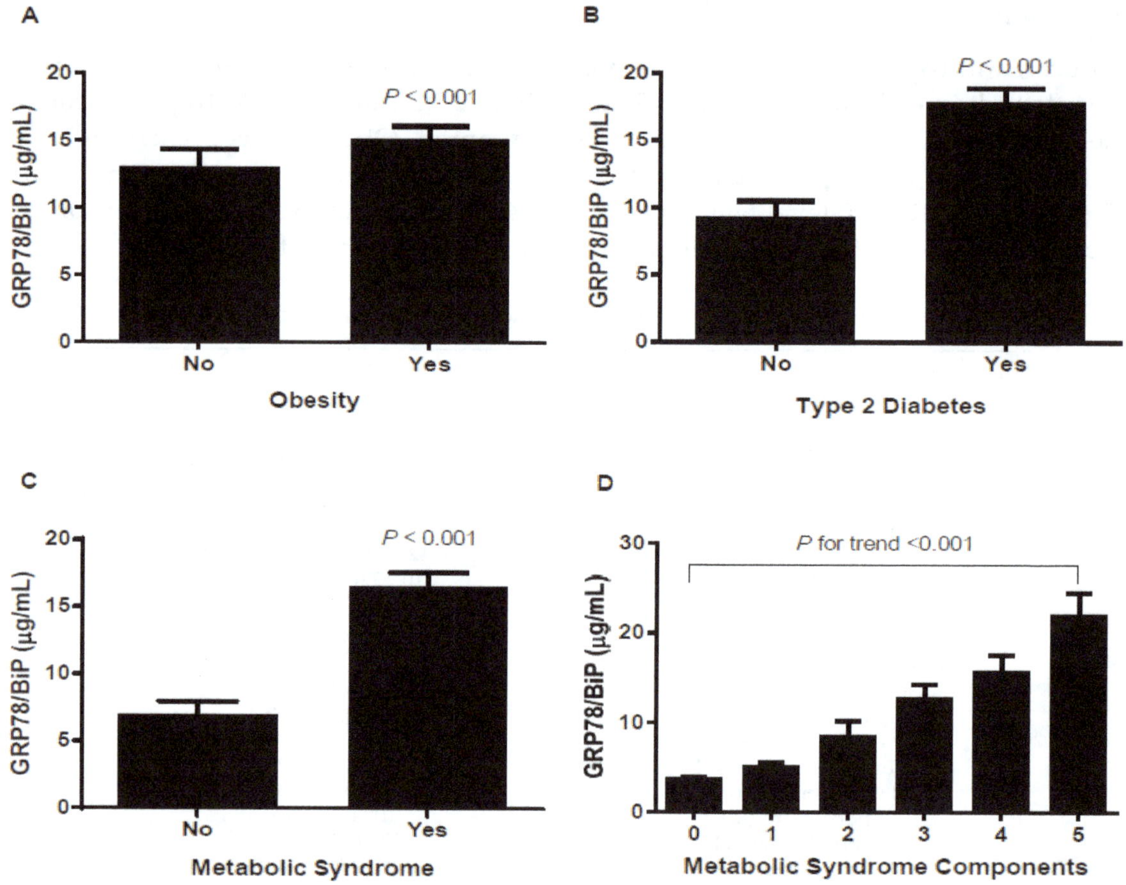

Figure 1. Circulating 78 kDa glucose-regulated protein/binding immunoglobulin protein (GRP78/BiP) levels according to obesity (**A**), type 2 diabetes (**B**), metabolic syndrome (**C**) and metabolic syndrome components (**D**). The results are expressed as the mean ± SEM. p values for group comparisons are reported for the age- and gender-adjusted ANCOVA test.

A logistic regression analysis revealed that the serum GRP78/BiP levels were associated with the presence of obesity, DM, and MS in the crude and in the gender- and age-adjusted model (model 1). After adjusting for other risk factors (model 2), GRP78/BiP levels remained directly associated with DM and MS (Supplemental Table S1).

3.3. *Associations of GRP78/BiP with the Clinical, Biochemical and Vascular Imaging Data*

The associations among GRP78/BiP and the clinical, anthropometric, and standard biochemical data and the adipokine and vascular values are shown in Table 2. Notably, GRP78/BiP was directly related to all adiposity indexes, including the BMI, standard lipids, lipoprotein levels, glucose concentrations, inflammation and adipokines, and was inversely related to apo A1 and HMW-adiponectin. The mean GRP78/BiP was also directly related to cIMT.

Table 2. Relationships between log-GRP78/BiP and continuous variables.

	Log GRP78/BiP	*p Value*	Log GRP78/BiP *	*p Value* *
Age	0.034	0.499	-	-
BMI	0.307	<0.001	-	-
Waist Circumference	0.269	<0.001	0.125	0.121
Systolic BP	0.394	<0.001	0.154	0.055
Diastolic BP	0.153	<0.001	0.122	0.129
Glucose	0.296	<0.001	−0.045	0.576
Total cholesterol	0.429	<0.001	0.156	0.052
LDL-C	0.351	<0.001	0.099	0.217
HDL-C	−0.011	0.830	0.038	0.637
Non-HDL-C	0.472	<0.001	0.176	0.028
Total triglycerides	0.392	<0.001	0.243	0.002
ApoB100	0.420	<0.001	0.169	0.035
ApoA1	−0.165	0.001	−0.137	0.088
Lp(a)	0.065	0.190	0.039	0.626
PCSK9	0.191	<0.001	0.077	0.340
hsCRP	0.256	<0.001	0.084	0.297
FABP4	0.141	0.005	0.104	0.195
FABP5	0.274	<0.001	0.095	0.236
HMW-Adiponectin	−0.176	0.001	−0.055	0.493
cIMT	0.165	0.003	0.244	0.002

GRP78/BiP = 78 kDa glucose-regulated protein/binding immunoglobulin protein; BMI = body mass index; BP = blood pressure; LDL-C = LDL cholesterol; HDL-C = HDL cholesterol; Non-HDL-C = non-HDL cholesterol; ApoB100 = apolipoprotein B100; ApoA1 = apolipoprotein A1, Lp(a) = lipoprotein a; PCSK9 = proprotein convertase subtilisin/kexin type 9; hsCRP = high-sensitivity C-reactive protein; FABP4 = fatty acid binding protein 4; FABP5 = fatty acid binding protein 5; HMW-adiponectin = high-molecular-weight adiponectin; cIMT = carotid intima–media thickness. *p* values for Spearman's correlations are reported. * *p* values corrected by age, gender and BMI.

After adjusting for age, gender, and BMI, the relationships that remained statistically significant with GRP78/BiP were cholesterol, non-HDL-C, triglycerides, apoB100 and cIMT ($p < 0.05$ for all comparisons) (Table 2).

Thereafter, a multivariate stepwise regression analysis was used to identify factors influencing circulating GRP78/BiP across obesity, DM, and MS. In the entire study population, gender, systolic blood pression, triglycerides, and cIMT were the determinants of circulating GRP78/BiP, accounting for 32.7% of the observed variance (Supplemental Table S2). Further analysis of obese individuals revealed that gender accounted for 15.4% of the variance observed in the circulating GRP78/BiP levels. In diabetic individuals, gender, BMI, triglycerides, and cIMT accounted for 25.3% of the variance. For MS, the determinants of circulating GRP78/BiP were gender, triglycerides, and cIMT, which accounted for 20.3% of the variance.

3.4. Associations Between GRP68/BiP and the Carotid Plaque Burden

Age- and gender-adjusted GRP78/BiP was higher in patients with carotid plaques (7.13 (4.56–12.63) μg/mL vs 11.8 (7.91–24.99) μg/mL, $p < 0.001$, $n = 316$, respectively) (Figure 2). GRP78/BiP was directly related to the carotid plaque presence (odds ratio OR, 95% confidence interval [CI] = 7.077 (3.357–14.922), $p < 0.001$) in the age- and gender-adjusted model. The direct association of GRP78/BiP with the presence of a plaque was significant in the patients with obesity (OR [CI] = 5.053 (1.716–14.876), $p = 0.003$), DM (OR [CI] = 6.296 (2.521–15.724), $p < 0.001$), and MS (OR [CI] = 5.109 (2.216–11.778), $p < 0.001$) (Supplemental Table S3).

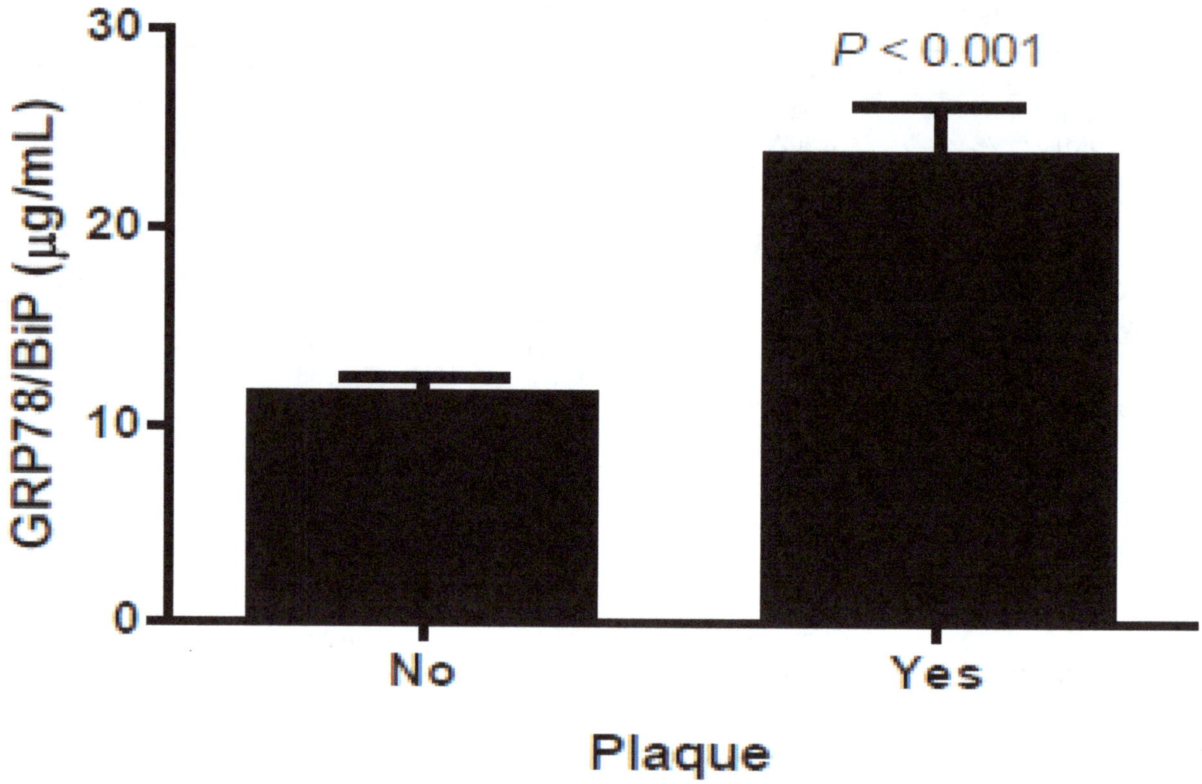

Figure 2. Circulating 78 kDa glucose-regulated protein/binding immunoglobulin protein (GRP78/BiP) levels according to the presence of atherosclerotic plaques. The results are expressed as the mean ± SEM. p values for group comparison are reported for the age- and gender-adjusted ANCOVA test.

3.5. GRP68/BiP and Prediabetes

GRP78/ BiP was increased in the subjects with prediabetes compared with the levels in the subjects with neither prediabetes nor diabetes (4.46 (3.22–8.66) μg/mL vs. 7.23 (4.54–13.96) μg/mL, $p < 0.001$, respectively). Additionally, a positive association was detected with the HOMA-IR ($r = 0.407$; $p < 0.001$, $n = 168$) that persisted after age and gender adjustment ($r = 0.231$; $p = 0.003$). In the patients with triglycerides < 2.26 mmol/L, GRP78/BiP was significantly higher in those with prediabetes and diabetes than in the controls, whereas the levels in the patients with high triglycerides (>2.26 mmol/L) were equally altered (Supplemental Figure S1).

3.6. Effect of Treatment on Circulating GRP78/BiP in DM Patients

The clinical characteristics of the patients participating in the intervention trial were previously published [24]. The median (25th percentile–75th percentiles) age was 58 (53–65) years, and 36.7% were women. Similar to the main study cohort, the age- and gender-matched GRP78/BiP levels were higher in the DM patients than in the control group ($p < 0.001$). Similar to those of the main study cohort, GRP78/BiP showed a direct association with triglycerides ($r = 0.581$; $p < 0.001$) and the cIMT ($r = 0.509$; $p = 0.016$, $n = 22$). Interestingly, in the DM patients, treatment with nicotinic acid for a 12-week period ($n = 26$) significantly reduced GRP78/BiP by 11% ($p = 0.038$) (Figure 3). This reduction was accompanied by the expected reduction in triglycerides (39%, $p = 0.003$). Treatment with fenofibrate ($n = 29$) also accounted for a significant reduction of triglycerides (32%, $p = 0.002$) but resulted in a non-significant reduction of GRP78/BiP ($p = 0.705$).

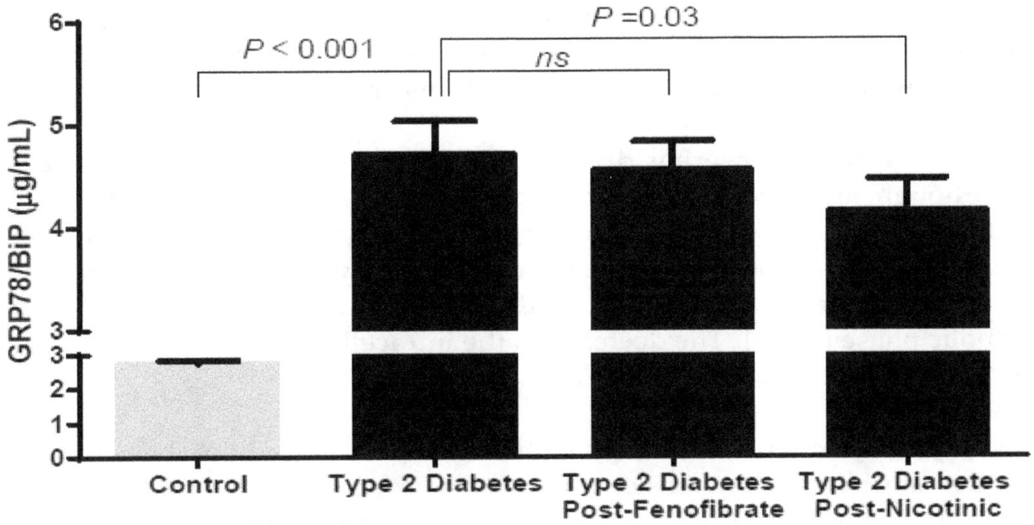

Figure 3. Circulating 78 kDa glucose-regulated protein/binding immunoglobulin protein (GRP78/BiP) in the control group and the type 2 diabetes patients before and after fenofibrate and nicotinic treatment in a validation cohort. The results are expressed as the mean ± SEM. p values for the group comparisons are reported for the age- and gender-adjusted ANCOVA test or paired Wilcoxon test.

4. Discussion

We communicate that the circulating GRP78/BiP levels are significantly increased in obese, DM, and MS patients. Higher GRP78/BiP concentrations are also associated with subclinical atherosclerosis. The data are robust enough to support the use of GRP78/BiP serum concentrations as a biomarker of metabolic and vascular derangements. The endoplasmic reticulum is a crucial subcellular organelle that is responsible for protein, lipid, glucose, and calcium metabolism. Conditions in which its physiological capacity is overwhelmed are referred to as ERS, in which a complex molecular reaction is activated and proteins are not properly processed due to the UPR [27]. GRP78/BiP is a cornerstone protein of this process [1]. It is physiologically located in the inner layer of the ER and maintains the localization of several proteins associated with the ERS response. In ERS situations, GRP78/BiP frees these proteins to counterbalance the UPR by reducing protein synthesis, increasing misfolded protein removal and improving the protein folding capacity. Increased extracellular delivery of GRP78/BiP occurs because of this process. According to the results of our and other studies [4], this increased secretion leads to higher circulating GRP78/BiP concentrations in humans. Thus, a high serum GRP78/BiP level should be interpreted as an ERS marker. Triglycerides and cholesterol esters are assembled in the ER. ER homeostasis is altered in the presence of a high amount of lipids, leading to ERS [28–30]. Therefore, our data showing an increased amount of a circulating protein associated with ERS in subjects with important alterations in intermediate metabolism are logical. According to our data, GRP78/BiP can be detected in the sera at very low levels, which increase in the presence of obesity, DM, and MS. Interestingly, a robust direct association exists between GRP78/BiP and cholesterol and triglycerides, suggesting that alterations in lipid metabolism are involved in ERS and the increase in circulating GRP78/BiP. This finding could be of interest, given that GRP78/BiP expression in vitro is associated with an increase in expression of the very low-density lipoprotein receptor [6], which is important in tissues with active fatty acid metabolism. In other words, the high fat pools in tissues involved in lipid metabolism, such as the liver and adipose tissue, would be at least partially responsible for ERS. This possibility is of interest in patients with normal triglyceride levels but signs of prediabetes or resistance to insulin; we observed that GRP78/BiP was already high in these patients, suggesting that other metabolic alterations might play a role in GRP78/BiP secretion.

On the other hand, inflammation is also associated with ERS [31]. This fact could also explain ERS in diabetes and obesity because they are associated to chronic subclinical inflammation. In our hands, GRP78/BiP was also correlated with the hsCRP concentration.

Interestingly, triglyceride-lowering drugs have different impacts on the GRP78/BiP plasma concentration, although, as expected, both drugs produced a significant triglyceride-lowering effect. Niacin but not fenofibrate induced a significant reduction of GRP78/BiP. The lipid-lowering effect of niacin is not completely understood but seems to be mediated by a decrease in adipose tissue lipolysis, which reduces the substrate for triglyceride synthesis in the liver, whereas fenofibrate acts mainly during the catabolic phase [32,33]. The decrease in the intracellular lipid burden mediated by niacin can most likely explain the observed differences.

An interesting observation of our study is the significant association between GRP78/BiP and the presence of subclinical atherosclerosis, particularly in those with carotid plaques. We have no elements to link a direct impact of GRP78/BiP with atherosclerotic pathogenesis, although the protein is expressed in macrophages, smooth muscle cells, and endothelial cells of atherosclerotic lesions in animal models [20]. We cannot exclude the possibility that high circulating GRP78/BiP levels are signaling individuals with more severe metabolic alterations, although the correlation between GRP78/BiP and carotid plaques is maintained after multiple adjustments.

Our work has some limitations. The cross-sectional design precludes obtaining causal relationships between GRP78/BiP and metabolic and vascular alterations. The prospective, randomized and controlled validation study was open, the sample size was small, and the study was not designed for this objective. However, the data obtained are in concordance with the results from the main part of the study and provide additional information on the reversibility of ERS.

In conclusion, the circulating GRP78/BiP levels are significantly increased in people with DM, obesity, and its associated metabolic alterations. The associated hyperlipidemia probably plays a role in ERS in these patients. GRP78/BiP was also associated with subclinical atherosclerosis. Taking all of these results together, our work supports the use of the circulating GRP78/BiP level as a marker of vascular and metabolic risk. Our data provide elements to bring derangement of a crucial cellular mechanism to the clinical setting.

Author Contributions: Conceptualization, J.G., N.P. and L.M.; Data curation, J.G., D.I., R.F., N.P. and L.M.; Formal analysis, J.G., J.-C.V. and L.M.; Funding acquisition, J.G. and L.M.; Investigation, J.G., C.R.-B., R.F., N.P. and L.M.; Methodology, J.G., C.R.-B., D.I., J.-C.V., M.H., R.R.-C., S.G.-E. and N.M.-M.; Supervision, J.G., C.R.-B., D.I. and L.M.; Writing—original draft, J.G., J.-C.V. and L.M.; Writing—review & editing, J.G., C.R.-B., D.I., J.-C.V. and L.M.

Acknowledgments: The authors thank the UVASMET in Sant Joan University Hospital for assistance and all patients who gave time to this study. The authors acknowledge the IISPV-BIOBANC for sample handling.

References

1. Pobre, K.F.R.; Poet, G.J.; Hendershot, L.M. The endoplasmic reticulum (ER) chaperone BiP is a master regulator of ER functions: Getting by with a little help from ERdj friends. *J. Biol. Chem.* **2019**, *294*, 2098–2108. [CrossRef] [PubMed]
2. Ozcan, U.; Cao, Q.; Yilmaz, E.; Lee, A.-H.; Iwakoshi, N.N.; Ozdelen, E.; Tuncman, G.; Görgün, C.; Glimcher, L.H.; Hotamisligil, G.S. Endoplasmic reticulum stress links obesity, insulin action, and type 2 diabetes. *Science* **2004**, *306*, 457–461. [CrossRef] [PubMed]

3. Fang, L.; Kojima, K.; Zhou, L.; Crossman, D.K.; Mobley, J.A.; Grams, J. Analysis of the Human Proteome in Subcutaneous and Visceral Fat Depots in Diabetic and Non-Diabetic Patients with Morbid Obesity. *J. Proteom. Bioinform.* **2015**, *8*, 133–141.

4. Khadir, A.; Kavalakatt, S.; Abubaker, J.; Cherian, P.; Madhu, D.; Al-Khairi, I.; Abu-Farha, M.; Warsame, S.; Elkum, N.; Dehbi, M.; et al. Physical exercise alleviates ER stress in obese humans through reduction in the expression and release of GRP78 chaperone. *Metabolism* **2016**, *65*, 1409–1420. [CrossRef] [PubMed]

5. Shiu, R.P.; Pouyssegur, J.; Pastan, I. Glucose depletion accounts for the induction of two transformation-sensitive membrane proteinsin Rous sarcoma virus-transformed chick embryo fibroblasts. *Proc. Natl. Acad. Sci. USA* **1977**, *74*, 3840–3844. [CrossRef]

6. Yang, D.; Gao, L.; Wang, T.; Qiao, Z.; Liang, Y.; Zhang, P. Hypoxia triggers endothelial endoplasmic reticulum stress and apoptosis via induction of VLDL receptor. *FEBS Lett.* **2014**, *588*, 4448–4456. [CrossRef]

7. Tsai, Y.-L.; Zhang, Y.; Tseng, C.-C.; Stanciauskas, R.; Pinaud, F.; Lee, A.S. Characterization and Mechanism of Stress-induced Translocation of 78-Kilodalton Glucose-regulated Protein (GRP78) to the Cell Surface. *J. Biol. Chem.* **2015**, *290*, 8049–8064. [CrossRef]

8. Mazaki, Y.; Higashi, T.; Onodera, Y.; Nam, J.-M.; Hashimoto, A.; Hashimoto, S.; Horinouchi, T.; Miwa, S. Endothelin type B receptor interacts with the 78-kDa glucose-regulated protein. *FEBS Lett.* **2019**, *593*, 644–651. [CrossRef]

9. Li, Z.; Zhuang, M.; Zhang, L.; Zheng, X.; Yang, P.; Li, Z. Acetylation modification regulates GRP78 secretion in colon cancer cells. *Sci. Rep.* **2016**, *6*, 30406. [CrossRef]

10. Li, R.; Yanjiao, G.; Wubin, H.; Yue, W.; Jianhua, H.; Huachuan, Z.; Rongjian, S.; Zhidong, L. Secreted GRP78 activates EGFR-SRC-STAT3 signaling and confers the resistance to sorafeinib in HCC cells. *Oncotarget* **2017**, *8*, 19354–19364.

11. Ma, X.; Guo, W.; Yang, S.; Zhu, X.; Xiang, J.; Li, H. Serum GRP78 as a Tumor Marker and Its Prognostic Significance in Non-Small Cell Lung Cancers: A Retrospective Study. *Dis. Markers* **2015**, *2015*, 814670. [CrossRef] [PubMed]

12. Aksoy, M.O.; Kim, V.; Cornwell, W.D.; Rogers, T.J.; Kosmider, B.; Bahmed, K.; Barrero, C.; Merali, S.; Shetty, N.; Kelsen, S.G. Secretion of the endoplasmic reticulum stress protein, GRP78, into the BALF is increased in cigarette smokers. *Respir. Res.* **2017**, *18*, 78. [CrossRef] [PubMed]

13. Back, S.H.; Kaufman, R.J. Endoplasmic reticulum stress and type 2 diabetes. *Annu. Rev. Biochem.* **2012**, *81*, 767–793. [CrossRef] [PubMed]

14. Nakatani, Y.; Kaneto, H.; Kawamori, D.; Yoshiuchi, K.; Hatazaki, M.; Matsuoka, T.; Ozawa, K.; Ogawa, S.; Hori, M.; Yamasaki, Y.; et al. Involvement of Endoplasmic Reticulum Stress in Insulin Resistance and Diabetes. *J. Biol. Chem.* **2005**, *280*, 847–851. [CrossRef]

15. Sharma, N.K.; Das, S.K.; Mondal, A.K.; Hackney, O.G.; Chu, W.S.; Kern, P.A.; Rasouli, N.; Spencer, H.J.; Yao-Borengasser, A.; Elbein, S.C. Endoplasmic reticulum stress markers are associated with obesity in nondiabetic subjects. *J. Clin. Endocrinol. Metab.* **2008**, *93*, 4532–4541. [CrossRef]

16. Boden, G.; Duan, X.; Homko, C.; Molina, E.J.; Song, W.; Perez, O.; Cheung, P.; Merali, S. Increase in Endoplasmic Reticulum Stress-Related Proteins and Genes in Adipose Tissue of Obese, Insulin-Resistant Individuals. *Diabetes* **2008**, *57*, 2438–2444. [CrossRef]

17. Ozcan, U.; Yilmaz, E.; Ozcan, L.; Furuhashi, M.; Vaillancourt, E.; Smith, R.O.; Görgün, C.Z.; Hotamisligil, G.S. Chemical chaperones reduce ER stress and restore glucose homeostasis in a mouse model of type 2 diabetes. *Science* **2006**, *313*, 1137–1140. [CrossRef]

18. Ye, R.; Jung, D.Y.; Jun, J.Y.; Li, J.; Luo, S.; Ko, H.J.; Kim, J.K.; Lee, A.S. Grp78 heterozygosity promotes adaptive unfolded protein response and attenuates diet-induced obesity and insulin resistance. *Diabetes* **2010**, *59*, 6–16. [CrossRef]

19. Gregor, M.F.; Yang, L.; Fabbrini, E.; Mohammed, B.S.; Eagon, J.C.; Hotamisligil, G.S.; Klein, S. Endoplasmic reticulum stress is reduced in tissues of obese subjects after weight loss. *Diabetes* **2009**, *58*, 693–700. [CrossRef]

20. Zhou, J.; Lhoták, S.; Hilditch, B.A.; Austin, R.C. Activation of the unfolded protein response occurs at all stages of atherosclerotic lesion development in apolipoprotein E-deficient mice. *Circulation* **2005**, *111*, 1814–1821. [CrossRef]

21. Cominacini, L.; Garbin, U.; Mozzini, C.; Stranieri, C.; Pasini, A.; Solani, E.; Tinelli, I.A.; Pasini, A.F. The atherosclerotic plaque vulnerability: Focus on the oxidative and endoplasmic reticulum stress in orchestrating the macrophage apoptosis in the formation of the necrotic core. *Curr. Med. Chem.* **2015**, *22*, 1565–1572. [CrossRef] [PubMed]
22. Myoishi, M.; Hao, H.; Minamino, T.; Watanabe, K.; Nishihira, K.; Hatakeyama, K.; Asada, Y.; Okada, K.; Ishibashi-Ueda, H.; Gabbiani, G.; et al. Increased Endoplasmic Reticulum Stress in Atherosclerotic Plaques Associated with Acute Coronary Syndrome. *Circulation* **2007**, *116*, 1226–1233. [CrossRef] [PubMed]
23. Feaver, R.E.; Hastings, N.E.; Pryor, A.; Blackman, B.R. GRP78 upregulation by atheroprone shear stress via p38-, alpha2beta1-dependent mechanism in endothelial cells. *Arterioscler. Thromb. Vasc. Biol.* **2008**, *28*, 1534–1541. [CrossRef] [PubMed]
24. Masana, L.; Cabré, A.; Heras, M.; Amigó, N.; Correig, X.; Martínez-Hervás, S.; Real, J.T.; Ascaso, J.F.; Quesada, H.; Julve, J.; et al. Remarkable quantitative and qualitative differences in HDL after niacin or fenofibrate therapy in type 2 diabetic patients. *Atherosclerosis* **2015**, *238*, 213–219. [CrossRef] [PubMed]
25. Levy, J.C.; Matthews, D.R.; Hermans, M.P. Correct homeostasis model assessment (HOMA) evaluation uses the computer program. *Diabetes Care* **1998**, *21*, 2191–2192. [CrossRef]
26. Touboul, P.-J.; Hennerici, M.G.; Meairs, S.; Adams, H.; Amarenco, P.; Bornstein, N.; Csiba, L.; Desvarieux, M.; Ebrahim, S.; Hernandez Hernandez, R.; et al. Mannheim Carotid Intima-Media Thickness and Plaque Consensus (2004–2006–2011). *Cerebrovasc. Dis.* **2012**, *34*, 290–296. [CrossRef]
27. Todd, D.J.; Lee, A.-H.; Glimcher, L.H. The endoplasmic reticulum stress response in immunity and autoimmunity. *Nat. Rev. Immunol.* **2008**, *8*, 663–674. [CrossRef]
28. Sozen, E.; Ozer, N.K. Impact of high cholesterol and endoplasmic reticulum stress on metabolic diseases: An updated mini-review. *Redox Biol.* **2017**, *12*, 456–461. [CrossRef]
29. Han, J.; Kaufman, R.J. The role of ER stress in lipid metabolism and lipotoxicity. *J. Lipid Res.* **2016**, *57*, 1329–1338. [CrossRef]
30. Balasus, D.; Way, M.; Fusilli, C.; Mazza, T.; Morgan, M.Y.; Cervello, M.; Giannitrapani, L.; Soresi, M.; Agliastro, R.; Vinciguerra, M.; et al. The association of variants in PNPLA3 and GRP78 and the risk of developing hepatocellular carcinoma in an Italian population. *Oncotarget* **2016**, *7*, 86791–86802. [CrossRef]
31. McGrath, K.C.Y.; Heather, A.K. Endoplasmic Reticulum Stress in Inflammatory Disease. *Endocrinology* **2012**, *153*, 2949–2952. [CrossRef] [PubMed]
32. Ali, A.H.; Mundi, M.; Koutsari, C.; Bernlohr, D.A.; Jensen, M.D. Adipose Tissue Free Fatty Acid Storage In Vivo: Effects of Insulin Versus Niacin as a Control for Suppression of Lipolysis. *Diabetes* **2015**, *64*, 2828–2835. [CrossRef] [PubMed]
33. Forcheron, F.; Cachefo, A.; Thevenon, S.; Pinteur, C.; Beylot, M. Mechanisms of the triglyceride- and cholesterol-lowering effect of fenofibrate in hyperlipidemic type 2 diabetic patients. *Diabetes* **2002**, *51*, 3486–3491. [CrossRef] [PubMed]

5

Effects of Caloric Intake and Aerobic Activity in Individuals with Prehypertension and Hypertension on Levels of Inflammatory, Adhesion and Prothrombotic Biomarkers

En-Young N. Wagner [1,2,3,*], Suzi Hong [1,4], Kathleen L. Wilson [1,4], Karen J. Calfas [4], Cheryl L. Rock [4], Laura S. Redwine [5], Roland von Känel [2] and Paul J. Mills [1,4]

[1] Department of Psychiatry, University of California, San Diego, CA 92093, USA; s1hong@ucsd.edu (S.H.); k8wilson@ucsd.edu (K.L.W.); pmills@ucsd.edu (P.J.M.)
[2] Department of Consultation-Liaison Psychiatry and Psychosomatic Medicine, University Hospital Zurich, 8091 Zurich, Switzerland; roland.vonkaenel@usz.ch
[3] Department of BioMedical Research, Inselspital, Bern University Hospital, 3010 Bern, Switzerland
[4] Department of Family Medicine and Public Health, University of California, San Diego, CA 92093, USA; kcalfas@ucsd.edu (K.J.C.); clrock@ucsd.edu (C.L.R.)
[5] College of Nursing, University of South Florida, Tampa, FL 33612, USA; lredwine@health.usf.edu
[*] Correspondence: en-young.wagner@dbmr.unibe.ch

Abstract: Background: Cardiopulmonary fitness and low calorie diets have been shown to reduce inflammation but few studies have been conducted in individuals with elevated blood pressure (BP) in a randomized intervention setting. Thereby, adhesion biomarkers, e.g., soluble intercellular adhesion molecule (sICAM)-3, have not been examined so far. Methods: Sixty-eight sedentary prehypertensive and mildly hypertensive individuals (mean age ± SEM: 45 ± 1 years; mean BP: 141/84 ± 1/1 mmHg) were randomized to one of three 12-week intervention groups: cardio training and caloric reduction, cardio training alone, or wait-list control group. Plasma levels of inflammatory, adhesion and prothrombotic biomarkers were assessed. In a second step, intervention groups were combined to one sample and multivariate regression analyses were applied in order to account for exercise and diet behavior changes. Results: There were no significant differences among the intervention groups. In the combined sample, greater caloric reduction was associated with a larger increase of sICAM-3 ($p = 0.026$) and decrease of C-reactive protein ($p = 0.018$) as a result of the interventions. More cardio training was associated with increases of sICAM-3 ($p = 0.046$) as well as interleukin-6 ($p = 0.004$) and a decrease of tumor necrosis factor-α ($p = 0.017$) levels. Higher BP predicted higher plasminogen activator inhibitor (PAI)-1 ($p = 0.001$), and greater fitness predicted lower PAI-1 levels ($p = 0.006$) after the intervention. Conclusions: In prehypertensive and hypertensive patients, plasma levels of the adhesion molecule sICAM-3 and inflammatory biomarkers have different response patterns to cardio training with and without caloric reduction. Such anti-inflammatory and anti-thrombotic effects may have implications for the prevention of atherothrombotic cardiovascular disease among individuals at increased risk.

Keywords: hypertension; prehypertension; exercise; diet; adhesion molecule; sICAM; soluble intercellular adhesion molecule; inflammatory markers; intervention

1. Introduction

The pathogenesis of hypertension seems to be more complex, as it is difficult to treat despite established antihypertensive drugs and longtime cardiovascular research. Hypertension (blood pressure (BP) ≥ 140/90 mmHg) is a highly prevalent disease among United States (U.S.) citizens with a well-known impact on numerous comorbid conditions and public-health related outcomes [1–3]. On a cellular level, it is established knowledge that individuals with hypertension exhibit elevated blood levels of cellular adhesion molecules [4–6] as well as inflammatory markers [7–15]. The reason for that is mainly seen in endothelial activation [12], which explains the tight linkage between elevated BP, chronic inflammatory processes including atherosclerosis and adverse health related outcomes [7,16]. So far, studies on the effects of human hypertension on adhesion molecules have been focusing on soluble intercellular adhesion molecule-1 (sICAM-1; sCD54) [4–6] while studies measuring sICAM-3, which is potentially much more important for immune response [17], are scarce.

In treating hypertension, lifestyle modifications including adopting a regular exercise regimen are key constituents of treatment [18,19]. This recommendation might also apply to prehypertension (BP > 120/80 and <140/90 mmHg), a risk factor for the development of hypertension. The effect achieved depends on both intensity and frequency of exercise [20–22], and BP reductions of up to 15 mmHg can be achieved without using antihypertensive drugs and thus avoiding their common side effects [23]. In overweight hypertensive subjects, a combined exercise and dietary weight-loss intervention was shown to lead to even greater reductions in BP than exercise alone [22].

Meanwhile, few studies have examined the relationship between exercise and inflammation in hypertensive patients. One of the few studies showed that exercise and/or exercise plus diet interventions lead to reductions in circulating interleukin (IL)-6 and C-reactive protein (CRP) levels in obese individuals [24]. In normotensive, healthy individuals, cross-sectional epidemiological studies have shown physical activity to be negatively associated with CRP, fibrinogen, and white blood cell count [25] and inflammatory markers, including tumor necrosis factor (TNF)-α and IL-6 and prothrombotic plasminogen activator inhibitor (PAI-1) were shown to be inversely related to physical activity levels [26–28]. Furthermore, our group has shown that physical activity level and fitness are inversely related to leukocyte adhesion molecule expression [29,30].

Guided by the above described effects observed in healthy individuals, the purpose of this study was to explore the relationship of a 12-week exercise (and diet) intervention and inflammation/cell adhesion in patients with prehypertension and hypertension by measuring circulating levels of CRP, IL-6, TNF-α, PAI-1, and sICAM-1 and sICAM-3 by taking relevant cardio-metabolic confounding factors (body mass index (BMI), physical inactivity) into account. Based on these data of a randomized controlled trial (RCT), our aim was to show for the first time in vivo that exercise has not only an impact on levels of inflammatory biomarkers, but also on levels of cellular adhesion molecules. Our main hypothesis was that, compared to a 12-week wait-list control group, the 12-week exercise intervention, and especially the 12-week exercise plus diet intervention, would result in greater reduction of inflammatory biomarkers and cell adhesion molecules pre to post intervention. Second, we expected that both intervention groups would show increased fitness levels and greater BP reduction and weight reduction as compared to the wait-list control group.

2. Methods

2.1. Ethical Approval and Informed Consent

Data is taken from a clinical trial on the effects of exercise and diet on inflammation in hypertensive individuals registered in a public registry (www.clinicaltrials.gov, ClinicalTrials.gov Identifier: NCT00338572). The University of California San Diego (UCSD) Institutional Review Board approved the study protocol, to which all participants signed a written informed consent. All procedures performed in studies involving human participants were in accordance with the ethical standards of the institutional and/or national research committee and with the 1964 Helsinki Declaration and its later amendments or comparable ethical standards. Participants were recruited from the local community through flyers, referrals from local doctor's offices and e-mail list serve distribution.

2.2. Data Source, Effect of Exercise and Diet on Inflammation in Hypertensive Individuals Trial

The data of the present secondary analysis is derived from a prospective, randomized controlled intervention study examining the effect of exercise and diet on inflammation in hypertensive individuals. That study was conducted in order to compare the effect of an exercise program versus a combined exercise and diet program on reducing inflammation in hypertensive individuals. Figure 1 shows the RCT CONSORT flow diagram for participants. Of 168 eligible people, 77 individuals chose not to enter the RCT. The 91 remaining participants were randomly assigned to one of three 12-week intervention groups: aerobic cardio training and caloric reduction, aerobic cardio training alone, or wait-list control group. Participants assigned to the wait-list group were controls for at least 12 weeks until they were allocated to one of the intervention groups (exercise alone or exercise plus "Dietary Approaches to Stop Hypertension" (DASH) group). Of these 91 subjects, 9 individuals did not complete the study for personal reasons, moving away from San Diego (n = 2), becoming too busy or starting a new job (n = 5), becoming ill (n = 2, colon rupture, neurological concerns), and 14 individuals were not reliable/cancelled.

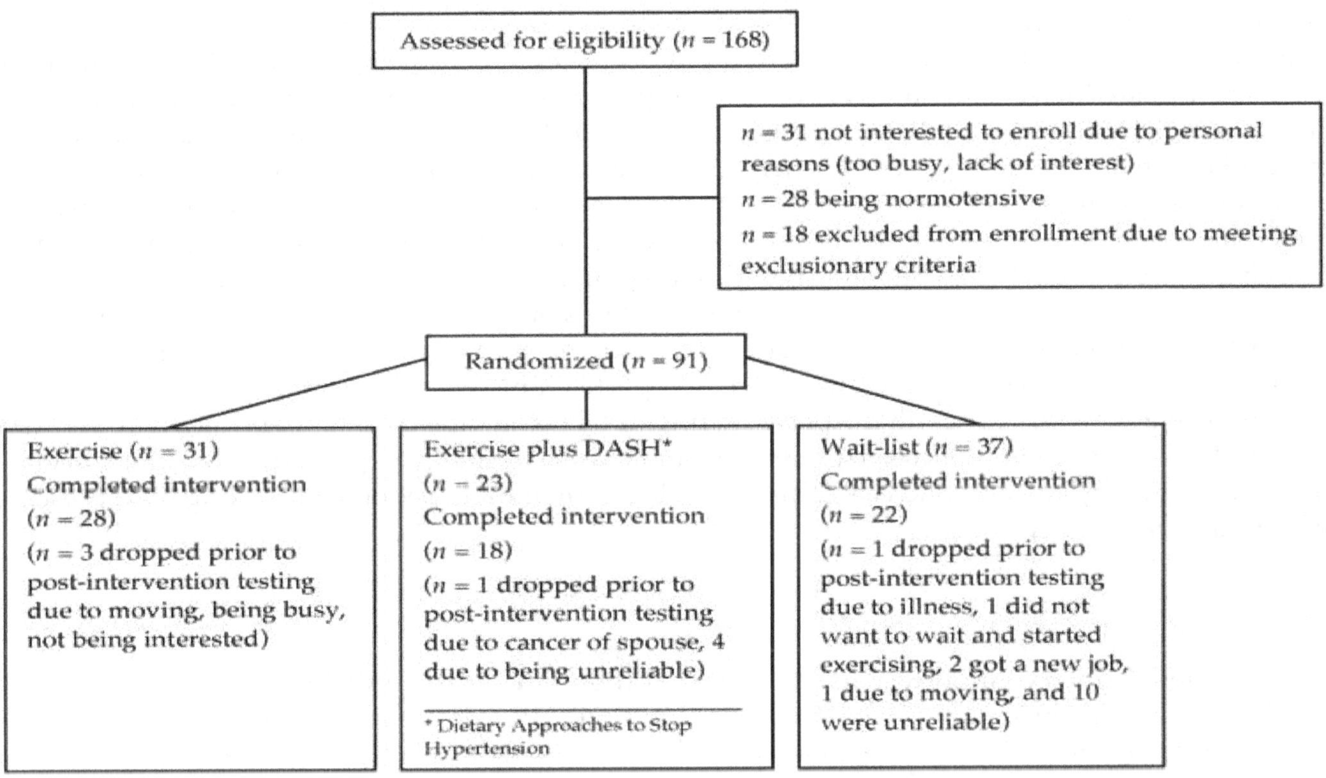

Figure 1. CONSORT flow diagram for participants.

The trial included relatively healthy, sedentary and non-medicated men and women (n = 91) between age 18 and 65 years with prehypertension (>120/80 but <140/90 mmHg) and stage 1 and 2 hypertension (≥140/90 but <180/110 mmHg), who were not on a current diet or had been participating in an exercise program within the past 6 months. The level of habitual physical activity was assessed using the Leisure Time Exercise Questionnaire (LTEQ) by Godin and Shepard [31] to confirm the sedentary status; individuals with LTEQ total scores above 40 were excluded. Major concomitant diseases were ruled out by blood sample, resting electrocardiogram and medical history. For each eligible participant, a trained technician or registered nurse obtained anthropometric data through standard procedures. Body weight, height and average resting BP (six measurements taken after a

15-min seated rest on two separate days using a Dinamap Compact BP® monitor (Critikon, Tempa, FL, USA)). Participants with values of high-sensitivity CRP >10 mg/L were excluded from the analyses, as values above this threshold are indicative of an acute infection.

2.3. Fitness Testing

Participants underwent a maximum oxygen intake (VO_{2peak}, mL/kg/min) treadmill exercise test to determine cardiorespiratory fitness using the standard Bruce protocol in which treadmill speed and grade were increased gradually from 1.7 mph and 10% grade every 3 min. Expired gas was analyzed by Sensormedics metabolic cart, Milano, Italy (Vmax software version 6-2A).

2.4. Aerobic Cardio Training

Since all participants were relatively sedentary at baseline, the training intervention was designed to increase exercise levels gradually to the ultimate physical activity goal: Five or more days per week of at least moderate-intensity cardiovascular physical activity (e.g., walking) for 30 to 60 min. Exercise intensity was individually adapted by the assessed heart rate (before and during exercise). Participants met with a certified personal trainer (study personnel) at the local YMCA 2 days a week for the entire 12-week intervention period. They shared with the trainer the fitness information. In-person sessions with a trainer were scheduled, as they are more likely to be completed than entirely home-based exercise and may increase the motivation for completion of the three sessions per week of exercise without a personal trainer. The sessions with the trainer included training in proper warm up, exercise and cool down and stretching. The participant was asked to do physical activity on his or her own (either in their home, neighborhood or at the YMCA) for three additional days per week. In addition to meeting a goal for the number of minutes of physical activity, participants were asked to increase incidental physical activity. To monitor their progress, participants were given a pedometer and asked to work up to an ultimate goal of an average of 10,000+ steps per day. We used the same pedometer (Omron®, Kyōto, Japan) throughout the study to warrant an adequate comparison. The inclusion of the pedometer and step goal helped to ensure that participants were not compensating for increased activity during their sessions with the personal trainer by being more sedentary throughout the rest of the day. The achievement of these goals ensured an increase in energy expenditure, which contributed to a negative energy balance. Subjects completed a log of their daily pedometer readings and presented them to the trainer each week.

2.5. Caloric Reduction

The dietary intervention was led by research dietitians at the Nutrition Services Core of the UCSD Medical Center General Clinical Research Center (GCRC) or Clinical and Translational Research Institute (CTRI). The core of the diet plan was based on the DASH clinical study [32,33]. This dietary pattern is high in fruits, vegetables, and low fat dairy foods, and low in saturated and total fat. It also is high in dietary fiber, potassium, calcium, and magnesium, and moderately high in protein. The dietary intervention aimed at reducing the individual energy intake by 500–1000 kcal/day taking into account lifestyle and dietary preferences of the participant [34]. In addition, concomitant behavioral strategies like conscious eating and stimulus control were trained. Thus, participants received intensive intervention approaches known to produce behavior change. Subjects in the experimental group met with registered dietitians and/or certified exercise trainers to establish initial dietary and physical activity goals. Regular meetings in person and by phone continued for the entire 12-week intervention. All subjects recorded their food (caloric intake in kilojoule) and provided the information to the study investigators. Diet adherence was assessed with three daily dietary recalls administered by the study dietician.

2.6. *Assessment of Inflammatory Biomarkers and Cellular Adhesion Molecules*

Fasting blood samples were collected within one week of, but at least two days after, the maximum exercise test at baseline. All assays were performed in the UCSD Clinical Research Biomarker Laboratory using commercially available immunoassay kits (R&D Systems products, Minneapolis, MN, or MSD Systems, Rockville, MD, USA). Intra- and inter-assay coefficients of variation (CV) were confirmed to be <5%. For subsequent statistical analyses, soluble ICAM-1 (sample size, 63), sICAM-3 (66), PAI-1 (68), CRP (62), IL-6 (65), and TNF-α (63) measures were log-transformed to normalize distributions with differing sample sizes reflecting missing biomarker data due to technical errors, etc., and we calculated the difference (Δ) from pre to post intervention levels for all biomarker measures by detracting the value before the intervention from the value after the intervention.

2.7. *Secondary Analysis of Trial Data*

According to the RCT protocol, $n = 18$ had been to the aerobic cardio training and caloric reduction intervention, $n = 28$ to the aerobic cardio training alone intervention and $n = 22$ to the wait-list control group. However, in reality, participants began modifying their exercise or diet behavior regardless of their intervention group assignment and modest group sizes limited statistical power. Therefore, we decided for a statistical approach with a secondary analysis of data from all 68 participants combined that may better warrant to indicate the actual behavior and inflammatory processes and consider the intervention effect described respectively.

Thus, a series of multivariate linear regression analyses were performed to examine the role of the different intervention elements (predictors). For the three predictors fitness, cardio training, and caloric intake, the differences (Δ) from pre to post intervention levels were used in the statistical analyses. We calculated these differences (Δ) by detracting the value before the intervention from the value after the intervention. Associations between the four predictors (BP, fitness, cardio training, and caloric intake) and outcomes (differences (Δ) from pre to post intervention levels of cellular adhesion molecules (sICAM-1, sICAM-3) and inflammatory biomarkers (CRP, IL-6, TNF-α)) were determined using multiple linear regression models, separately for each of the five outcome variables. Results were considered statistically significant at $p \leq 0.05$. We did not adjust p-values for multiple comparisons, as the main primary outcome was CRP; however, as we examined the potential interaction among inflammatory, adhesion and prothrombic markers, we defined one primary outcome marker in each of these three biomarker domains playing different roles in CVD: CRP for inflammation, sICAM-1 for adhesion molecules, and PAI-1 for prothrombotic factors. All other outcomes (IL-6, TNF, sICAM-3) were secondary (Il-6 and TNF) or exploratory (sICAM-3, as no study so far has been investigating sICAM-3).

For the associations between each of the predictors and inflammatory marker outcome levels, two models of increasing complexity were computed: in Model 1 we adjusted for (prehypertensive or hypertensive) BP and sociodemographic factors (age, gender) only, and in Model 2 we additionally adjusted for the other remaining predictors in one complete regression model (Table 1). Only the significant results of the five statistical models are shown for a better overview (Table 1). For our second hypothesis, mean pre and post intervention BP, fitness levels, and weight of the three groups were compared to each other. All statistical analyses were performed using IBM® SPSS® version 22.0 statistical software package (IBM Corporation, New York, NY, USA).

Table 1. First step [a] and final [b] multivariate regression analyses between inflammatory biomarkers and intervention elements (predictors) in the studied pre- and hypertensive participants.

Predictor	Δ [c] Outcome [d]	β	p [e]
SBP [e]	Δ PAI-1 ($n = 62$)	[a] 0.415 [b] 0.427	0.003 0.001

Table 1. *Cont.*

Predictor	Δ [c] Outcome [d]	β	p [e]
Δ Fitness (VO_{2peak})	Δ PAI-1 (n = 62)	[a] −0.369	0.004
		[b] −0.392	0.006
Δ Caloric intake	Δ sICAM-3 (n = 63)	[a] −0.363	0.014
		[b] −0.332	0.026
	Δ CRP (n = 63)	[a] 0.317	0.025
		[b] 0.342	0.018
Δ Cardio training [f]	Δ sICAM-3 (n = 63)	[a] 0.314	0.037
		[b] 0.301	0.046
	Δ IL-6 (n = 66)	[a] 0.403	0.005
		[b] 0.415	0.004
	Δ TNF-α (n = 68)	[a] −0.337	0.018
		[b] −0.357	0.017

[a] The first step regression model included predictor, age, gender, and the difference from pre to post intervention biomarker level, and systolic blood pressure (except for systolic blood pressure as predictor). [b] The final model included the first step model and additionally the other predictors, and the difference from pre to post intervention body mass index level. [c] Δ, value difference from pre to post intervention level: We calculated the difference from pre to post intervention levels by detracting the value before the intervention from the value after the intervention. [d] PAI, plasminogen activator inhibitor; sICAM, soluble intercellular adhesion molecule; CRP, C-reactive protein; IL, interleukin; TNF-α, tumor necrosis factor-alpha. [e] SBP, systolic blood pressure. [f] Cardio training, moderate aerobic cardio training: total minutes during 12-week-intervention. [e] $p < 0.05$.

3. Results

3.1. Study Sample

The baseline demographic, metabolic and health behavior characteristics of all study participants (n = 68) included in the statistical analyses are displayed in Table 2. In the combined 68 participants, 22 subjects had reduced caloric intake and exercised regularly. These 22 participants had an average daily caloric reduction of 673 ± 594 calories (mean ± SEM) and had on average exercised 22.9 ± 2.8 h during the 12-week intervention (on average 114.5 ± 14 min per week). The intensity of aerobic cardio training of the hypertensive patients did not differ significantly from that of the prehypertensive patients (p = 0.18). Subjects who exercised regularly but had no caloric reduction (n = 38) had spent on average 21.1 ± 2.0 h on training during the 12-week intervention (on average 105.5 ± 10 min per week). Thirteen % of the participants were current smokers based on self-report.

Table 2. Demographic, metabolic and health behavior characteristics of the study participants before the intervention.

Variable	n [a]	Mean ± SEM and Range in Parentheses or Percentage Value
Prehypertension/Hypertension	68	44.1%/55.9%
Systolic blood pressure, mmHg	68	141 ± 1 (124–174)
Diastolic blood pressure, mmHg	68	84 ± 1 (69–102)
Heart rate, beats/min	68	75 ± 1 (53.0–99)
Age, years	68	45 ± 1 (25–60)
Gender, male/female	68	45%/55%
Body mass index, kg/m^2	67	30.8 ± 0.5 (22.4–38.8)
Glucose, mg/dL	64	89 ± 1 (59–120)
Total cholesterol/HDL-cholesterol ratio	63	4.8 ± 0.2 (0.5–10.8)
Smoking	68	13%
Concomitant medication	68	0%
Leisure time exercise questionnaire	65	11.7 ± 1.2 (0.0–35.0)
VO_{2peak} [b] (mL/kg/min)	68	27.9 ± 0.9 (15.0–54.0)

Table 2. *Cont.*

Variable	n [a]	Mean ± SEM and Range in Parentheses or Percentage Value
Inflammatory measures before the intervention	n [c]	
C-reactive protein, mg/L	63	2.8 (1.1–7.1)
Interleukin-6, pg/mL	66	2.7 (1.2–4.3)
Tumor necrosis factor-α, pg/mL	68	2.7 (1.2–4.1)
Plasminogen activator inhibitor-1, ng/mL	62	41.1 (21.4–61.2)
Soluble intercellular adhesion molecule-1, ng/mL	65	306.8 (239.3–374.1)
Soluble intercellular adhesion molecule-3, ng/mL	63	2.6 (2.2–3.2)

Data are given as mean ± standard error of the mean (SEM) (range) or percentage values. Inflammatory measures are given as medians (interquartile range). [a] n, number of subjects included. [b] VO_{2peak}, peak oxygen consumption. [c] n, number of subjects who provided biomarker's measurement before and after the intervention.

3.2. *Blood Pressure Classification before and after Intervention*

After the intervention the mean SBP reduction for hypertensive subjects (n = 34) with 10.1 ± 2.6 mmHg was greater than the prehypertensive subjects (n = 25) with 4.4 ± 1.3 mmHg but not significantly so ($p = 0.06$). However, the average SBP of the hypertensive patients (n = 34; mean ± SEM: 148.1 ± 1.6 mmHg) decreased to the prehypertensive level of 137.9 ± 2.3 mmHg.

3.3. *Cellular Adhesion Molecules and Inflammatory Biomarker Associations with Elevated Blood Pressure, Fitness and Obesity in the 68 Participants*

We calculated Pearson's correlations to examine the associations of the soluble intercellular adhesion molecules and inflammatory biomarkers with BP, BMI, and fitness before the intervention. CRP was negatively correlated with fitness ($r = -0.308$; $p < 0.05$) and positively with BMI ($r = 0.327$; $p < 0.01$). IL-6 was negatively associated with fitness ($r = -0.311$; $p < 0.05$) and positively associated with SBP ($r = 0.310$; $p < 0.05$). TNF-α was negatively correlated with SBP ($r = -0.364$; $p < 0.01$). Soluble ICAM-1 was negatively associated with fitness ($r = -0.242$; $p < 0.05$) and was positively associated with CRP ($r = 0.414$; $p < 0.01$) but not with BP. Soluble ICAM-3 had no associations with BP, BMI, fitness or sICAM-1.

3.4. *Behavioral Change by Intervention Elements, Change of BMI and Fitness and Its Role in Inflammation in All Participants with Elevated Blood Pressures*

The higher the SBP the higher were PAI-1 levels (β = 0.427; $p = 0.001$), and the more the fitness level had improved during the intervention the lower were PAI-1 levels (β = −0.392; $p < 0.01$) after the intervention (Table 1). Aerobic cardio training was a significant independent predictor of sICAM-3, IL-6, and TNF-α levels after controlling for sociodemographic variables and SBP in a first step regression model (Table 1), meaning the greater the amount of total moderate exercise was, the higher were the levels of sICAM-3 and IL-6, and the lower were the levels of TNF-α (Table 1) after the intervention. From earlier analyses [35,36], BMI decreased in the exercise groups, and fitness increased in those groups. These results remained statistically significant, even after adjusting for changes in BMI, fitness, and caloric reduction in the final model (sICAM-3 (β = 0.301; $p < 0.05$), IL-6 (β = 0.415; $p < 0.01$), and TNF-α (β = −0.357; $p < 0.05$); Table 1). Caloric reduction (to reduce caloric intake) predicted significantly higher sICAM-3 (β = −0.332; $p < 0.05$) and lower CRP (β = 0.342; $p < 0.05$) levels in the first step and final model (Table 1).

4. Discussion

We examined the differential effects of aerobic cardio training and caloric reduction on inflammatory, adhesion and prothrombotic biomarkers in prehypertensive and hypertensive subjects. Our study adds to the existent body of literature in the context of behavioral (aerobic exercise and diet) intervention and hypertension for inflammatory biomarker outcomes. The more comprehensive approach of lifestyle changes including exercise and diet behavior change of this 12-week-intervention study might explain the differential changes of inflammatory (CRP, IL-6, TNF-α) and prothrombotic (PAI-1), and adhesion (sICAM-1 and -3) biomarkers.

The key finding is that aerobic cardio training and/or caloric reduction had differential effects on IL-6 and adhesion molecule sICAM-3 in vivo. In particular, the latter finding is novel showing a prospective association between exercise and caloric reduction respectively and sICAM-3 levels. Thereby, this is the first study to our knowledge that shows that aerobic exercise has not only an impact on inflammatory biomarkers but also on levels of cellular adhesion molecules. Until now, it was unclear how they might interact, although it is well known that aerobic exercise reduces inflammatory processes.

The increase of sICAM-3 and IL-6 in subjects with elevated BP was independently predicted by the intensity of aerobic cardio training and caloric reduction. We think that this finding may be initially counter-intuitive but is important for the following reasons: First, this finding is consistent with prior studies, which showed that exercise was associated with a significant increase in IL-6 [37,38]. In this study, however, increased IL-6 levels after intervention and its positive correlation with both exercise levels and caloric reduction may be explained by potentially anti-inflammatory effects of IL-6 [39]. IL-6 is a pleiotropic cytokine released by skeletal myocytes under contraction, mediating anti-inflammatory effects by stimulating the production of anti-inflammatory cytokines and suppression of TNF-α production [39] with all these mechanisms concurring with the results of this study. Second, this is the first study to highlight the potential role of sICAM-3 in vascular inflammatory effects of exercise and/or diet intervention among prehypertensive and hypertensive subjects. To date, studies on the effects of human hypertension on adhesion molecules have been focusing on sICAM-1 levels, which are increased in hypertensive individuals [4–6]. Soluble ICAM-1 levels reflect ICAM-1 expression on activated endothelial cells [40] and are associated with the degree of atherosclerosis [41]. Although ICAM-1 and ICAM-3 share a similar immunoglobulin-like structure and amino acid identity of about 48%, with the greatest homology observed in domains 2 and 3 [42], their differential pattern of expression and cellular distribution suggest a different functional role [42]. The interactions of ICAM-1 and ICAM-3 with lymphocyte function-associated antigen (LFA)-1 are integral to the normal functioning of the immune system [42]. ICAM-3 is expressed on resting leucocytes and is potentially the most important ligand for LFA-1 in the initiation of the immune response because the expression of ICAM-1 on resting leucocytes is low [17]. Although sICAM-3 binds to LFA-1 with an affinity approximately nine-times weaker than sICAM-1, sICAM-1 and sICAM-3 compete with each other for binding to LFA-1 [42]. As we did not find changes in sICAM-1 levels post interventions in this study, we speculate that the increase in sICAM-3 levels as a result of changes in exercise and/or diet behavior in this study may exhibit a "buffer" for the sICAM-1 function, potentially leading to down-regulating vascular endothelial inflammation. It is not fully understood whether the increase of sICAM-3 by cardio training and caloric reduction in prehypertensive and hypertensive subjects reflects a cardio-protective mechanism. Given the lack of knowledge in the vascular function of sICAM-3 and its implications as a vascular inflammatory biomarker, a follow-up investigation is necessary to examine its vascular action and interactions separate of or in conjunction with other better-known vascular endothelial markers such as sICAM-1.

Another relevant potential underlying pathway in hypertension, metabolic syndrome, dyslipidaemia, and abdominal obesity, is the dysregulation of the hypothalamic–pituitary–adrenal (HPA) axis leading to catecholamine activation of β-adrenergic receptors (β-ARs) [43]. This may lead to altered leukocyte/endothelial binding, endothelial injury with up-regulation of endothelial ICAM-1 expression and increase of inflammatory cytokines [44]. In this context, regular aerobic exercise has also been shown to enhance β-AR sensitivity in the context of age-related decline in adrenergic responsiveness, i.e., increase of total peripheral resistances, which is a relevant factor underlying hypertension, atherosclerosis, and vascular insufficiency [45,46].

This study has a number of limitations. First, a weakness of the experimental design of this study is the lack of healthy BP controls. Thus, we are unable to determine whether the inflammatory, adhesion, and prothrombotic factors measured were indeed elevated in our sample of individuals with hypertension and prehypertension as compared with healthy individuals, and whether the changes induced by diet and exercise in these factors are at the level of clinical benefits. Second, a randomized and controlled trial of 12-week intervention of health behavior change was proven challenging and resulted in modest group sizes, limiting statistical power. More importantly, few significant differences found among intervention groups led us to scrutinize the actual changes in exercise and diet behavior. In reality, in spite of our best efforts to avoid "cross-contamination" between health behaviors, participants naturally began modifying their exercise or diet behavior regardless of their intervention group assignment. Some participants assigned to wait-list control condition also began to change their health behavior. Although troubling for behavior intervention trials, this kind of behavior is not particularly surprising, as exercise and healthy diet behaviors tend to co-occur [47]. It was revealed also particularly challenging to prohibit study volunteers who exhibit "readiness" to change their health behavior from doing so to follow randomization to a wait-list control group in a trial such as this. Therefore, as aforementioned, we collapsed all groups into one sample and applied multivariate regression analyses to the whole sample in order to account for exercise and diet behavior changes in practice during the intervention period. Third, regarding the dietary intervention, we have to mention that we did not differ short supply chain (SSC) from long supply chain (LSC) food included in the DASH [48]. A recent cross-sectional study found that only individuals adhering to the Mediterranean diet with an SSC had a significantly reduced prevalence of metabolic syndrome compared to those with an LSC [48]. Further, recent studies have shown that inflammatory effects of food parameters exist with a high variability [49] due to either a different genetic pattern or to diverse genetic–environmental interactions, and potential interactions (synergism, antagonism) among food parameters. However, as previously proposed, such a "dietary inflammatory index" ought to be advanced further [49]. Another intervention group, diet alone, may have contributed to important additional information. Fourth, our study did not explore the role of gender in the potentially differing effects of exercise and/or diet on inflammatory or prothrombotic markers, which was beside the primary aim of the study and limited by a limited sample size. Future studies should investigate the effect of gender not only on the intervention effects but also such behavior changes.

In summary, regular exercise and caloric reduction in individuals at risk of essential hypertension may have differential effects on biomarkers of CVD risk which may have clinical implications for the prevention of atherothrombotic cardiovascular disease. Assessments of the actual behavioral changes above and beyond intervention group assignment appear to be important. Nonetheless, the evidence of beneficial effects of regular physical activity on CV health and prevention of CVD risk, including BP, lipid levels and glucose tolerance [50] needs to be highlighted.

Author Contributions: Conceptualization, S.H., K.J.C., C.L.R., R.v.K. and P.J.M.; methodology, E.-Y.N.W., S.H., K.L.W. and P.J.M.; software, E.-Y.N.W.; formal analysis, E.-Y.N.W., S.H. and R.v.K.; investigation, all authors; resources, S.H., R.v.K., E.-Y.N.W. and P.J.M.; data curation, K.L.W.; writing—original draft preparation, E.-Y.N.W.; writing—review and editing, all authors; visualization, E.-Y.N.W. and S.H.; supervision, E.-Y.N.W., S.H. and P.J.M.; project administration, E.-Y.N.W., S.H. and P.J.M.; funding acquisition, P.J.M. All authors have read and agreed to the published version of the manuscript.

Acknowledgments: Special thanks to the dedicated personal trainers and staff at the Mission Valley YMCA and La Jolla YMCA. This work had been submitted posthumously for Karen Calfas whose scientific contribution to the field and public health impact she has made are greatly appreciated and honored.

References

1. Vasan, R.S.; Beiser, A.; Seshadri, S.; Larson, M.G.; Kannel, W.B.; D'Agostino, R.B.; Levy, D. Residual lifetime risk for developing hypertension in middle-aged women and men: The framingham heart study. *JAMA* **2002**, *287*, 1003–1010. [CrossRef] [PubMed]
2. Retta, T.M.; Randall, O.S. Hypertension and concomitant diseases: A guide for evidence-based therapy. *J. Natl. Med. Assoc.* **2004**, *96*, 450–460.
3. Goetzel, R.Z.; Long, S.R.; Ozminkowski, R.J.; Hawkins, K.; Wang, S.; Lynch, W. Health, absence, disability, and presenteeism cost estimates of certain physical and mental health conditions affecting U.S. employers. *J. Occup. Environ. Med.* **2004**, *46*, 398–412. [CrossRef] [PubMed]
4. DeSouza, C.A.; Dengel, D.R.; Macko, R.F.; Cox, K.; Seals, D.R. Elevated levels of circulation cell adhesion molecule in uncomplicated essential hypertension. *Am. J. Hypertens.* **1997**, *10*, 1335–1341. [CrossRef]
5. de Faria, A.P.; Ritter, A.M.; Sabbatini, A.R.; Corrêa, N.B.; Brunelli, V.; Modolo, R.; Moreno, H. Deregulation of soluble adhesion molecules in resistant hypertension and its role in cardiovascular remodeling. *Circ. J.* **2016**, *80*, 1196–1201. [CrossRef] [PubMed]
6. Komatsu, S.; Panes, J.; Russell, J.M.; Anderson, D.C.; Muzykantov, V.R.; Miyasaka, M.; Granger, D.N. Effects of chronic arterial hypertension on constitutive and induced intercellular adhesion molecule-1 expression in vivo. *Hypertension* **1997**, *29*, 683–689. [CrossRef]
7. Ross, R. Atherosclerosis—An inflammatory disease. *N. Engl. J. Med.* **1999**, *340*, 115–126. [CrossRef]
8. Raggi, P.; Genest, J.; Giles, J.T.; Rayner, K.J.; Dwivedi, G.; Beanlands, R.S.; Gupta, M. Role of inflammation in the pathogenesis of atherosclerosis and therapeutic interventions. *Atherosclerosis* **2018**, *276*, 98–108. [CrossRef]
9. Chae, C.U.; Lee, R.T.; Rifai, N. Blood pressure and inflammation in apparently healthy men. *Hypertension* **2001**, *38*, 399–403. [CrossRef]
10. Peeters, A.C.; Netea, M.G.; Janssen, M.C.; Kullberg, B.J.; Van der Meer, J.W.; Thien, T. Pro-inflammatory cytokines in patients with essential hypertension. *Eur. J. Clin. Invest.* **2001**, *31*, 31–36. [CrossRef]
11. Mirhafez, S.R.; Mohebati, M.; Feiz Disfani, M.; Saberi Karimian, M.; Ebrahimi, M.; Avan, A.; Eslami, S.; Pasdar, A.; Rooki, H.; Esmaeili, H.; et al. An imbalance in serum concentrations of inflammatory and anti-inflammatory cytokines in hypertension. *J. Am. Soc. Hypertens.* **2014**, *8*, 614–623. [CrossRef]
12. Ridker, P.M.; Buring, J.E.; Cook, N.R.; Rifai, N. C-reactive protein, the metabolic syndrome, and risk of incident cardiovascular events: An 8-year follow-up of 14719 initially healthy American women. *Circulation* **2003**, *107*, 391–397. [CrossRef] [PubMed]
13. Horvei, L.D.; Grimnes, G.; Hindberg, K.; Mathiesen, E.B.; Njølstad, I.; Wilsgaard, T.; Brox, J.; Braekkan, S.K.; Hansen, J.B. C-reactive protein, obesity, and the risk of arterial and venous thrombosis. *J. Thromb. Haemost.* **2016**, *14*, 1561–1571. [CrossRef] [PubMed]
14. Hashimoto, H.; Kitagawa, K.; Hougaku, H.; Etani, H.; Hori, M. Relationship between C-reactive protein and progression of early carotid atherosclerosis in hypertensive subjects. *Stroke* **2004**, *35*, 1625–1630. [CrossRef] [PubMed]
15. Schillaci, G.; Pirro, M.; Gemelli, F.; Pasqualini, L.; Vaudo, G.; Marchesi, S.; Siepi, D.; Bagaglia, F.; Mannarino, E. Increased C-reactive protein concentrations in never-treated hypertension: The role of systolic and pulse pressures. *J. Hypertens.* **2003**, *21*, 1841–1846. [CrossRef]
16. Ridker, P.M.; Hennekens, C.H.; Roitman-Johnson, B.; Buring, J.E.; Grodstein, F. Plasma concentration of soluble intercellular adhesion molecule 1 and risks of future myocardial infarction in apparently healthy men. *Lancet* **1998**, *351*, 88–92. [CrossRef]
17. Fawcett, J.; Holness, C.L.; Needham, L.A.; Turley, H.; Gatter, K.C.; Mason, D.Y.; Simmons, D.L. Molecular cloning of ICAM-3, a third ligand for LFA-1, constitutively expressed on resting leukocytes. *Nature* **1992**, *360*, 481–484. [CrossRef]
18. Whelton, S.P.; Chin, A.; Xin, X. Effect of aerobic exercise on blood pressure: A meta-analysis of randomized, controlled trials. *Ann. Intern. Med.* **2002**, *136*, 493–503. [CrossRef]
19. Chobanian, A.V.; Bakris, G.L.; Black, H.R.; Cushman, W.C.; Green, L.A.; Izzo, J.L., Jr.; Jones, D.W.; Materson, B.J.; Oparil, S.; Wright, J.T., Jr.; et al. Seventh report of the joint national committee on prevention, detection, evaluation, and treatment of high blood pressure. *Hypertension* **2003**, *42*, 1206–1252. [CrossRef]
20. Bacon, S.L.; Sherwood, A.; Hinderliter, A.; Blumenthal, J.A. Effects of exercise, diet and weight loss on high blood pressure. *Sports Med.* **2004**, *34*, 307–316. [CrossRef]

21. Lesniak, K.T.; Dubbert, P.M. Exercise and hypertension. *Curr. Opin. Cardiol.* **2001**, *16*, 356–359. [CrossRef] [PubMed]
22. Carroll, S.; Dudfield, M. What is the relationship between exercise and metabolic abnormalities? A review of the metabolic syndrome. *Sports Med.* **2004**, *34*, 371–418. [CrossRef] [PubMed]
23. Bremner, A.D. Antihypertensive medication and quality of life—Silent treatment of a silent killer? *Cardiovasc. Drugs. Ther.* **2002**, *16*. [CrossRef] [PubMed]
24. Nicklas, B.J.; You, T.; Pahor, M. Behavioural treatments for chronic systemic inflammation: Effects of dietary weight loss and exercise training. *CMAJ* **2005**, *172*, 1199–1209. [CrossRef] [PubMed]
25. Geffken, D.F.; Cushman, M.; Burke, G.L.; Polak, J.F.; Sakkinen, P.A.; Tracy, R.P. Association between physical activity and markers of inflammation in a healthy elderly population. *Am. J. Epidemiol.* **2001**, *153*, 242–250. [CrossRef]
26. Pischon, T.; Hankinson, S.E.; Hotamisligil, G.S.; Rifai, N.; Rimm, E.B. Leisure-time physical activity and reduced plasma levels of obesity-related inflammatory markers. *Obes. Res.* **2003**, *11*, 1055–1064. [CrossRef]
27. von Känel, R.; Hong, S.; Pung, M.A.; Mills, P.J. Association of blood pressure and fitness with levels of atherosclerotic risk markers pre-exercise and post-exercise. *Am. J. Hypertens.* **2007**, *20*, 670–675. [CrossRef]
28. DeSouza, C.A.; Jones, P.P.; Seals, D.R. Physical activity status and adverse age-related differences in coagulation and fibrinolytic factors in women. *Arterioscler. Thromb. Vasc. Biol.* **1998**, *18*, 362–368. [CrossRef]
29. Mills, P.J.; Hong, S.; Redwine, L.; Carter, S.M.; Chiu, A.; Ziegler, M.G.; Dimsdale, J.E.; Maisel, A.S. Physical fitness attenuates leukocyte-endothelial adhesion in response to acute exercise. *J. Appl. Physiol.* **2006**, *101*, 785–788. [CrossRef]
30. Hong, S.; Johnson, T.A.; Farag, N.H.; Guy, H.J.; Matthews, S.C.; Ziegler, M.G. Attenuation of T lymphocyte demargination and adhesion molecule expression in response to moderate exercise in fit versus non-fit individuals. *J. Appl. Physiol.* **2005**, *98*, 1057–1063. [CrossRef]
31. Godin, G.; Shephard, R.J. A simple method to assess exercise behavior in the community. *Can. J. Appl. Sport. Sci.* **1985**, *10*, 141–146. [PubMed]
32. Phillips, K.M.; Stewart, K.K.; Karanja, N.M.; Windhauser, M.M.; Champagne, C.M.; Swain, J.F.; Lin, P.H.; Evans, M.A. Validation of diet composition for the dietary approaches to stop hypertension trial. DASH collaborative research group. *J. Am. Diet. Assoc.* **1999**, *99*, S60–S68. [CrossRef]
33. Zimmerman, E.; Wylie-Rosset, J. Nutrition therapy for hypertension. *Curr. Diab. Report.* **2003**, *3*, 404–411. [CrossRef]
34. Expert Panel on the Identification, Evaluation, and Treatment of Overweight in Adults. Clinical guidelines on the identification, evaluation, and treatment of overweight and obesity in adults: Executive summary. *Am. J. Clin. Nutr.* **1998**, *68*, 899–917. [CrossRef] [PubMed]
35. Edwards, K.M.; Wilson, K.L.; Sadja, J.; Ziegler, M.G.; Mills, P.J. Effects on blood pressure and autonomic nervous system function of a 12-week exercise or exercise plus DASH-diet intervention in individuals with elevated blood pressure. *Acta Physiol. (Oxf.)* **2011**, *203*, 343–350. [CrossRef] [PubMed]
36. Sadja, J.; Tomfohr, L.; Jiménez, J.A.; Edwards, K.M.; Rock, C.L.; Calfas, K.; Mills, P.J. Higher physical fatigue predicts adherence to a 12-week exercise intervention in women with elevated blood pressure. *Health Psychol.* **2012**, *31*, 156–163. [CrossRef] [PubMed]
37. Mills, P.J.; Maisel, A.S.; Ziegler, M.G.; Dimsdale, J.E.; Carter, S.; Kennedy, B.; Woods, V.L., Jr. Peripheral blood mononuclear cell-endothelial adhesion in human hypertension following exercise. *J. Hypertens.* **2000**, *18*, 1801–1806. [CrossRef] [PubMed]
38. Chen, N.G.; Abbasi, F.; Lamendola, C.; McLaughlin, T.; Cooke, J.P.; Tsao, P.S.; Reaven, G.M. Mononuclear cell adherence to cultured endothelium is enhanced by hypertension and insulin resistance in healthy nondiabetic volunteers. *Circulation* **1999**, *100*, 940–943. [CrossRef]
39. Pedersen, B.K. IL-6 Signalling in exercise and disease. *Biochem. Soc. Trans.* **2007**, *35*, 1295–1297. [CrossRef]
40. Leeuwenberg, J.F.; Smeets, E.F.; Neefjes, J.J.; Shaffer, M.A.; Cinek, T.; Jeunhomme, T.M.; Ahern, T.J.; Buurman, W.A. E-selectin and intercellular adhesion Molecule-1 are released by activated human endothelial cells in vitro. *Immunology* **1992**, *77*, 543–549.
41. Rohde, L.E.; Lee, R.T.; Rivero, J.; Jamacochian, M.; Arroyo, L.H.; Briggs, W.; Rifai, N.; Libby, P.; Creager, M.A.; Ridker, P.M. Circulating cell adhesion molecules are correlated with ultrasound-based assessment of carotid atherosclerosis. *Arterioscler. Thromb. Vasc. Biol.* **1998**, *18*, 1765–1770. [CrossRef] [PubMed]

42. Woska, J.R., Jr.; Morelock, M.M.; Jeanfavre, D.D.; Caviness, G.O.; Bormann, B.J.; Rothlein, R. Molecular comparison of soluble intercellular adhesion molecule (SICAM)-1 and SICAM-3 binding to lymphocyte function-associated antigen. *J. Biol. Chem.* **1998**, *273*, 4725–4733. [CrossRef]
43. Ciccarelli, M.; Santulli, G.; Pascale, V.; Trimarco, B.; Iaccarino, G. Adrenergic receptors and metabolism: Role in development of cardiovascular disease. *Front. Physiol.* **2013**, *4*, 265. [CrossRef] [PubMed]
44. Schedlowski, M.; Hosch, W.; Oberbeck, R.; Benschop, R.; Jacobs, R.; Raab, H.; Schmidt, R. Catecholamines modulate human NK cell circulation and function via spleen-independent ß2-adrenergic mechanisms. *J. Immunol.* **1996**, *156*, 93–99. [PubMed]
45. Santulli, G.; Ciccarelli, M.; Trimarco, B.; Iaccarino, G. Physical activity ameliorates cardiovascular health in elderly subjects: The functional role of the β adrenergic system. *Front. Physiol.* **2013**, *4*, 20. [CrossRef] [PubMed]
46. Gambardella, J.; Morelli, M.B.; Wang, X.J.; Santulli, G. Pathophysiological mechanisms underlying the beneficial effects of physical activity in hypertension. *J. Clin. Hypertens. (Greenwich)* **2020**. [CrossRef]
47. Hong, S.; Bardwell, W.A.; Natarajan, L.; Flatt, S.W.; Rock, C.L.; Newman, V.A.; Madlensky, L.; Mills, P.J.; Dimsdale, J.E.; Thomson, C.A.; et al. Correlates of physical activity levels in breast cancer survivors participating in the women's healthy eating and living (WHEL) study. *Breast Cancer Res. Treat.* **2007**, *101*, 225–232. [CrossRef]
48. Santulli, G.; Pascale, V.; Finelli, R.; Visco, V.; Giannotti, R.; Massari, A.; Morisco, C.; Ciccarelli, M.; Illario, M.; Iaccarino, G.; et al. We are what we eat: Impact of food from short supply chain on metabolic syndrome. *J. Clin. Med.* **2019**, *8*, 2061. [CrossRef] [PubMed]
49. Gambardella, J.; Santulli, G. Integrating diet and inflammation to calculate cardiovascular risk. *Atherosclerosis* **2016**, *253*, 258–261. [CrossRef]
50. Grøntved, A.; Koivula, R.W.; Johansson, I.; Wennberg, P.; Østergaard, L.; Hallmans, G.; Renström, F.; Franks, P.W. Bicycling to work and primordial prevention of cardiovascular risk: A cohort study among swedish men and women. *J. Am. Heart Assoc.* **2016**, *5*, e004413. [CrossRef]

6

Association of Trimethylamine, Trimethylamine N-oxide and Dimethylamine with Cardiovascular Risk in Children with Chronic Kidney Disease

Chien-Ning Hsu [1,2], Guo-Ping Chang-Chien [3,4], Sufan Lin [3,4], Chih-Yao Hou [5], Pei-Chen Lu [6] and You-Lin Tain [6,7,*]

1 Department of Pharmacy, Kaohsiung Chang Gung Memorial Hospital, Kaohsiung 833, Taiwan; chien_ning_hsu@hotmail.com
2 School of Pharmacy, Kaohsiung Medical University, Kaohsiung 807, Taiwan
3 Center for Environmental Toxin and Emerging-Contaminant Research, Cheng Shiu University, Kaohsiung 833, Taiwan; guoping@csu.edu.tw (G.-P.C.-C.); linsufan2003@gmail.com (S.L.)
4 Super Micro Mass Research and Technology Center, Cheng Shiu University, Kaohsiung 833, Taiwan
5 Department of Seafood Science, National Kaohsiung University of Science and Technology, Kaohsiung 811, Taiwan; chihyaohou@gmail.com
6 Department of Pediatrics, Kaohsiung Chang Gung Memorial Hospital and College of Medicine, Chang Gung University, Kaohsiung 833, Taiwan; alexiellu@gmail.com
7 Institute for Translational Research in Biomedicine, Kaohsiung Chang Gung Memorial Hospital and Chang Gung University, College of Medicine, Kaohsiung 833, Taiwan
* Correspondence: tainyl@cgmh.org.tw

Abstract: Chronic kidney disease (CKD) is associated with high risk for cardiovascular disease (CVD). Gut microbiota-dependent metabolites trimethylamine (TMA), trimethylamine N-oxide (TMAO), and dimethylamine (DMA) have been linked to CKD and CVD. We examined whether these methylamines are correlated with cardiovascular risk in CKD children. A total of 115 children and adolescents with CKD stage G1–G4 were enrolled in this cross-sectional study. Children with CKD stage G2–G4 had higher plasma levels of DMA, TMA, and TMAO, but lower urinary levels of DMA and TMAO than those with CKD stage G1. Up to 53% of CKD children and adolescents had blood pressure (BP) abnormalities on 24-h ambulatory BP monitoring (ABPM). Plasma TMA and DMA levels inversely associated with high BP load as well as estimated glomerular filtration rate (eGFR). Additionally, CKD children with an abnormal ABPM profile had decreased abundance of phylum *Cyanobacteria*, genera *Subdoligranulum*, *Faecalibacterium*, *Ruminococcus*, and *Akkermansia*. TMA and DMA are superior to TMAO when related to high BP load and other CV risk factors in children and adolescents with early-stage CKD. Our findings highlight that gut microbiota-dependent methylamines are related to BP abnormalities and CV risk in pediatric CKD. Further studies should determine whether these microbial markers can identify children at risk for CKD progression.

Keywords: ambulatory blood pressure monitoring; cardiovascular disease; children; chronic kidney disease; dimethylamine; gut microbiota; hypertension; trimethylamine; trimethylamine N-oxide

---

1. Introduction

Chronic kidney disease (CKD) is associated with high risk for cardiovascular disease (CVD), not just for adults but also for children [1,2]. Even though overt CVD barely presents in children, the process of atherosclerosis can originate in early life. Therefore, heightened efforts are needed to identify CKD children at higher risk for CVD during their lifetimes to develop effective interventions for preemption [3]. Several noninvasive procedures, such as 24-h ambulatory blood pressure monitoring (ABPM) [4], ambulatory arterial stiffness index (AASI) [5], and left ventricular mass [6], are available to evaluate risk for CVD in children with CKD.

Gut microbiome has been identified as a source of pathogenic mediators in CKD [7]. Certain gut microbiota-derived metabolites have been shown to correlate with CVD in patients with CKD [8,9]. Among them, trimethylamine N-oxide (TMAO) has attracted increasing notoriety recently as a causative factor in various CVD. Emerging evidence has linked higher blood levels of TMAO with a higher risk of CVD [10].

TMAO production is a two-step process. The first step involves the liberation of trimethylamine (TMA) from dietary precursors (e.g., choline and carnitine) by gut microbes. In the second step, TMA is oxidized to TMAO by hepatic flavin-containing monooxygenases (FMOs). Both TMAO and TMA can be subsequently converted to dimethylamine (DMA). Thus, the plasma TMAO-to-TMA ratio may reflect FMO activity, while DMA-to-TMAO ratio is related to TMAO-metabolizing activity.

Although plasma levels of TMAO, TMA, and DMA are all increased in uremic patients [11], little attention has been paid to understand the role of their levels and combined ratios in the development of CVD in children with early-stage CKD. Because TMAO, TMA, and DMA are all tightly linked to each other and because all these methylamines are excreted into urine [12], we assume that simultaneous analysis of their combined ratios in the plasma and urine may provide more information to reflect the TMA–TMAO metabolic pathway. Thus, we assessed the association between CVD assessments, microbial markers, and TMA–TMAO metabolic pathway in early pediatric CKD.

2. Materials and Methods

2.1. Study Population

This is a cross-sectional study of 115 children and adolescents with CKD who were enrolled in the Kaohsiung Chang Gung Memorial Hospital from January 2019 to December 2019. Human subjects review board approval was obtained from the Institution Review Board and Ethics Committee of Chang Gung Medical Foundation, Taoyuan, Taiwan (Permit number: 201701735A3C501). Our study protocol was conducted in accordance with the 1964 Helsinki Declaration and its later amendments. Written informed consent was obtained from all participants. CKD is defined as abnormal kidney structure or function lasting more than three months [13]. We calculated estimated glomerular filtration rate (eGFR) with the Schwartz formula according to body height and blood creatinine (Cr) level [14]. Kidney damage included proteinuria, urine sediment abnormalities, or structural abnormalities and was detected by histology or imaging. Participants were categorized according to eGFR (mL/min/1.73 m^2): G1 ≥90, G2 60–89, G3 30–59, or G4 15–29. The causes of kidney diseases were divided to two categories: Congenital anomalies of the kidney and urinary tract (CAKUT) or non-CAKUT. CAKUT structural anomalies ranged from renal agenesis, kidney hypo-/dysplasia, horseshoe kidney, duplex collecting system, multi-cystic kidney dysplasia, posterior urethral valves, and ureter abnormalities [15]. Patients were excluded from the study if they (1) had a history of congenital heart disease; (2) were already documented as being pregnant; (3) had eGFR <15 mL/min/1.73 m^2 or were on dialysis maintenance, or had ever received renal transplantation; (4) were unable to cooperate with CV assessment.

2.2. Biochemical Analysis

Fasting plasma and spot urine samples were stored at −80 °C until analysis. We directed the family to have their children avoid excessive intake of foods rich in choline and carnitine (e.g., eggs, fish, or red meat) for 1 week before blood and urine sampling. Blood urea nitrogen (BUN), creatinine, total cholesterol, low-density lipoprotein (LDL), triglyceride, sodium, potassium, calcium, phosphate, uric acid, glucose, hemoglobin, hematocrit, and urine total protein-to-creatinine ratio were measured by the hospital central laboratory as described previously [16].

2.3. *Liquid Chromatography–Mass Spectrometry (LC–MS/MS) Analysis*

We analyzed plasma and urinary concentrations of DMA, TMA, and TMAO by LC–MS/MS analysis using an Agilent 6410 Series Triple Quadrupole mass spectrometer (Agilent Technologies, Wilmington, DE, USA) equipped with an electrospray ionization source [16]. The multiple-reaction-monitoring mode was set up using characteristic precursor-product ion transitions to detect m/z 46.1→30, m/z 60.1→44.1, and m/z 76.1→58.1, for DMA, TMA, and TMAO, respectively. Separation was performed in the Agilent Technologies 1200 HPLC system consisting of an autosampler and a binary pump. Chromatographic separation was performed on a SeQuant ZIC-HILIC column (150 × 2.1 mm, 5 μm; Merck KGaA, Darmstadt, Germany) protected by an Ascentis C18 column (2 cm × 4 mm, 5 μm; Merck KGaA, Darmstadt, Germany). Diethylamine was added to samples as an internal standard. The mobile phase containing methanol with 15mmol/L ammonium formate (phase A) and acetonitrile (phase B) was used at a ratio of 20:80 (phase A: phase B), with the flow rate set as 0.3–1 mL/min. The urinary concentration of each methylamine was corrected for urine Cr concentration, which was represented in ng/mg Cr.

2.4. *Blood Pressure Measurement and Echocardiography*

Participants were instructed to measure office blood pressure (BP) at the clinic visit after a 5 min rest with at least 1 min between recordings. The mean value was used for calculations. The 24-h ABPM data were collected for subjects aged 6–18 years, handled by an experienced specialist nurse as described previously [16]. We used the Oscar II monitoring device (SunTech Medical, Morrisville, NC) to measure BP and pulse rate at 20-min intervals over 24 h. The participants and their parents were requested to complete a diary of sleeping and waking times, as well as activities that may influence BP measurements. An abnormal ABPM profile was defined as (1) awake, asleep, systolic, or diastolic BP loads ≥95th percentile based on gender and height using ABPM reference data [17]; (2) awake, asleep, systolic or diastolic BP load ≥25%; and (3) asleep decrease of BP load <10% compared with average awake BP load. Next, the ambulatory arterial stiffness index (AASI) is an index derived from 24-h ABPM for the evaluation of arterial stiffness [5]. The AASI was defined as 1 minus the regression slope of diastolic BP (DBP) on systolic BP (SBP) [18]. Echocardiographic examination was performed with commercially available machines (Philips IE33 system, Philips, Bothell, WA, USA). The left ventricular (LV) mass was calculated using images obtained in the parasternal long-axis or short-axis view of the left ventricle by M-mode echocardiography. The LV mass index (LVMI) was obtained by indexing LV mass to height$^{2.7}$ [19].

2.5. *Analysis of Gut Microbiota Composition*

Metagenomic DNA was extracted from frozen fecal samples. Simple centrifugation processing was carried out to remove impurity, proteins, and other organic compounds. As described previously [16], all polymerase chain-reaction amplicons were mixed together with the Biotools Co., Ltd. (Taipei, Taiwan) for sequencing using an Illumina Miseq platform (Illumina, CA, USA). Amplicons were prepared according to the 16S Metagenomics Sequencing Library Preparation protocol (Illumina, CA, USA), and sequenced using the variable V3–V4 regions of the 16S rRNA gene with the Illumina MiSeq platform (Illumina, CA, USA) in paired-end mode with 600-cycle sequencing reagent. The sequences were analyzed using QIIME version 1.9.1. A median of 116,776 raw sequencing reads and 79,067 effective tag sequences per sample was obtained, respectively. Sequences with a distance-based similarity of 97% or greater were grouped into operational taxonomic units (OTUs) using the USEARCH algorithm. The phylogenetic relationships were determined based on a representative sequence alignment using Fast-Tree. Shannon's index accounting for both abundance and evenness of the taxa present was analyzed by QIIME version 1.9.1. We evaluated the β-diversity changes in gut microbiota across groups by the Partial Least Squares Discriminant Analysis (PLS-DA) and the weighted or unweighted UniFrac distances. To determine the significantly differential taxa, we applied linear discriminant analysis effect size (LEfSe) to compare samples between groups. The LEfSe uses linear discriminant analysis (LDA) to estimate the effect size of each differentially abundant feature. The threshold of the linear discriminant was set to 3.

2.6. Statistical Analysis

Continuous variables were expressed with the median (25th–75th percentile), and categorical variables were indicated by number (%). The Mann–Whitney U test or Chi-square test was used to test the differences in variables between children with normal and abnormal ABPM. The associations between variables were examined using Spearman's correlation coefficient. A linear regression model was performed, followed by the stepwise multivariable analyses integrating relevant parameters to explain BP load, AASI, and LV mass. A value of $p < 0.05$ was considered statistically significant. Analyses were performed using the Statistical Package for the Social Sciences (SPSS) software 14.0 (Chicago, IL, USA).

3. Results

Characteristics of the study subjects are shown in Table 1. A total of 115 children and adolescents with CKD were enrolled in this study, including 79 G1 subjects (68.7%), 27 G2 subjects (23.5%), seven G3 subjects (6.1%), and two G4 subjects (1.7%). The median age was 11.3 years. Our study population had a slight preponderance of males (M:F = 1.4:1). The median eGFR was 100.7 mL/min/1.73 m^2, demonstrating most participants were in the early stage of CKD. The major cause of CKD was due to CAKUT (66.1%). Among them, 49 cases (42.6%) had office BP exceeding the 95th percentile for age, gender, and height. As illustrated in Table 1, in terms of biochemical parameters, most patients were well controlled for common complications of CKD. Thirty-one patients (27%) displayed proteinuria. There was a trend toward moderate hyperlipidemia: 23 (20%) and 10 (9%) patients were above the upper normal limit of 200 and 130 mg/dL for total cholesterol and triglyceride, respectively. Moreover, 20 patients (17%) had hyperuricemia. Neither severe anemia nor hyperkalemia was observed.

Table 1. Descriptive statistics for clinical, anthropometric, and biomedical characteristics of 115 study participants.

Characteristics	
Age, years	11.3 (7.2–15.5)
Male	67 (58.3%)
CKD staging	
Stage G1	79 (68.7%)
Stage G2	27 (23.5%)
Stage G3	7 (6.1%)
Stage G4	2 (1.7%)
CAKUT	76 (66.1%)
Hypertension (by office BP)	49 (42.6%)
Body height, percentile	50 (25–75)
Body weight, percentile	50 (15–85)
Systolic blood pressure, mmHg	112 (101–122)
Diastolic blood pressure, mmHg	71 (66–80)
Body mass index, kg·m^{-2}	17.9 (15.2–21.5)
Blood urea nitrogen, mg/dL	13 (10–15)
Creatinine, mg/dL	0.58 (0.46–0.77)
eGFR, mL/min/1.73 m^2	100.7 (82.3–113.4)
Urine total protein-to-creatinine ratio, mg/g	62.7 (33.9–176.9)
Hemoglobin, g/dL	13.3 (12.7–14.1)
Hematocrit, %	40.5 (38.5–43)
Total cholesterol, mg/dL	169 (144–197)
Low-density lipoprotein, mg/dL	93 (74–118)
Triglyceride, mg/dL	70 (51–92)
Uric acid, mg/dL	5.2 (4.3–6.7)
Sodium, mEq/L	140 (139–141)
Potassium, mEq/L	4.3 (4.2–4.6)
Calcium, mg/dL	9.8 (9.6–10.1)
Phosphate, mg/dL	4.6 (4.2–5)

Data are medians (25th, 75th percentile) or n (%). CAKUT = Congenital anomalies of the kidney and urinary tract.

Table 2 summarizes the results of cardiovascular assessments in children and adolescents with CKD: 75 patients (65%) aged 6–18 years had undergone 24-h ABPM. In total, 53% (40/75) of them had at least one BP load abnormality. Among them, seven (9%), seven (9%), and eight patients (11%) had SBP or DBP load ≥95th percentile at 24-h, awake, and asleep stages, respectively. Additionally, there were 23 patients (31%) with BP load ≥25% and 31 patients (41%) with a non-dipping nocturnal BP profile. CKD children with stage G2–G4 had a higher awake SBP load than that in CKD stage 1. Moreover, the cases with asleep BP ≥95th percentile and BP load ≥25% were greater in CKD stage G2–G4 vs. stage G1 group. The AASI and LV mass were higher in children with CKD stage G2–G4 than those with stage G1. However, LVMI was not different between the two groups.

Table 2. Cardiovascular assessments in children and adolescents with chronic kidney disease (CKD) stage G1–G4.

CKD Stage	G1	G2–G4
24-h ABPM	N = 48	N = 27
Awake SBP load (%)	6.5 (0–13)	15 (1–36) *
Asleep SBP load (%)	8.5 (0–25.3)	21 (6–69)
Awake DBP load (%)	2 (0–6)	3 (0–10)
Asleep DBP load (%)	9 (0–18.8)	7 (0–41)
Abnormal ABPM profile (with any of the following abnormalities)	23 (48%)	17 (63%)
Average 24-h BP >95th percentile	2 (4%)	5 (19%)
Average awake BP >95th percentile	2 (4%)	5 (19%)
Average asleep BP >95th percentile	2 (4%)	6 (22%) *
BP load ≥25%	10 (21%)	13 (48%) *
Nocturnal decrease of BP <10%	18 (38%)	13 (48%)
AASI	0.33 (0.21–0.45)	0.41 (0.33–0.57) *
Left ventricular mass (g)	74.6 (54.6–102)	96 (51.8–141.3) *
LVMI (g/m$^{2.7}$)	30.8 (25.2–37.1)	32.7 (28.4–36.3)

Data are medians (25th, 75th percentile) or n (%). * $p < 0.05$ by the Chi-square test or the Mann–Whitney *U*-test. ABPM = 24-h ambulatory blood pressure monitoring. AASI = ambulatory arterial stiffness index. LVMI = left ventricular mass index.

We next analyzed methylamines in the plasma and urine. Children with CKD stage G2–G4 had higher plasma levels of DMA, TMA, and TMAO compared to those with CKD stage 1 (Table 3). Conversely, urinary levels of DMA and TMAO were lower in patients with CKD stage G2–G4 vs. stage G1. However, both TMAO-to-TMA and DMA-to-TMAO ratios in the plasma and urine did not differ between the two groups. Additionally, fractional excretion of DMA, TMA, and TMAO was comparable between CKD children with stage G1 and stage G2–G4.

Using data pooled from all subjects, correlations between plasma and urinary methylamine levels and CV risk factors were analyzed (Table 4). We observed that urinary DMA level was negatively correlated with awake SBP load ($r = -0.235$, $p = 0.043$), asleep SBP load ($r = -0.289$, $p = 0.012$), awake DBP load ($r = -0.288$, $p = 0.012$), and LV mass ($r = -0.554$, $p < 0.001$). Additionally, LV mass exhibited negative correlations with urinary TMA ($r = -0.226$, $p = 0.016$) and TMAO levels ($r = -0.324$, $p < 0.001$). In CKD children and adolescents, there were significantly inverse correlations between eGFR and plasma DMA ($r = -0.718$, $p < 0.001$), TMA ($r = -0.371$, $p < 0.001$), and TMAO ($r = -0.283$, $p = 0.002$) (Figure 1).

Table 3. Plasma and urinary levels of dimethylamine (DMA), trimethylamine (TMA), and trimethylamine N-oxide (TMAO) in children and adolescents with CKD stage G1–G4.

CKD Stage	G1	G2–G4
	N = 73	N = 36
Plasma level, ng/ml		
DMA	91 (81.7–104.8)	124.4 (107.7–147.4) *
TMA	100.8 (83.9–123.1)	112.6 (105.2–138.6) *
TMAO	170.5 (112.9–232.7)	245.7 (129.6–477.1) *
TMAO-to-TMA ratio	1.56 (1.05–2.33)	2.11 (1.17–4.33)
DMA-to-TMAO ratio	0.57 (0.4–0.86)	0.45 (0.34–1)
Urine level, ng/mg Cr		
DMA	222.2 (164.7–281.3)	196.8 (123.8–243.2) *
TMA	3.18 (2.46–5.75)	2.96 (1.44–6.62)
TMAO	271.1 (167.3–417.8)	183.8 (107.5–291.6) *
TMAO-to-TMA ratio	87.5 (55.8–113.7)	68.7 (38.2–112.9)
DMA-to-TMAO ratio	0.84 (0.55–1.15)	0.89 (0.51–1.48)
Fractional excretion of DMA	44.2 (30.2–61.2)	48.8 (36.9–69.6)
Fractional excretion of TMA	1.6 (1.13–2.84)	1.87 (1.13–4.99)
Fractional excretion of TMAO	82.3 67.9–96.8)	81.3 (61–92.1)

Data are medians (25th, 75th percentile). * $p < 0.05$ by the Mann–Whitney *U*-test. DMA = dimethylamine; TMA = trimethylamine; TMAO = trimethylamine N-oxide.

Table 4. Correlation between plasma and urinary methylamines and cardiovascular risk factors in children with CKD stage G1–G4.

CV Risk Factors	Awake SBP Load		Asleep SBP Load		Awake DBP Load		Asleep DBP Load		LV Mass	
	r	*p*	*r*	*p*	*r*	*p*	*r*	*p*	*r*	*p*
Plasma										
DMA	0.144	0.221	0.141	0.232	0.117	0.32	0.039	0.74	0.059	0.534
TMA	0.115	0.329	0.133	0.26	−0.029	0.807	0.137	0.244	0.093	0.326
TMAO	0.113	0.339	−0.018	0.879	0.088	0.457	−0.08	0.945	0.024	0.797
Urine										
DMA	−0.235	0.043 *	−0.289	0.012 *	−0.288	0.012 *	−0.022	0.854	−0.554	<0.001 *
TMA	0.212	0.067	0.07	0.548	0.105	0.368	0.131	0.261	−0.226	0.016 *
TMAO	0.043	0.716	−0.223	0.055	0.013	0.91	0.003	0.980	−0.324	<0.001 *

*$p < 0.05$ by Spearman's correlation coefficient. DMA = dimethylamine; TMA = trimethylamine; TMAO = trimethylamine N-oxide.

As illustrated in Table 5, associations between methylamines and CV risk were further examined in a multivariate linear regression model. To specify the exact role of each methylamine biomarker in CV risk, a multivariate linear regression model using the stepwise selection was applied for age, sex, eGFR, and other methylamines. In the best predictive model ($r = 0.479$, $p < 0.001$), office DBP was associated with urinary TMA ($p = 0.009$) as well as plasma TMA level ($p = 0.02$), controlling for age. Urine DMA-to-TMAO ratio was inversely associated with office DBP controlling for age ($r = 0.441$, $p < 0.001$). A positive association between plasma TMA level and awake DBP was found in the adjusted regression model ($r = 0.283$, $p = 0.015$). Additionally, plasma TMA level was associated with asleep DBP (p = 0.036), controlling for age. We also found that urine DMA-to-TMAO ratio had a negative association with LV mass controlling for age and sex ($r = 0.771$, $p < 0.001$). Furthermore, an inverse association between plasma DMA-to-TMAO ratio and LVMI was found in the adjusted regression model controlling for eGFR and sex ($r = 0.465$, $p < 0.001$).

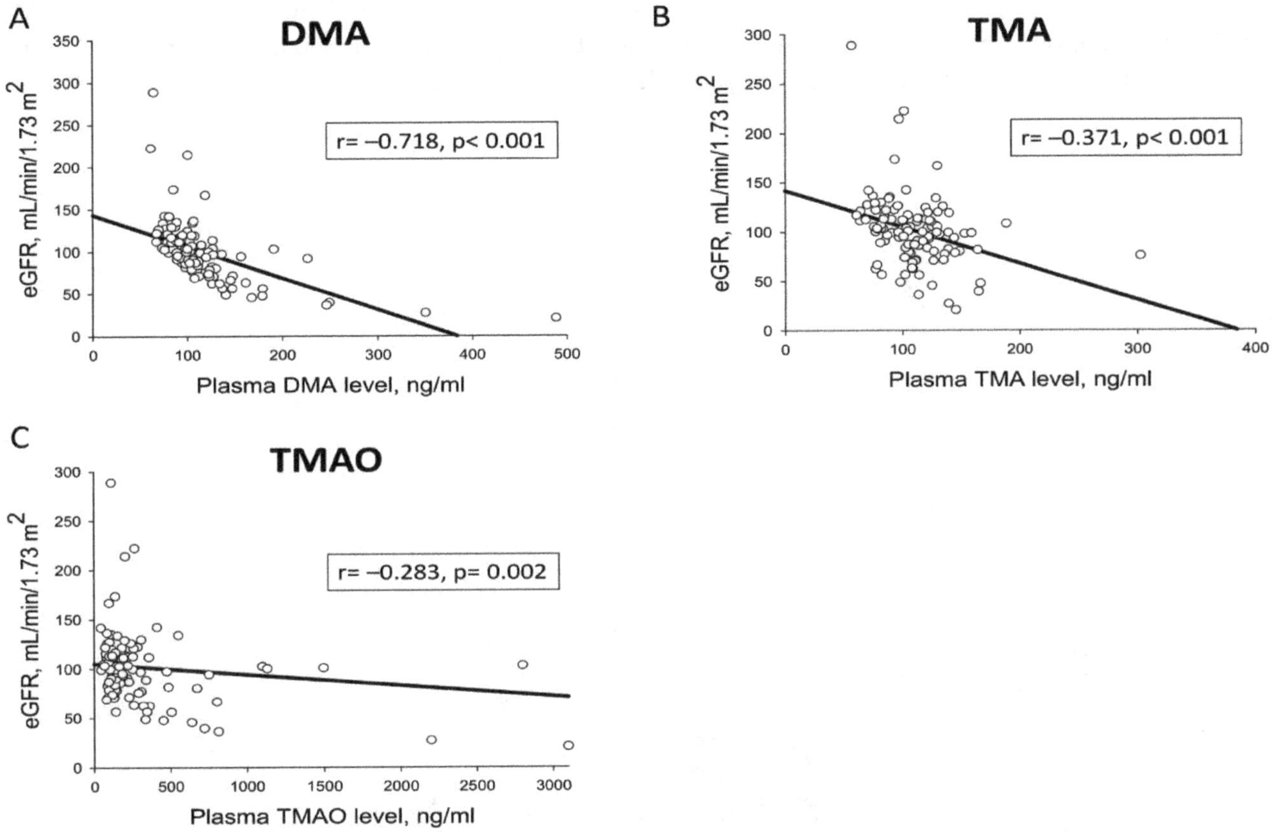

Figure 1. Correlation of plasma (**A**) DMA, (**B**) TMA, and (**C**) TMAO levels (ng/mL) with estimated glomerular filtration rate (eGFR) (ml/min/1.73m^2) by Spearman's correlation coefficient. DMA = dimethylamine; TMA = trimethylamine; TMAO = trimethylamine N-oxide.

Table 5. Adjusted regression model estimates of the association between plasma and urinary methylamines and cardiovascular risk factors in children with CKD stage G1–G4.

Dependent Variable	Explanatory Variable	Adjusted [a]		Model	
		Beta	*p* Value	*r*	*p* Value
Office DBP	Urine TMA	−0.227	0.009	0.479	<0.001
	Plasma TMA	0.202	0.02		
	Urine DMA-to-TMAO ratio	−0.221	0.012	0.441	<0.001
Awake DBP	Plasma TMA	0.283	0.015	0.283	0.015
Asleep DBP	Plasma TMA	0.232	0.036	0.423	0.001
LV mass	Urine DMA-to-TMAO ratio	−0.148	0.018	0.771	<0.001
LVMI	Plasma DMA-to-TMAO ratio	−0.218	0.012	0.465	<0.001

DMA = dimethylamine; TMA = trimethylamine; TMAO = trimethylamine N-oxide. LVMI = left ventricular mass index. [a] Adjusted for age, sex, eGFR, and other methylamines.

We further analyzed the composition of the gut microbiota. We determined α-diversity as the mean species richness, quantified by the Shannon index, and found that there was no significant difference between CKD children with normal vs. abnormal ABPM (Figure 2A; $p = 0.723$). The β-diversity was measured by calculating the unweighted UniFrac distances between each pair of samples, and the unweighted UniFrac distance matrix was measured and visualized using a partial least squares discriminant analysis (PLS-DA) analysis. The score plots of PLS-DA analysis showed that two groups were well separated (Figure 2B). The unweighted UniFrac results differed from the normal, and the abnormal ABPM group reached significance ($p = 0.005$). At the phylum level, we observed that the main phyla were *Firmicutes*, *Actinobacteria*, *Proteobacteria*, *Bacteroidetes*, and *Verrucomicrobia*

(Figure 2C). Although several phyla showed lower abundance in the abnormal vs. normal ABPM group (Figure 2D), only phylum *Cyanobacteria* reached the significance ($p < 0.05$; Figure 2E). Moreover, the *Firmicutes* to *Bacteroidetes* ratio was comparable between two groups.

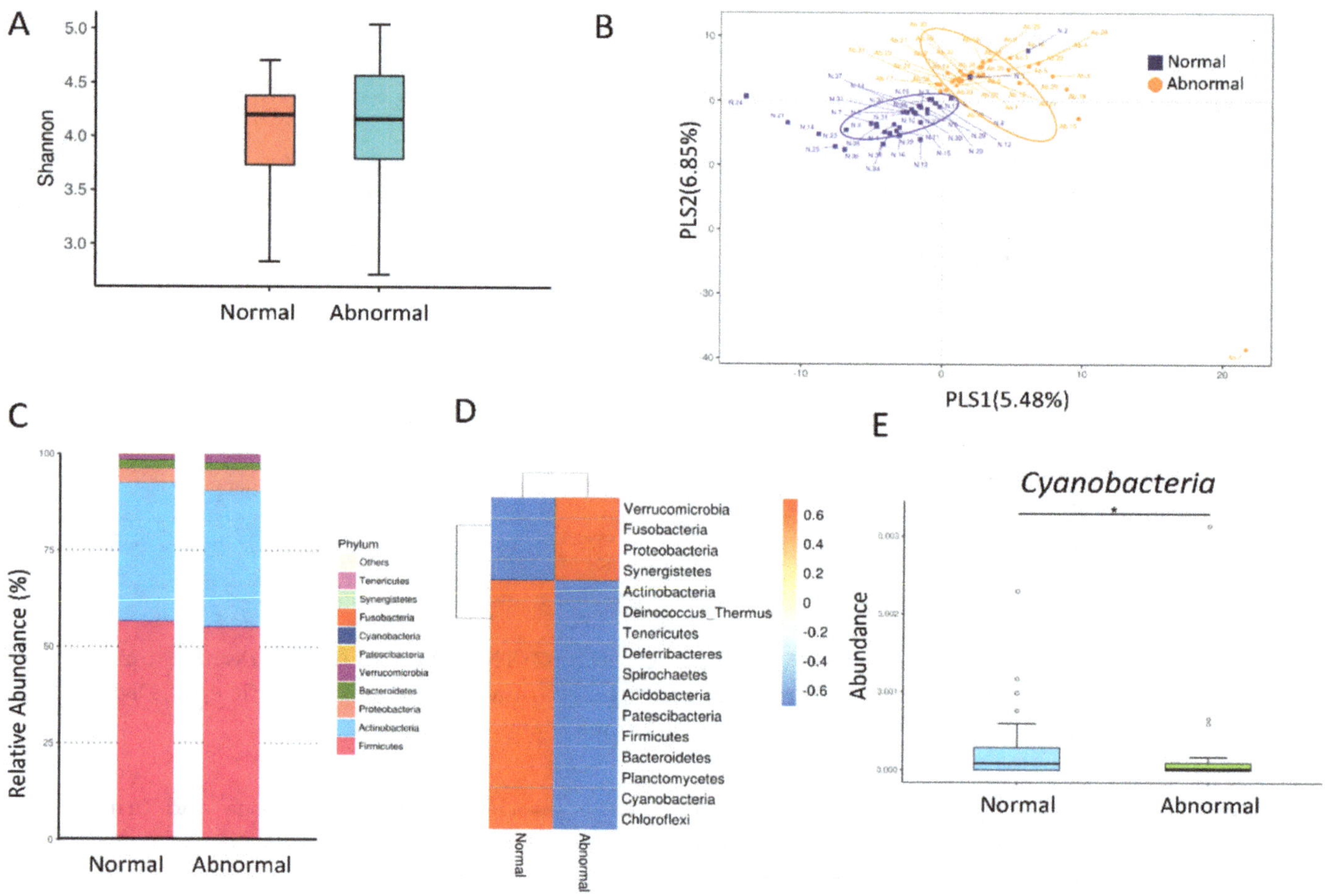

Figure 2. (**A**) Fecal bacterial α-diversity in CKD children with normal and abnormal ABPM represented by the Shannon's diversity indexes. (**B**) β-diversity changes in gut microbiota between CKD children with normal and abnormal ABPM by the partial least squares discriminant analysis (PLS-DA). (**C**) Relative abundance of top 10 phyla of the gut microbiota between the normal and abnormal ABPM group. (**D**) Heat map of 16S rRNA gene sequencing analysis of gut microbiome at the phylum level. (**E**) The abundance of phylum *Cyanobacteria* in CKD children with normal vs. abnormal ABPM. The asterisk indicates $p < 0.05$.

At the genus level (Figure 3A), the abundances of most top 10 genera were not different between the normal and abnormal ABPM group, except genera *Subdoligranulum* ($p = 0.034$) and *Ruminococcus* ($p = 0.033$). Finally, we ran the LEfSe algorithm to identify metagenomic biomarkers (Figure 3B). Our results identified that genera *Subdoligranulum*, *Holdemanella*, and *Actinomyces* are detected by LEfSe with a high LDA score (more than three orders of magnitude), reflecting marked higher abundance in the normal ABPM group. In contrast, the abnormal ABPM group had decreased abundance of genera *Faecalibacterium* and *Akkermansia*. Additionally, the abnormal ABPM group showed a decreased abundance of genera *Providencia* (Figure 3C), *Gemella* (Figure 3D), and *Peptosreptoccocus* (Figure 3E) (all $p < 0.05$).

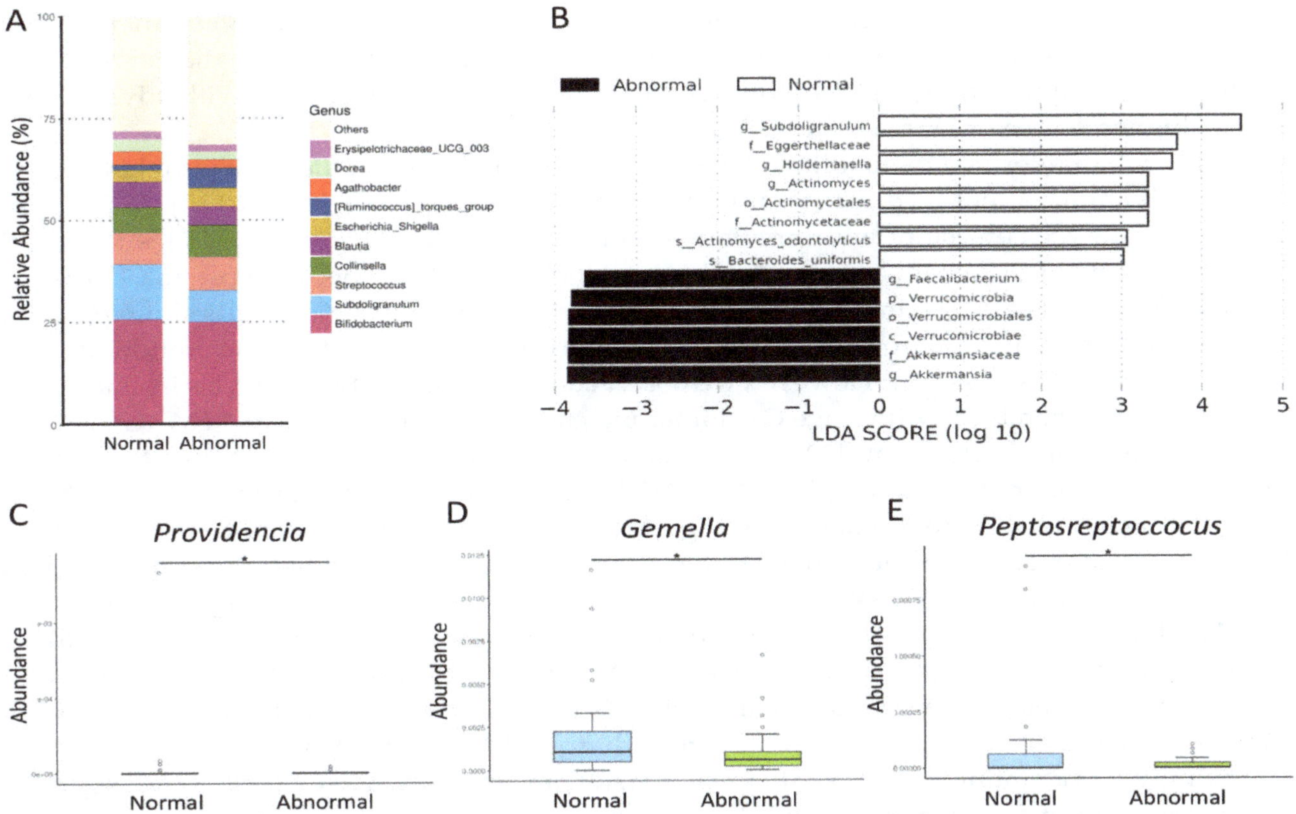

Figure 3. (**A**) Relative abundance of top 10 genera of the gut microbiota in CKD children with normal and abnormal ABPM group. (**B**) Linear discriminant analysis effect size (LEfSe) to identify the taxa that were significantly different between normal vs. abnormal ABPM group. The threshold of the linear discriminant was set to 3. (**C**) The abundance of genus *Providencia*, (**D**) *Gemella*, and (**E**) *Peptosreptoccocus* in CKD children with normal vs. abnormal ABPM. The asterisk indicates $p < 0.05$.

4. Discussion

To the best of our knowledge, this study is the first to evaluate the association between gut microbiota-dependent methylamines and CV risk in early-stage pediatric CKD. The key findings are (1) children with CKD stage G2–G4 had higher plasma levels of DMA, TMA, and TMAO, but lower urinary levels of DMA and TMAO compared to those with CKD stage G1; (2) plasma TMA and DMA levels were not only inversely associated with high BP load, but also eGFR; (3) CKD children with abnormal and normal ABPM associated into two distinct enterotypes; (4) CKD children with an abnormal ABPM profile had decreased abundance of phylum *Cyanobacteria*, genera *Subdoligranulum*, *Faecalibacterium*, *Ruminococcus*, and *Akkermansia*; and (5) TMA and DMA are superior to TMAO related to CV risk in early-stage CKD children.

In the current study, more than half of CKD children exhibited BP abnormalities on ABPM. Our data showed the cases with nocturnal hypertension and increased BP load were greater in children with CKD stage G2–G4 than those with stage G1. Of note is that up to 48% of children with CKD stage G1 had BP abnormalities on ABPM. Our findings are consistent with previous reports wherein hypertension is extremely prevalent in CKD children, even in an early stage [20–23]. The present study supported the notion that ABPM is superior to office BP in identifying children with BP abnormalities [24]. As expected, the severity of CKD is associated with certain markers of CV risk, like AASI and LV mass in the current study. AASI, an index of arterial stiffness, has been proposed as a surrogate marker to predict CV morbidity and mortality [18]. Our previous report demonstrated that high AASI is related to BP abnormalities in CKD children, even in an early stage [23]. The present results showed AASI was higher in children with CKD stage G2–G4 than those with stage G1, which ties well with the previous study in that high AASI worsens GFR decline in adult CKD patients [25]. Left ventricular hypertrophy is an index of target organ damage as well as a risk factor for CVD in adult CKD patients [26]. In keeping with previous studies showing that LV mass is greater in CKD children on dialysis and ABPM correlates with LV hypertrophy in CKD children [6,27,28], we observed children with advanced CKD displayed higher degree of LV mass and BP abnormalities.

Gut microbiota-derived metabolites TMAO, TMA, and DMA from dietary methylamines have recently gained much attention due to their high association with CV risk [8–10,29,30]. In the present study, our results are consistent with previous reported data in CKD adults [31,32], showing that TMAO is increased in CKD with a weak inverse correlation ($r = -0.283$) between plasma TMAO level and eGFR. Our results are also in agreement with a previous report in CKD adults showing urinary excretion is a dominant route for TMAO elimination with a steady fractional excretion of TMAO, regardless of the CKD stages [32]. However, we observed lower urinary TMAO levels in children with CKD stage G2–G4 than those with stage G1. Either increased or decreased urinary TMAO levels have been reported in adult CKD patients [32,33]. Conflicting results are likewise seen in this study showing that decreased urinary but increased plasma TMAO levels in children with advanced-stage CKD may represent reduced renal excretion of circulating TMAO or increased local renal TMAO metabolism. Although observational and experimental studies suggest a positive correlation between high plasma TMAO levels and increased CV risk [10], data are contradictory and the underlying mechanism is not yet validated [34]. Therefore, it is debated whether TMAO is harmful or beneficial for CV health. Our data showed no significant association between TMAO and most CV surrogate markers, except that urinary TMAO level had a negative correlation with LV mass. Therefore, whether plasma and urinary TMAO may aid in predicting CVD in early-stage pediatric CKD awaits further elucidation.

Strikingly, less attention has been paid to the TMAO precursor TMA in CV risk. TMA is generated by the metabolism of gut microbes using dietary precursors such as choline or carnitine [34]. Like TMAO, TMA is considered as a uremic toxin [29]. Results from this study identified plasma TMA level is increased in CKD children, which is in accordance with data from CKD adults [29,35]. Children with stage G2–G4 had higher plasma TMA levels than those with stage G1. There was also a trend towards a higher plasma TMAO-to-TMA ratio, an index of FMO activity, in this group. Taking into account that plasma TMA and TMAO levels both are simultaneously elevated in children with advanced CKD, our data suggest their increases could be due to increased gut bacterial production and TMA-to-TMAO conversion. Of note, eGFR exhibited a stronger correlation with the TMA than with TMAO. Additionally, TMAO and BP abnormalities were unrelated, whereas plasma TMA level was positively correlated with awake DBP, asleep DBP, and office DBP. Our findings suggest the superiority for the TMA over TMAO as a cardiovascular risk index in children with early-stage CKD.

Another important result of this study is the description of an inverse association between plasma DMA level and cardiovascular risk. Since we found a strong inverse association between plasma DMA level and eGFR, high plasma level but low urinary level of DMA in advanced CKD is possible due to decreased renal excretion. On the other hand, both TMAO and TMA can be metabolized to DMA. It is presumably that an increased plasma DMA level in children with advanced CKD is due to, at least in part, increased gut microbiota-derived TMA and TMAO production. Our previous study showed that urine DMA level was negatively associated with asleep BP load in CKD children [36]. In the present study, we further confirm that urinary DMA level is inversely associated with awake SBP load, asleep SBP load, awake DBP load, and LV mass. These findings suggest that DMA is superior to TMAO in predicting CV risk in early-stage pediatric CKD. On the other hand, our data demonstrated that DMA-to-TMAO ratio, but not TMAO, in the plasma and urine related to several CV risk markers. Given that phases of TMAO synthesis and metabolism happens simultaneously and that DMA-to-TMAO is considered as an index of TMAO-metabolizing activity, data from this study suggest that measures of the combined ratio instead of individual methylamine (i.e., DMA, TMA, and TMAO) may provide us a better understanding of TMA-TMAO metabolic pathway on CVD in CKD children. On the other hand, a previous study demonstrated that the presence of gut microbes might not be essential for DMA production as its excretion is the same in germ-free and control animals [37]. Therefore, DMA might be produced from other endogenous pathways. Indeed, DMA is also a derivative of nitric oxide (NO) metabolism [38]. Asymmetric dimethylarginine (ADMA), an endogenous inhibitor of NO synthase, can be metabolized by dimethylarginine dimethylaminohydrolase to generate DMA and citrulline [38]. Noteworthily, DMA can come from the TMA–TMAO pathway as well the ADMA–NO pathway, and TMAO and ADMA both are uremic toxins related to cardiovascular risk [34,39]. Whether DMA links two pathways together to play a role in the development of hypertension in CKD awaits further elucidation.

In the current study, CKD children with abnormal and normal ABPM associated into two distinct enterotypes, represented by β-diversity changes. Our data support the notion that gut microbiota is linked to the development of hypertension [40,41]. At the phylum level, the abundance of *Cyanobacteria* was lower in the abnormal vs. normal ABPM group. This finding is in line with an animal study showing that minocycline-treated Dahl salt-sensitive rats developed hypertension related to a decrease in *Cyanobacteria* [42]. Although the *Firmicutes*-to-*Bacteroidetes* ratio has been linked to hypertension [41], we did not find the difference of this ratio between CKD children with normal and abnormal ABPM profile. The reason is possibly because we analyzed gut microbiota in CKD children preceding hypertension onset but not in the stage of established hypertension. According to our data, CKD children with abnormal ABPM group had decreased abundance of genera *Subdoligranulum*, *Faecalibacterium*, *Ruminococcus*, and *Akkermansia*. Low abundance of genera *Subdoligranulum* and *Faecalibacterium* has been identified as a microbial marker in adult hypertensive patients [40,43]. *Ruminococcus* abundance was shown to be deficient in hypertension mice [40]. *Akkermansia* is known as a beneficial gut microbe [44]. Overall, these observations suggest that these certain bacteria populations might have beneficial cardiovascular properties in CKD children to halt the development of hypertension. Moreover, CKD children with abnormal ABPM had decreased abundance of genera *Providencia*, *Gemella*, and *Peptosreptoccocus*. Interestingly, these genera of bacteria have been reported to be involved in TMA production [45]. Thus, whether these microbes play a crucial role on the development of hypertension via mediating the TMA–TMAO metabolic pathway in children with early-stage CKD deserves further clarification. Of note is that a key factor in determining gut microbiota composition is the type of diet in patients with CKD [46]. Since the Mediterranean diet that is rich in fiber has been proven to reduce cardiovascular risk [47], it can be speculated that high-fiber dietary intervention might be an efficient way to control microbiota to further prevent CVD in CKD children [48,49].

This study has several limitations that should be acknowledged. First, a low number of CKD children from one hospital would not be representative of an entire population. Multicenter studies of large numbers of patients may be required to elucidate the true relationship. Second, we presented the associations between certain microbes and BP abnormalities but we do not reveal the pathophysiological mechanism by which those specific microbes contribute to the TMA–TMAO pathway and hypertension. Third, our data might not be applicable to other populations for ethnic reasons. Lastly, there remains a lack of reference for AASI and LVMI to define a cut-off value to indicate normal versus abnormal in a pediatric population. We also did not recruit non-CKD controls because children with CKD stage G1 were served as the controls to compare the differences of BP abnormalities and methylamines levels between two different levels of renal function (i.e., CKD stage G1 vs. stage G2–G4). Although age was different between the two groups, we adjusted the age factor in the multivariate linear regression model.

5. Conclusions

Our study in early-stage CKD children demonstrates the associations between gut microbiota-dependent methylamines and BP abnormalities assessed by ABPM. Our results cast a new light on the link between the TMA–TMAO metabolic pathway, gut microbiota, and cardiovascular risk in CKD children. As hypertension and CKD both can originate from early life, early identification of microbial markers related to cardiovascular risk may aid in developing the ideal intervention to improve cardiovascular outcomes in pediatric CKD.

Author Contributions: C.-N.H.: contributed to concept generation, data interpretation, drafting of the manuscript, critical revision of the manuscript and approval of the article; G.-P.C.-C.: contributed to methodology and approval of the article; S.L.: contributed to methodology and approval of the article; C.-Y.H.: contributed to methodology and approval of the article; P.-C.L.: contributed to data interpretation, critical revision of the manuscript and approval of the article; Y.-L.T.: contributed to concept generation, data interpretation, drafting of the manuscript, critical revision of the manuscript and approval of the article. All authors have read and agreed to the published version of the manuscript.

Acknowledgments: We would like to thank the Super Micro Mass Research and Technology Center and the Center for Environmental Toxin and Emerging-Contaminant Research, Cheng Shiu University, Kaohsiung for technical support.

References

1. Go, A.S.; Chertow, G.M.; Fan, D.; McCulloch, C.E.; Hsu, C.Y. Chronic kidney disease and the risks of death, cardiovascular events, and hospitalization. *N. Engl. J. Med.* **2004**, *351*, 1296–1305. [CrossRef]
2. Weaver, D.J.; Mitsnefes, M. Cardiovascular Disease in Children and Adolescents with Chronic Kidney Disease. *Semin. Nephrol.* **2018**, *38*, 559–569. [CrossRef] [PubMed]
3. Ingelfinger, J.R.; Kalantar-Zadeh, K.; Schaefer, F.; World Kidney Day Steering Committee. World Kidney Day 2016: Averting the legacy of kidney disease-focus on childhood. *Pediatr. Nephrol.* **2016**, *31*, 343–348. [CrossRef] [PubMed]
4. Urbina, E.M.; Williams, R.V.; Alpert, B.S.; Collins, R.T.; Daniels, S.R.; Hayman, L.; Jacobson, M.; Mahoney, L.; Mietus-Snyder, M.; Rocchini, A.; et al. Noninvasive assessment of subclinical atherosclerosis in children and adolescents: Recommendations for standard assessment for clinical research: A scientific statement from the American Heart Association. *Hypertension* **2009**, *54*, 919–950. [PubMed]
5. Taal, M.W. Arterial stiffness in chronic kidney disease: An update. *Curr. Opin. Nephrol. Hypertens.* **2014**, *23*, 169–173. [CrossRef] [PubMed]
6. Kupferman, J.C.; Aronson Friedman, L.; Cox, C.; Flynn, J.; Furth, S.; Warady, B.; Mitsnefes, M. CKiD Study Group. BP control and left ventricular hypertrophy regression in children with CKD. *J. Am. Soc. Nephrol.* **2014**, *25*, 167–174. [CrossRef]
7. Ramezani, A.; Raj, D.S. The gut microbiome, kidney disease, and targeted interventions. *J. Am. Soc. Nephrol.* **2014**, *25*, 657–670. [CrossRef]
8. Meijers, B.; Jouret, F.; Evenepoel, P. Linking gut microbiota to cardiovascular disease and hypertension: Lessons from chronic kidney disease. *Pharmacol. Res.* **2018**, *133*, 101–107. [CrossRef]
9. Jovanovich, A.; Isakova, T.; Stubbs, J. Microbiome and Cardiovascular Disease in CKD. *Clin. J. Am. Soc. Nephrol.* **2018**, *13*, 1598–1604. [CrossRef]
10. Schiattarella, G.G.; Sannino, A.; Toscano, E.; Giugliano, G.; Gargiulo, G.; Franzone, A.; Trimarco, B.; Esposito, G.; Perrino, C. Gut microbe-generated metabolite trimethylamine-N-oxide as cardiovascular risk biomarker: A systematic review and dose-response meta-analysis. *Eur. Heart J.* **2017**, *38*, 2948–2956. [CrossRef]
11. Duranton, F.; Cohen, G.; De Smet, R.; Rodriguez, M.; Jankowski, J.; Vanholder, R.; Argiles, A.; European Uremic Toxin Work Group. Normal and pathologic concentrations of uremic toxins. *J. Am. Soc. Nephrol.* **2012**, *23*, 1258–1270. [CrossRef] [PubMed]
12. Smith, J.L.; Wishnok, J.S.; Deen, W.M. Metabolism and excretion of methylamines in rats. *Toxicol. Appl. Pharmacol.* **1994**, *125*, 296–308. [CrossRef] [PubMed]
13. Kidney Disease: Improving Global Outcomes (KDIGO) CKD Work Group. KDIGO 2012 clinical practice guideline for the evaluation and management of chronic kidney disease. *Kidney Int. Suppl.* **2013**, *3*, 1–150.
14. Schwartz, G.J.; Muñoz, A.; Schneider, M.F.; Mak, R.H.; Kaskel, F.; Warady, B.A.; Furth, S.L. New equations to estimate GFR in children with CKD. *J. Am. Soc. Nephrol.* **2009**, *20*, 629–637. [CrossRef] [PubMed]
15. Renkema, K.Y.; Winyard, P.J.; Skovorodkin, I.N.; Levtchenko, E.; Hindryckx, A.; Jeanpierre, C.; Weber, S.; Salomon, R.; Antignac, C.; Vainio, S.; et al. Novel perspectives for investigating congenital anomalies of the kidney and urinary tract (CAKUT). *Nephrol. Dial. Transplant.* **2011**, *26*, 3843–3851. [CrossRef]

16. Hsu, C.N.; Lu, P.C.; Lo, M.H.; Lin, I.C.; Chang-Chien, G.P.; Lin, S.; Tain, Y.L. Gut Microbiota-Dependent Trimethylamine N-Oxide Pathway Associated with Cardiovascular Risk in Children with Early-Stage Chronic Kidney Disease. *Int. J. Mol. Sci.* **2018**, *19*, 3699. [CrossRef]
17. Kollias, A.; Stergiou, W.E.; Witte, K.; Soergelm, M.; Mehls, O.; Schaefer, F. German Working Group on Pediatric Hypertension. Distribution of 24-h ambulatory blood pressure in children: Normalized reference values and role of body dimensions. *J. Hypertens.* **2002**, *20*, 1995–2007.
18. Kollias, A.; Stergiou, G.S.; Dolan, E.; O'Brien, E. Ambulatory arterial stiffness index: A systematic review and meta-analysis. *Atherosclerosis* **2012**, *224*, 291–301. [CrossRef]
19. Daniels, S.R.; Kimball, T.R.; Morrison, J.A.; Khoury, P.; Meyer, R.A. Indexing left ventricular mass to account for differences in body size in children and adolescents without cardiovascular disease. *Am. J. Cardiol.* **1995**, *76*, 699–701. [CrossRef]
20. Flynn, J.T.; Mitsnefes, M.; Pierce, C.; Cole, S.R.; Parekh, R.S.; Furth, S.L.; Warady, B.A. Chronic Kidney Disease in Children Study Group: Blood pressure in children with chronic kidney disease: A report from the Chronic Kidney Disease in Children study. *Hypertension* **2008**, *52*, 631–637. [CrossRef]
21. Wühl, E.; Trivelli, A.; Picca, S.; Litwin, M.; Peco-Antic, A.; Zurowska, A.; Testa, S.; Jankauskiene, A.; Emre, S.; Caldas-Afonso, A.; et al. ESCAPE Trial Group: Strict blood-pressure control and progression of renal failure in children. *N. Engl. J. Med.* **2009**, *361*, 1639–1650.
22. Chou, H.H.; Lin, C.Y.; Chiou, Y.H.; Tain, Y.L.; Wang, Y.F.; Wang, H.H.; Chiou, Y.Y. Clinical characteristics and prevalence of complications of chronic kidney disease in children: The Taiwan Pediatric Renal Collaborative study. *Pediatr. Nephrol.* **2016**, *31*, 1113–1120. [CrossRef] [PubMed]
23. Hsu, C.N.; Lu, P.C.; Lo, M.H.; Lin, I.C.; Tain, Y.L. The association between nitric oxide pathway, blood pressure abnormalities, and cardiovascular risk profile in pediatric chronic kidney disease. *Int. J. Mol. Sci.* **2019**, *20*, 5301. [CrossRef] [PubMed]
24. Graves, J.W.; Althaf, M.M. Utility of ambulatory blood pressure monitoring in children and adolescents. *Pediatr. Nephrol.* **2006**, *21*, 1640–1652. [CrossRef]
25. Eriksen, B.O.; Stefansson, V.T.N.; Jenssen, T.G.; Mathisen, U.D.; Schei, J.; Solbu, M.D.; Wilsgaard, T.; Melsom, T. High Ambulatory Arterial Stiffness Index Is an Independent Risk Factor for Rapid Age-Related Glomerular Filtration Rate Decline in the General Middle-Aged Population. *Hypertension* **2017**, *69*, 651–659. [CrossRef] [PubMed]
26. K/DOQI Workgroup. K/DOQI clinical practice guidelines for cardiovascular disease in dialysis patients. *Am. J. Kidney Dis.* **2005**, *45*, S1–S153.
27. Robinson, R.F.; Nahata, M.C.; Sparks, E.; Daniels, C.; Batisky, D.L.; Hayes, J.R.; Mahan, J.D. Abnormal left ventricular mass and aortic distensibility in pediatric dialysis patients. *Pediatr. Nephrol.* **2005**, *20*, 64–68. [CrossRef]
28. Mitsnefes, M.; Flynn, J.; Cohn, S.; Samuels, J.; Blydt-Hansen, T.; Saland, J.; Kimball, T.; Furth, S.; Warady, B.; CKiD Study Group. Masked hypertension associates with left ventricular hypertrophy in children with CKD. *J. Am. Soc. Nephrol.* **2010**, *21*, 137–144. [CrossRef]
29. Jaworska, K.; Hering, D.; Mosieniak, G.; Bielak-Zmijewska, A.; Pilz, M.; Konwerski, M.; Gasecka, A.; Kapłon-Cieślicka, A.; Filipiak, K.; Sikora, E.; et al. TMA, A Forgotten Uremic Toxin, but Not TMAO, Is Involved in Cardiovascular Pathology. *Toxins* **2019**, *11*, 490. [CrossRef]
30. Kuo, H.C.; Hsu, C.N.; Huang, C.F.; Lo, M.H.; Chien, S.J.; Tain, Y.L. Urinary arginine methylation index associated with ambulatory blood pressure abnormalities in children with chronic kidney disease. *J. Am. Soc. Hypertens.* **2012**, *6*, 385–392. [CrossRef] [PubMed]
31. Stubbs, J.R.; House, J.A.; Ocque, A.J.; Zhang, S.; Johnson, C.; Kimber, C.; Schmidt, K.; Gupta, A.; Wetmore, J.B.; Nolin, T.D.; et al. Serum Trimethylamine-N-Oxide is Elevated in CKD and Correlates with Coronary Atherosclerosis Burden. *J. Am. Soc. Nephrol.* **2016**, *27*, 305–313. [CrossRef] [PubMed]
32. Pelletier, C.C.; Croyal, M.; Ene, L.; Aguesse, A.; Billon-Crossouard, S.; Krempf, M.; Lemoine, S.; Guebre-Egziabher, F.; Juillard, L.; Soulage, C.O. Elevation of Trimethylamine-N-Oxide in Chronic Kidney Disease: Contribution of Decreased Glomerular Filtration Rate. *Toxins* **2019**, *11*, 635. [CrossRef] [PubMed]
33. Posada-Ayala, M.; Zubiri, I.; Martin-Lorenzo, M.; Sanz-Maroto, A.; Molero, D.; Gonzalez-Calero, L.; Fernandez-Fernandez, B.; de la Cuesta, F.; Laborde, C.M.; Barderas, M.G.; et al. Identification of a urine metabolomics signature in patients with advanced-stage chronic kidney disease. *Kidney Int.* **2014**, *85*, 103–111. [CrossRef] [PubMed]

34. Velasquez, M.T.; Ramezani, A.; Manal, A.; Raj, D.S. Trimethylamine N-Oxide: The Good, the Bad and the Unknown. *Toxins* **2016**, *8*, 326. [CrossRef] [PubMed]
35. Storino, G.; Moraes, C.; Saldanha, J.; Mafra, D. Cardiovascular mortality in chronic kidney patients: The role of uremic toxins. *Int. J. Cardiovasc. Sci.* **2015**, *28*, 327–334. [CrossRef]
36. Zeisel, S.H.; DaCosta, K.A.; Fox, J.G. Endogenous formation of dimethylamine. *Biochem. J.* **1985**, *232*, 403–408. [CrossRef]
37. Lin, I.C.; Hsu, C.N.; Lo, M.H.; Chien, S.J.; Tain, Y.L. Low urinary citrulline/arginine ratio associated with blood pressure abnormalities and arterial stiffness in childhood chronic kidney disease. *J. Am. Soc. Hypertens.* **2016**, *10*, 115–123. [CrossRef]
38. Tain, Y.L.; Hsu, C.N. Toxic dimethylarginines: Asymmetric dimethylarginine (ADMA) and symmetric dimethylarginine (SDMA). *Toxins* **2017**, *9*, 92. [CrossRef]
39. Hsu, C.N.; Tain, Y.L. Regulation of Nitric Oxide Production in the Developmental Programming of Hypertension and Kidney Disease. *Int. J. Mol. Sci.* **2018**, *20*, 681. [CrossRef]
40. Li, J.; Zhao, F.; Wang, Y.; Chen, J.; Tao, J.; Tian, G.; Wu, S.; Liu, W.; Cui, Q.; Geng, B.; et al. Gut microbiota dysbiosis contributes to the development of hypertension. *Microbiome* **2017**, *5*, 14. [CrossRef]
41. Galla, S.; Chakraborty, S.; Cheng, X.; Yeo, J.; Mell, B.; Zhang, H.; Mathew, A.V.; Vijay-Kumar, M.; Joe, B. Disparate effects of antibiotics on hypertension. *Physiol. Genomics* **2018**, *50*, 837–845. [CrossRef]
42. Yang, T.; Santisteban, M.M.; Rodriguez, V.; Li, E.; Ahmari, N.; Carvajal, J.M.; Zadeh, M.; Gong, M.; Qi, Y.; Zubcevic, J.; et al. Gut dysbiosis is linked to hypertension. *Hypertension* **2015**, *65*, 1331–1340. [CrossRef] [PubMed]
43. Kim, S.; Goel, R.; Kumar, A.; Qi, Y.; Lobaton, G.; Hosaka, K.; Mohammed, M.; Handberg, E.M.; Richards, E.M.; Pepine, C.J.; et al. Imbalance of gut microbiome and intestinal epithelial barrier dysfunction in patients with high blood pressure. *Clin. Sci. (Lond.)* **2018**, *132*, 701–718. [CrossRef] [PubMed]
44. Cani, P.D.; de Vos, W.M. Next-Generation Beneficial Microbes: The Case of Akkermansia muciniphila. *Front. Microbiol.* **2017**, *8*, 1765. [CrossRef] [PubMed]
45. Nelson, T.M.; Borgogna, J.L.; Brotman, R.M.; Ravel, J.; Walk, S.T.; Yeoman, C.J. Vaginal biogenic amines: Biomarkers of bacterial vaginosis or precursors to vaginal dysbiosis? *Front. Physiol.* **2015**, *6*, 253. [CrossRef] [PubMed]
46. Koppe, L.; Fouque, D.; Soulage, C.O. The Role of Gut Microbiota and Diet on Uremic Retention Solutes Production in the Context of Chronic Kidney Disease. *Toxins* **2018**, *10*, 155. [CrossRef] [PubMed]
47. Estruch, R.; Ros, E.; Salas-Salvado, J.; Covas, M.I.; Corella, D.; Aros, F.; Gómez-Gracia, E.; Ruiz-Gutiérrez, V.; Fiol, M.; Lapetra, J.; et al. Primary prevention of cardiovascular disease with a Mediterranean diet. *N. Engl. J. Med.* **2013**, *368*, 1279–1290. [CrossRef]
48. Sonnenburg, J.L.; Bäckhed, F. Diet-microbiota interactions as moderators of human metabolism. *Nature* **2016**, *535*, 56–64. [CrossRef]
49. Zhang, C.; Yin, A.; Li, H.; Wang, R.; Wu, G.; Shen, J.; Zhang, M.; Wang, L.; Hou, Y.; Ouyang, H.; et al. Dietary Modulation of Gut Microbiota Contributes to Alleviation of Both Genetic and Simple Obesity in Children. *EBioMedicine* **2015**, *2*, 968–984. [CrossRef]

7

Severity of Coronary Atherosclerosis and Risk of Diabetes Mellitus

Iginio Colaiori [1,†], Raffaele Izzo [2,†], Emanuele Barbato [2,*], Danilo Franco [2], Giuseppe Di Gioia [1,2], Antonio Rapacciuolo [2], Jozef Bartunek [1], Costantino Mancusi [2], Maria Angela Losi [2], Teresa Strisciuglio [2], Maria Virginia Manzi [2], Giovanni de Simone [2], Bruno Trimarco [2] and Carmine Morisco [2]

1 Cardiovascular Research Center Aalst OLV Hospital, 9300 Aalst, Belgium
2 Department of Advanced Biomedical Sciences, University of Naples Federico II, 80100 Napoli, Italy
* Correspondence: emanuele.barbato@unina.it
† These authors equally contributed to the manuscript.

Abstract: Background: Cardio-vascular target organ damage predicts the onset of type 2 diabetes mellitus (DM) in hypertensive patients. Whether an increased incidence of DM is also in relation to the severity of coronary atherosclerosis is unknown. Objective: We evaluated the onset of DM in relation to the extent and severity of coronary atherosclerosis, using the SYNTAX (Synergy between Percutaneous Coronary Intervention with Taxus and Cardiac Surgery) score (SS), in patients with stable angina or acute coronary syndromes, referred for coronary angiography (CA). Methods: Non-diabetic patients that underwent CA for the first time were included, and the SS was computed. Predictors of DM onset in low, medium, and high SSs were investigated. Results: Five hundred and seventy patients were included, and the mean SS was 6.3 ± 7.6. During a median follow-up of 79 months (interquartile range (IQR): 67–94), 74 patients (13%) developed DM. The risk of DM onset was significantly higher in the patients with a medium or high SS (hazard ratio (HR)—95% confidence interval (CI): 16 (4–61), $p < 0.0001$; and 30 (9–105), $p < 0.0001$, vs low SS, respectively), even after adjustment for obesity, history of hypertension, impaired fasting glucose, and cardiovascular therapy. Conclusions: The severity and extent of the coronary atherosclerosis, evaluated by the SS, is a strong and independent predictor of the development of DM in patients, referred to CA.

Keywords: coronary artery disease; diabetes mellitus; atherosclerosis; coronary angiography

---

1. Introduction

Type 2 diabetes mellitus (DM) and cardiovascular (CV) disease are closely correlated. DM is associated with a two- to four-fold increased risk of coronary artery disease (CAD) and stroke [1]. On the other hand, CV diseases are the main causes of death and disability among patients with DM [2]. Furthermore, DM is associated with more extensive coronary atherosclerosis [3], and worse outcomes in acute coronary syndromes [4]. The association with coronary atherosclerosis spans from early stages of glucose intolerance to overt DM [5–7]. We previously demonstrated, in hypertensive patients, that uncontrolled blood pressure is associated with a two-fold increased risk of diabetes onset [8]. In addition, hypertension-mediated target organ damage (e.g., carotid atherosclerosis and left ventricular hypertrophy) is a significant predictor of DM onset, independently of the baseline metabolic profile, anti-hypertensive therapy, and other significant covariates [9]. Thus, a well-characterized phenotype of hypertensive patients, carrying features suggestive of a high atherosclerotic burden, places patients at a higher risk for developing DM during follow-up. However, at this time, there is no direct demonstration that atherosclerosis exposes patients to a higher risk of DM development with a dose-response pattern. Identifying patients with an increased risk of DM, in the setting of patients referred to Cat Labs for coronary angiography (CA), might be of paramount importance in terms of cardiovascular prevention [10]. Therefore, the early identification of individuals with established coronary artery disease at risk of type 2 DM could be further assessed for the severity of atherosclerosis, even before the clinical appearance of the disease, in order to promote the aggressive management of the metabolic profile in these patients.

Accordingly, we investigated whether the extension and severity of CAD diagnosed during CA might be predictive of the future onset of DM.

2. Research Design and Methods

2.1. Patients

We screened all of the consecutive patients who underwent CA at the Cardiovascular Center Aalst (Belgium), between 1 January 2009 and 31 December 2009. The exclusion criteria were as follows: previous coronary angiogram, history of myocardial infarction or coronary artery bypass graft, or the diagnosis of pre-existing diabetes. All patients signed informed consent for CA and for data collection before the procedure. During the index hospital admission for CA, the blood pressure (BP), heart rate (HR), body mass index (BMI), fasting glucose, glycated hemoglobin (HbA1c), lipid profile, and kidney function were routinely assessed for each patient. All of the patients underwent trans-thoracic echocardiogram (TTE), analyzed offline by one expert reader under the supervision of a senior consultant, using dedicated work-stations (Echo-PAC Clinical Workstation Software, GE Healthcare, Horten, Norway).

The SYNTAX (Synergy between Percutaneous Coronary Intervention with Taxus and Cardiac Surgery) score (SS) was calculated for all of the patients by two interventional cardiologists blinded to the baseline clinical characteristics, procedural data, and clinical outcomes. Each coronary lesion with more than a 50% diameter stenosis in vessels of at least 1.5 mm, by visual estimation, was scored separately using the SS algorithm from the related website [11]. To assess the intra-observer reproducibility, angiograms were re-analyzed by the same interventional cardiologist eight weeks after the first analysis. The investigator remained blinded to the results of the first analysis. After the first admission for CA (index procedure), patients were assessed for incidence of type 2 diabetes in all of the subsequent follow-up visits or laboratory exams at the Cardiovascular Center of Aalst. To standardize the follow-up (FU), we analyzed the ambulatory visits and laboratory data every 6 months, until the last FU.

2.2. Primary Endpoint

The primary endpoint of the study was the incidence of type 2 DM after index hospitalization. Diabetes was defined according to the 2018 American Diabetes Association (ADA) criteria, as follows: fasting plasma glucose of 126 mg/dL (7.0 m mol/L) or hemoglobin A1C of 6.5% (48 mmol/mol) [12]. To accurately date the first diagnosis of diabetes, we carefully checked on the initiation of anti-diabetic therapies, and on the laboratory data at the occasion of the outpatient clinic visit. The onset of diabetes was adjudicated based on the earliest evidence of ADA criteria at the follow-up.

2.3. Measurements and Definitions

Obesity was defined as a BMI of 30 kg/m^2. According to the ADA criteria, impaired fasting glucose (IFG) was considered when the fasting plasma glucose was between 101 and 125 mg/dL. The systolic and diastolic blood pressure (BP) was measured by standard aneroid sphygmomanometer after 5 min rest in the supine position. Three BP measurements were obtained in the sitting position, at 2 min intervals. The averages of these measurements were used for the analysis. Hypertension is defined as office systolic blood pressure (SBP) values of 140 mmHg, and/or diastolic BP (DBP) values of 90 mmHg, according to the European Society of Cardiology (ESC) guidelines [13]. We defined peripheral vascular disease (PVD) as disease documented by a vascular imaging study (including a Computed tomography (CT) scan, ultrasound, peripheral angiography, and magnetic resonance imaging (MRI) that was significant enough for the patient to be referred for elective vascular surgery or percutaneous intervention.

2.4. Statistical Analysis

The data were analyzed using IBM SPSS Statistics (version 25.0; SPSS, IBM, Armonk, NY, US), and expressed as mean ± 1 standard deviation (SD). The variables that were not normally distributed were log-transformed. The study population was divided into quartiles of SS. For the exploratory statistics, we considered the two lowest quartiles as low-risk SS (group 1); the third one, corresponding to the median of distribution, as moderate-risk SS (group 2); and the highest one, corresponding to the 75th percentile of the distribution, as high-risk SS (group 3). Analysis of variance (ANOVA) was used to compare the baseline characteristics of the three groups of patients according to SS. Under the assumption of increasing abnormalities from group 1 to group 3, polynomial linear and quadratic contrasts were used to estimate the trend. The $\chi 2$ distribution was used to compare the categorical variables, with the Monte Carlo simulation in order to obtain exact p-values.

The incidence of diabetes in relation to the three groups of SS was assessed using three models of Cox regression analysis, as follows: (a) in the first model, age, gender, and metabolic profile were included; (b) in the second model, the echo parameters and classes of drugs were included; (c) in the third model, the dosages (low vs high dosages) of the statins (i.e., patients on rosuvastatine ≥20 mg/die or atorvastatine ≥40 mg/die were considered as high dosage) were included. A two-tailed p-value of <0.05 was used to reject the null hypothesis.

3. Results

3.1. Patients

Within the study period, 570 non-diabetic (mean age 65 ± 10 years; 69% males) patients fulfilled the inclusion and exclusion criteria, and were included in this analysis. Table 1 shows the demographic and clinical characteristics of the patients stratified by SS. In the patient population, the included SSs were as follows: SS low, 0 to ≤4; SS medium, >4 to ≤10; and SS high, >10. The patients in the high SS were older, and showed a lower heart rate and left ventricular ejection fraction. The basal fasting plasma glucose was found to be progressively higher among the patients with medium and high SS, while the lipid profile was more favorable in the medium SS. Table 2 shows the medical therapy at discharge from the index hospitalization. All four classes of medications considered in the analysis were prescribed more frequently in patients with a higher SS.

Table 1. Baseline demographic and clinical characteristics of participants stratified by SYNTAX score (SS).

	Low SS (n = 295)	Medium SS (n = 151)	High SS (n = 124)	p (for trend)
Age (years)	65.5 ± 10.4	63.9 ± 10.5	67.1 ± 10.3	0.045
Sex (male/female %)	68.8/31.2	72.8/27.2	74.2/25.8	NS
Smokers (%)	47.5	53.0	48.4	NS
Hypertensives (%)	67.5	76.8	75.8	NS
BMI (Kg/m^2)	27.1 ± 4.5	27.2 ± 4.3	27.3 ± 5.4	NS
Systolic BP (mmHg)	133.3 ± 22.0	128.8 ± 17.1	133.2 ± 19.4	NS
Diastolic BP (mmHg)	69.5 ± 11.4	69.3 ± 10.6	69.3 ± 11.3	NS
HR (bpm)	67.7 ± 12.2	66.9 ± 11.9	64.6 ± 8.7	0.048
Ejection Fraction (%)	67.9 ± 16.0	64.9 ± 14.0	61.6 ± 15.4	0.001
Fasting plasma glucose (mg/dL)	83.8 ± 13.2	85.6 ± 13.4	94.7 ± 13.5	0.0001
HbA1c (mmol/mol)	40.5 ± 8.7	40.4 ± 7.3	41.0 ± 7.5	NS
Total cholesterol (mg/dL)	172.6 ± 44.2	154.4 ± 36.6	156.0 ± 41.6	0.0001
LDL cholesterol (mg/dL)	91.8 ± 39.0	77.8 ± 31.4	81.1 ± 34.7	0.001
HDL cholesterol (mg/dL)	52.2 ± 16.8	51.0 ± 17.9	46.4 ± 14.5	0.01
Triacylglycerols (mg/dL)	147.3 ± 83.0	124.4 ± 67.4	146.1 ± 87.2	0.044

Table 1. *Cont.*

	Low SS (n = 295)	Medium SS (n = 151)	High SS (n = 124)	p (for trend)
GFR_{EPI} (mL/min/1.73 m^2)	64.7 ± 28.3	70.5 ± 25.6	64.3 ± 24.8	NS
CRP (mg/L)	27.7 ± 77.1	15.9 ± 34.0	28.7 ± 67.5	NS
IFG (%)	12.5	15.2	36.3	0.0001

BMI = body mass index; BP = blood pressure; HR = heart rate; HbA1C = hemoglobin glycated A1C; LDL = low density lipoprotein; HDL = high density lipoprotein; GFR = glomerular filtration rate; CRP = C-reactive protein; IFG = impaired fasting glucose; NS = not significant.

Table 2. Classes of drugs prescribed at the discharge.

	Low SS (n = 295)	Medium SS (n = 151)	High SS (n = 124)	p
CCB (%)	2.7	8.6	14.5	<0.0001
β-blockers (%)	20.0	37.7	42.7	<0.0001
Statins (%)	39.0	76.8	83.9	<0.0001
Statins low dose (%)	32.5	58.3	64.5	<0.0001
Statins high dose (%)	6.5	18.5	19.4	<0.0001
Anti-RAS (%)	29.5	27.2	46.8	0.001

SS = SYNTAX score; CCB = calcium channel blockers; RAS = renin angiotensin system.

3.2. Follow-Up

During a median follow-up of 79 months (interquartile range (IQR): 67–94), 74 (13%) patients developed DM. The incidence of diabetes was significantly higher in the patients with a high SS (41%), than in patients with a medium (12%) and low SS (2%; p for trend < 0.0001; Figure 1). In the Cox regression analysis (Table 3), the predictors of DM onset during follow-up had higher baseline values of fasting plasma glucose (HR = 1.043; (95% CI 1.011–1.075); $p < 0.008$), medium SS (HR = 6.630; (95% CI 2.394–18.358); $p < 0.0001$), and high SS (HR = 14.789; (95% CI 5.796–37.737); $p < 0.0001$). The three curves (Figure 2) started to separate after 48–52 months from the index hospitalization, and further diverged after five years of follow-up. In the second Cox regression analysis performed by including the ejection fraction, heart rate, and the drugs prescribed (Table 4), the predictors of the new onset of DM were as follows: use of statins (HR = 6.953; (95% CI 1.618–29.880); $p = 0.009$), an anti-renin angiotensin system (RAS; HR = 3.338; (95% CI 1.917–5.812); $p = 0.0001$), medium SS (HR = 6.022; (95% CI 1.714–21.158); $p = 0.005$), and high SS (HR = 13.140; (95% CI 3.857–44.738); $p < 0.0001$) was further reinforced (Table 4). In the last model (Table 5), including the dosage of statins, the independent predictors of DM were a low dose of statins (HR = 8.631; (95% CI 2.017–36.931); $p = 0.004$), a high dose of statins (HR = 8.158; (95% CI 1.764–37.728); $p = 0.007$), anti-RAS (HR = 3.637; (95% CI 2.151–6.6.151); $p < 0.0001$), medium SS (HR = 3.505; (95% CI 1.274–9.644); $p = 0.015$), and high SS (HR = 8.906; (95% CI 3.404–23.296); $p = 0.0001$).

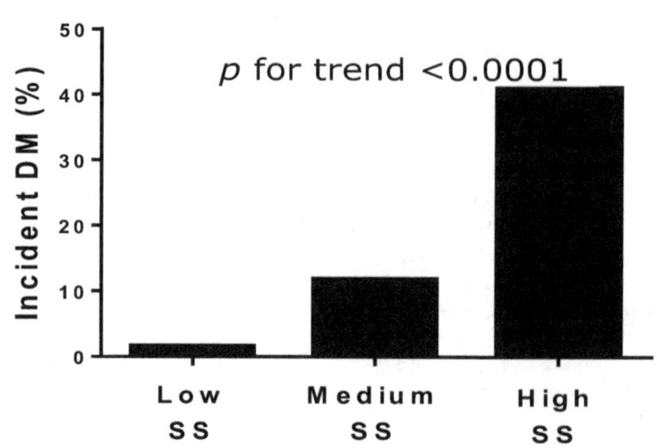

Figure 1. Rate of type 2 diabetes mellitus (DM) in the three SYNTAX score (SS) levels.

Table 3. Results of Cox regression, including the age, gender, and metabolic profile.

Predictors	Sig.	HR	95.0% CI	
			Lower	−Upper
Sex (1 male/2 female)	0.583	1.163	0.679	−1.993
Age (years)	0.085	1.026	0.996	−1.056
Fasting plasma glucose (mg/dL)	0.008	1.043	1.011	−1.075
LDL Cholesterol (mg/dL)	0.323	1.130	0.535	−2.385
IFG (y)	0.749	7.865	2.817	−21.959
Medium SS	0.000	6.630	2.304	−18.358
High SS	0.000	14.789	5.796	−37.737

Abbreviations as in Table 1. CI = confidence interval.

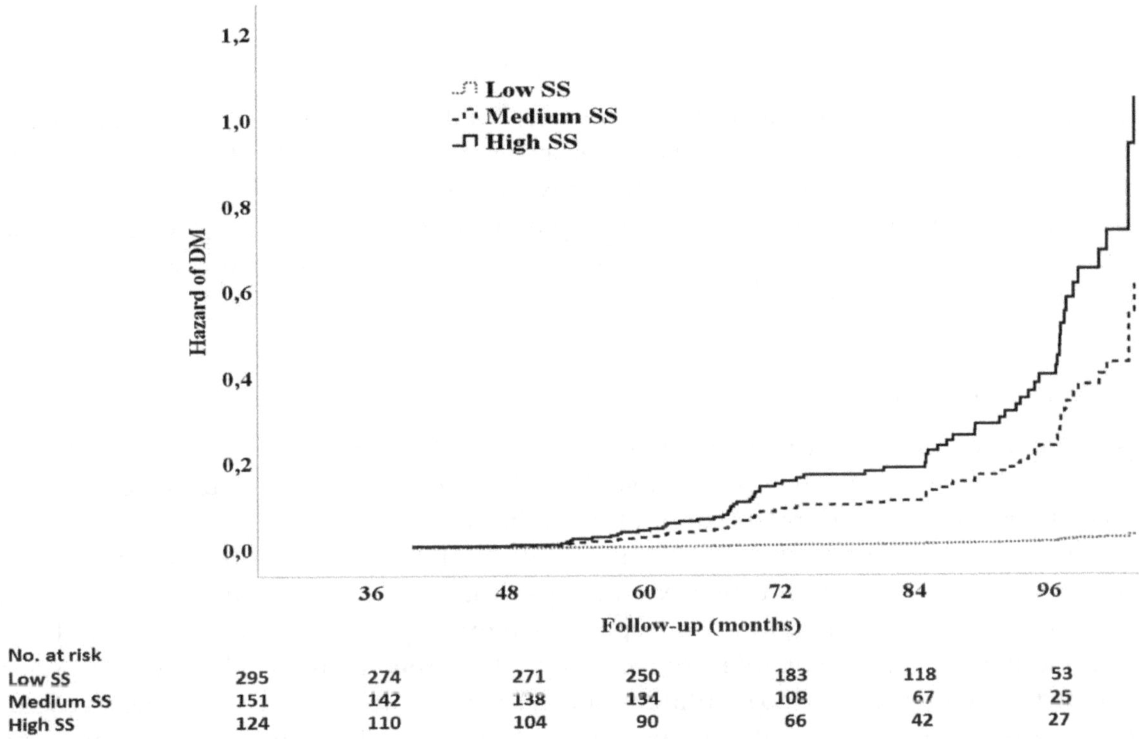

Figure 2. Cox regression time to event analysis for type 2 diabetes mellitus onset, in the function of the three SS levels.

Table 4. Results of Cox regression including ejection fraction, heart rate, and classes of drugs.

Predictors	Sig	HR	95.0% CI	
			Lower	−Upper
Ejection Fraction (%)	0.698	0.996	0.978	−1.015
HR (bpm)	0.128	1.021	0.994	−1.048
CCB (*y*)	0.549	0.215	0.643	−2.296
B-blockers (*y*)	0.416	1.223	0.753	−1.986
Statins (*y*)	0.009	6.953	1.618	−29.880
Anti RAS (*y*)	0.000	3.338	1.917	−5.812
Medium SS	0.005	6.022	1.714	−21.158
High SS	0.000	13.140	3.857	−44.768

Abbreviations as in Tables 1 and 2.

In patients who developed DM, no significant differences were detected in the incidence of major adverse cardiovascular events (i.e., death, myocardial infarction, or coronary revascularization) among the three SS subgroups ($p = 0.418$).

Table 5. Results of the COX regression, including the classes of drugs and statins dosage.

Predictors	Sig	HR	95.0% CI	
			Lower	Upper
CCB (y)	0.387	1.314	0.708	−2.440
B-blockers (y)	0.390	1.238	0.761	−2.013
Statins low dose (y)	0.004	8.631	2.017	−36.931
Statins high dose (y)	0.007	8.158	1.764	−37.728
Anti RAS (y)	0.0001	3.637	2.151	−6.151
Medium SS	0.015	3.505	1.274	−9.644
High SS	0.0001	8.906	3.404	−23.296

Abbreviations as in Tables 1 and 2.

4. Discussion

In non-diabetic patients, our study demonstrates, for the first time, a significant association between the severity and extent of coronary atherosclerosis, assessed by the SS, with the future development of type 2 DM. Compared with patients with low SS, those with medium or high values exhibited an 8-fold and 10-fold higher risk for developing type 2 DM during follow-up, an association that was independent of potential confounders, including initial metabolic profile, age, anthropometric and hemodynamic characteristics, and medications.

Vascular and Metabolic Disease

Our results parallel previous studies challenging the paradigm that type 2 DM normally precedes and portends to a higher risk of developing vascular atherosclerosis [14,15], although they provide direct evidence of this reverse temporal relation. Our results are consistent with findings in patients with essential hypertension, in whom both resistant hypertension [8] and left ventricular hypertrophy [9] precede the onset of type 2 DM. Our findings extend to patients with coronary artery disease (CAD), the evidence of this reverse temporal relation. We hypothesize that a possible vicious circle might be at the basis of this phenomenon. It is reasonable to speculate that the mechanisms relating atherosclerosis to the later onset of DM might be related to insulin resistance, rather than directly to a hyperglycaemic state. However, as the present study was not designed to explore the pathogenic mechanisms underlying the association between SS and the development of diabetes, the insulin sensitivity in our study population remained unexplored. Insulin resistance is a common pathogenic background for both DM and atherosclerosis [16,17]. Insulin resistance plays a mechanistic role, along with other risk factors, in the development of vascular damage and the occurrence of cardiovascular events (four) [18,19]. In particular, insulin resistance-mediated endothelial dysfunction (an early step of atherosclerosis) [20] has been proposed as a pathogenic mechanism of DM [21]. In turn, the presence of an extensive vascular atherosclerosis might facilitate the onset and maintenance of the insulin resistance state. This vicious circle can well explain how CV damage, instead of being a consequence, could progress, together with the development of DM.

Our results cannot exclude the possibility that sub-clinical DM was already present at the time of the index CA in patients who clinically manifested the disease during follow-up. As matter of fact, endothelial dysfunction precedes and predicts incident diabetes, supporting the hypothesis that vascular disease might precede pancreatic beta-cell failure, determining the shift from insulin resistance to diabetes [22]. Moreover, endothelial dysfunction and impaired nitric oxide-mediated vasodilatation have also been suggested to directly lead to reduced insulin delivery to skeletal muscles, resulting in peripheral insulin resistance and hyper-glycaemia [23].

It is of note that patients with medium or high SS manifested type 2 DM after a subclinical phase of nearly four years from the index CA. As SS was evaluated cross-sectionally, this study does not clarify whether the association between the magnitude of coronary atherosclerosis and the development of type 2 DM is a time-dependent or atherosclerotic-dependent phenomenon. However, the latter seems to play an important role, considering that the rate of DM increases with increasing the SS category (Figure 1).

The evidence that patients with more than a low SS have a much higher risk of incident type 2 DM is of clinical importance. It implies that these patients, in addition to their regular cardiovascular follow-up, require tailored management in terms of metabolic risk, including attention to pharmacological therapy. In particular, it has been demonstrated that a high-dose regimen with statins was associated with an increased risk of new-onset DM [24,25]. In keeping with these findings, we found that statin intake was significantly associated with more complex coronary artery disease, and was predictive of an increased rate of DM.

In terms of the choice of revascularization strategies, the knowledge of the higher risk of development of type 2 diabetes in patients with more than a low SS might favor surgical over percutaneous interventions, after taking into account the anatomical features of the CAD and the clinical conditions of the patient [26].

5. Conclusions

Our study demonstrates that the extension and severity of coronary atherosclerosis is a strong predictor of development of type 2 DM. This finding advocates the need for developing dedicated management strategies in patients with severe coronary artery disease, taking into account the risk of late metabolic impairment following the index coronary intervention.

Author Contributions: Conceptualization, I.C., R.I., C.M., and E.B.; methodology, E.B., M.A.L., J.B., and C.M.; validation, A.R., G.d.S., B.T., and J.B.; investigation, G.D.G., T.S., D.F., and M.V.M.; data curation, M.V.M., I.C., G.D.G., and T.S.; original draft preparation, I.C., R.I., C.M., and T.S.; writing (review and editing), I.C., D.F., R.I., and E.B.; supervision, A.R., B.T., C.M., E.B., and M.A.L.

Acknowledgments: T.S. and G.D.G. received a grant from the Cardiopath PhD program. R.I. and C.M. were recipients of University FEDERICO II financial support, annuity 2016.

References

1. Colhoun, H.M.; Betteridge, D.J.; Durrington, P.N.; Hitman, G.A.; Neil, H.A.; Livingstone, S.J.; Thomason, M.J.; Mackness, M.I.; Charlton-Menys, V.; Fuller, J.H.; et al. Primary prevention of cardiovascular disease with atorvastatin in type 2 diabetes in the Collaborative Atorvastatin Diabetes Study (CARDS): Multicentre randomised placebo-controlled trial. *Lancet* **2004**, *364*, 685–696. [CrossRef]
2. Wang, L.C.C.; Hess, C.N.; Hiatt, W.R.; Goldfine, A.B. Clinical Update: Cardiovascular Disease in Diabetes Mellitus: Atherosclerotic Cardiovascular Disease and Heart Failure in Type 2 Diabetes Mellitus Mechanisms, Management, and Clinical Considerations. *Circulation* **2016**, *133*, 2459–2502. [CrossRef] [PubMed]
3. Ryden, L.; Grant, P.J.; Anker, S.D.; Berne, C.; Cosentino, F.; Danchin, N.; Deaton, C.; Viigimaa, M.; Vlachopoulos, C.; Xuereb, R.G.; et al. Task Force on diabetes p-d, cardiovascular diseases of the European Society of C, European Association for the Study of D, ESC guidelines on diabetes, pre-diabetes, and cardiovascular diseases developed in collaboration with the EASD-summary. *Diabetes Vasc. Dis. Res.* **2014**, *11*, 133–173.
4. Deedwania, P.; Kosiborod, M.; Barrett, E.; Ceriello, A.; Isley, W.; Mazzone, T.; Raskin, P. American Heart Association Diabetes Committee of the Council on Nutrition PA, Metabolism: Hyperglycemia and acute coronary syndrome: A scientific statement from the American Heart Association Diabetes Committee of the Council on Nutrition, Physical Activity, and Metabolism. *Circulation* **2008**, *117*, 1610–1619. [PubMed]
5. Harris, M.I.; Klein, R.; Welborn, T.A.; Knuiman, M.W. Onset of NIDDM occurs at least 4-7 year before clinical diagnosis. *Diabetes Care* **1992**, *15*, 815–819. [CrossRef] [PubMed]

6. Hu, F.B.; Stampfer, M.J.; Haffner, S.M.; Solomon, C.G.; Willett, W.C.; Manson, J.E. Elevated risk of cardiovascular disease prior to clinical diagnosis of type 2 diabetes. *Diabetes Care* **2002**, *25*, 1129–1134. [CrossRef] [PubMed]
7. Acar, B.; Ozeke, O.; Karakurt, M.; Ozen, Y.; Ozbay, M.B.; Unal, S.; Karanfil, M.; Yayla, C.; Cay, S.; Maden, O.; et al. Association of Prediabetes with Higher Coronary Atherosclerotic Burden Among Patients with First Diagnosed Acute Coronary Syndrome. *Angiology* **2018**. [CrossRef]
8. Izzo, R.; Simone, G.; Chinali, M.; Iaccarino, G.; Trimarco, V.; Rozza, F.; Giudice, R.; Trimarco, B.; Luca, N. Insufficient control of blood pressure and incident diabetes. *Diabetes Care* **2009**, *32*, 845–850. [CrossRef]
9. Izzo, R.; Simone, G.; Trimarco, V.; Gerdts, E.; Giudice, R.; Vaccaro, O.; Luca, N.; Trimarco, B. Hypertensive target organ damage predicts incident diabetes mellitus. *Eur. Heart J.* **2013**, *34*, 3419–3426. [CrossRef]
10. Gillies, C.L.; Abrams, K.R.; Lambert, P.C.; Cooper, N.J.; Sutton, A.J.; Hsu, R.T.; Khunti, K. Pharmacological and lifestyle interventions to prevent or delay type 2 diabetes in people with impaired glucose tolerance: Systematic review and meta-analysis. *Bmj* **2007**, *334*, 299. [CrossRef]
11. Serruys, P.W.; Onuma, Y.; Garg, S.; Sarno, G.; Brand, M.; Kappetein, A.P.; Dyck, N.; Mack, M.; Holmes, D.; Feldman, T.; et al. Assessment of the SYNTAX score in the Syntax study. *EuroIntervention* **2009**, *5*, 50–56. [CrossRef] [PubMed]
12. American, D.A. Classification and Diagnosis of Diabetes: Standards of Medical Care in Diabetes-2018. *Diabetes Care* **2018**, *41*, S13–S27. [CrossRef] [PubMed]
13. Williams, B.; Mancia, G.; Spiering, W.; Agabiti, R.E.; Azizi, M.; Burnier, M.; Clement, D.L.; Coca, A.; Simone, G.; Dominiczak, A.; et al. ESC/ESH Guidelines for the management of arterial hypertension. *Eur. Heart J.* **2018**, *39*, 3021–3104. [CrossRef] [PubMed]
14. Gioia, D.G.; Scarsini, R.; Strisciuglio, T.; Biase, C.; Zivelonghi, C.; Franco, D.; Bruyne, B.; Ribichini, F.; Barbato, E. Correlation between Angiographic and Physiologic Evaluation of Coronary Artery Narrowings in Patients with Aortic Valve Stenosis. *Am. J. Cardiol.* **2017**, *120*, 106–110. [CrossRef] [PubMed]
15. Xaplanteris, P.; Ntalianis, A.; Bruyne, B.; Strisciuglio, T.; Pellicano, M.; Ciccarelli, G.; Milkas, A.; Barbato, E. Coronary lesion progression as assessed by fractional flow reserve (FFR) and angiography. *EuroIntervention* **2018**, *14*, 907–914. [CrossRef]
16. Olefsky, J.; Farquhar, J.W.; Reaven, G. Relationship between fasting plasma insulin level and resistance to insulin-mediated glucose uptake in normal and diabetic subjects. *Diabetes* **1973**, *22*, 507–513. [CrossRef] [PubMed]
17. Howard, G.; O'Leary, D.H.; Zaccaro, D.; Haffner, S.; Rewers, M.; Hamman, R.; Selby, J.V.; Saad, M.F.; Savage, P.; Bergman, R. Insulin sensitivity and atherosclerosis. The Insulin Resistance Atherosclerosis Study (IRAS) Investigators. *Circulation* **1996**, *93*, 1809–1817. [CrossRef]
18. Fournier, S.; Toth, G.G.; Bruyne, B.; Johnson, N.P.; Ciccarelli, G.; Xaplanteris, P.; Milkas, A.; Strisciuglio, T.; Bartunek, J.; Vanderheyden, M.; et al. Six-Year Follow-Up of Fractional Flow Reserve-Guided Versus Angiography-Guided Coronary Artery Bypass Graft Surgery. *Circ. Cardiovasc. Interv.* **2018**, *11*, e006368. [CrossRef]
19. Morisco, C.; Lembo, G.; Trimarco, B. Insulin resistance and cardiovascular risk: New insights from molecular and cellular biology. *Trends Cardiovasc. Med.* **2006**, *16*, 183–188. [CrossRef]
20. Carrizzo, A.; Izzo, C.; Oliveti, M.; Alfano, A.; Virtuoso, N.; Capunzo, M.; Pietro, P.; Calabrese, M.; Simone, E.; Sciarretta, S.; et al. The Main Determinants of Diabetes Mellitus Vascular Complications: Endothelial Dysfunction and Platelet Hyperaggregation. *Int. J. Mol. Sci.* **2018**, *19*, 2968. [CrossRef]
21. Tooke, J.E. Microvascular function in human diabetes. A physiological perspective. *Diabetes* **1995**, *44*, 721–726. [CrossRef]
22. Ferrannini, E. Insulin resistance versus insulin deficiency in non-insulin-dependent diabetes mellitus: Problems and prospects. *Endocr. Rev.* **1998**, *19*, 477–490. [CrossRef]
23. Balletshofer, B.M.; Rittig, K.; Enderle, M.D.; Volk, A.; Maerker, E.; Jacob, S.; Matthaei, S.; Rett, K. Haring HU: Endothelial dysfunction is detectable in young normotensive first-degree relatives of subjects with type 2 diabetes in association with insulin resistance. *Circulation* **2000**, *101*, 1780–1784. [CrossRef]

24. Preiss, D.; Seshasai, S.R.; Welsh, P.; Murphy, S.A.; Ho, J.E.; Waters, D.D.; DeMicco, D.A.; Barter, P.; Cannon, C.P.; Sabatine, M.S.; et al. Risk of incident diabetes with intensive-dose compared with moderate-dose statin therapy: A meta-analysis. *Jama* **2011**, *305*, 2556–2564. [CrossRef]
25. Izzo, R.; Simone, G.; Trimarco, V.; Giudice, R.; Marco, M.; Renzo, G.; Luca, N.; Trimarco, B. Primary prevention with statins and incident diabetes in hypertensive patients at high cardiovascular risk. *Nutr. Metab. Cardiovasc. Dis. NMCD* **2013**, *23*, 1101–1106. [CrossRef]
26. Farkouh, M.E.; Domanski, M.; Sleeper, L.A.; Siami, F.S.; Dangas, G.; Mack, M.; Yang, M.; Cohen, D.J.; Rosenberg, Y.; Solomon, S.D.; et al. Strategies for multivessel revascularization in patients with diabetes. *New Engl. J. Med.* **2012**, *367*, 2375–2384. [CrossRef]

8

Angiopoietins, Vascular Endothelial Growth Factors and Secretory Phospholipase A_2 in Ischemic and Non-Ischemic Heart Failure

Gilda Varricchi [1,2,3,4,*], Stefania Loffredo [1,2,3,4,*], Leonardo Bencivenga [1,5], Anne Lise Ferrara [1,2,3], Giuseppina Gambino [1], Nicola Ferrara [1], Amato de Paulis [1,2,3], Gianni Marone [1,2,3,4] and Giuseppe Rengo [1,6]

1 Department of Translational Medical Sciences, University of Naples Federico II, 80100 Naples, Italy; leonardobencivenga@gmail.com (L.B.); Anneliseferrara@gmail.com (A.L.F.); pina.gambino@gmail.com (G.G.); nicferra@unina.it (N.F.); depaulis@unina.it (A.d.P.); marone@unina.it (G.M.); giuseppe.rengo@unina.it (G.R.)
2 Center for Basic and Clinical Immunology Research (CISI), University of Naples Federico II, 80100 Naples, Italy
3 World Allergy Organization (WAO), Center of Excellence, 80100 Naples, Italy
4 Institute of Experimental Endocrinology and Oncology "G. Salvatore" (IEOS), National Research Council (CNR), 80100 Naples, Italy
5 Department of Advanced Biomedical Sciences, University of Naples Federico II, 80100 Naples, Italy
6 Istituti Clinici Scientifici Maugeri SpA Società Benefit, Via Bagni Vecchi, 1, 82037 Telese BN, Italy
* Correspondence: gildanet@gmail.com (G.V.); stefanialoffredo@hotmail.com (S.L.)

Abstract: Heart failure (HF) is a growing public health burden, with high prevalence and mortality rates. In contrast to ischemic heart failure (IHF), the diagnosis of non-ischemic heart failure (NIHF) is established in the absence of coronary artery disease. Angiopoietins (ANGPTs), vascular endothelial growth factors (VEGFs) and secretory phospholipases A_2 ($sPLA_2s$) are proinflammatory mediators and key regulators of endothelial cells. In the present manuscript, we analyze the plasma concentrations of angiogenic (ANGPT1, ANGPT2, VEGF-A) and lymphangiogenic (VEGF-C, VEGF-D) factors and the plasma activity of $sPLA_2$ in patients with IHF and NIHF compared to healthy controls. The concentrations of ANGPT1, ANGPT2 and their ratio significantly differed between HF patients and healthy controls. Similarly, plasma levels of VEGF-D and $sPLA_2$ activity were higher in HF as compared to controls. Concentrations of ANGPT2 and the ANGPT2/ANGPT1 ratio (an index of vascular permeability) were increased in NIHF patients. VEGF-A and VEGF-C concentrations did not differ among the three examined groups. Interestingly, VEGF-D was selectively increased in IFH patients compared to controls. Plasma activity of $sPLA_2$ was increased in IHF and NIHF patients compared to controls. Our results indicate that several regulators of vascular permeability and smoldering inflammation are specifically altered in IHF and NIHF patients. Studies involving larger cohorts of these patients will be necessary to demonstrate the clinical implications of our findings.

Keywords: angiopoietins; heart failure; VEGFs; $sPLA_2$; IHF; NIHF

---

1. Introduction

Heart failure (HF) represents a growing public health burden with an estimated prevalence in Europe and United States ranging from 0.4% to 2% [1]. Based on left ventricle ejection fraction (EF), HF recognizes three different classes: HF with a reduced EF (HFrEF with an EF < 40%); HF with a mild-range EF (HFmEF with an EF between 40% and 49%), and HF with a preserved EF

(HFpEF with an EF ≥ 50%) [2]. Although classification systems for HF causes are largely debated, within HFrEF ischemic heart disease represents the most common cause of myocardial injury and ventricular dysfunction, leading in a significant percentage of cases to post-ischemic heart failure (IHF). Non-ischemic HF (NIHF), which accounts for less than 50% of HFrEF cases, comprises all the remaining heterogeneous HF etiologies ranging from valvular diseases to toxic damage, up to metabolic conditions and genetic cardiomyopathies [3]. In a significant percentage (≅ 30%) of HF patients, the etiology remains undetermined, and the syndrome is referred to as "idiopathic HF" [4]. Identification of these diverse etiologies may be obtained through a complex diagnostic workup, frequently without a relevant therapeutic implication. Neurohormonal and inflammatory activation are widely recognized as playing a pivotal role in HF onset and progression, irrespective of etiology [5]. Despite advances in management and therapies, the prognosis in HF patients remains poor, thus a deeper knowledge of the molecular mechanisms involved in the complex HF pathophysiology are needed for the identification of novel therapeutic targets and biomarkers to stratify prognosis and drive decision-making processes [6]. To this aim, several investigations have focused their attention on inflammatory and neurohormonal molecules.

The angiopoietin (ANGPT) family is an important group of factors, specific for vascular endothelium, whose functions are mediated through two tyrosine kinase receptors, Tie1 and Tie2 [7]. The ANGPT-Tie ligand-receptor system exerts a key role in regulating vascular integrity [8,9]. Beside their roles in the modulation of angiogenesis [10,11] and lymphangiogenesis [12,13], ANGPTs also regulate inflammation in several disorders, including cardiovascular diseases [9,14,15]. Angiopoietin-1 (ANGPT1), produced by peri-endothelial mural cells (pericytes) [16] and immune cells [17,18], is a potent agonist of Tie2 receptor on endothelial cells [11,19]. ANGPT1 is an anti-inflammatory molecule [20] that maintains vascular integrity [21,22]. ANGPT2, stored in Weibel–Palade bodies in endothelial cells [23], is rapidly released in response to various stimuli [24]. ANGPT2 is considered a pro-inflammatory molecule [25,26] and inhibits ANGPT1/Tie2 interaction [10,27], resulting in vascular instability and leakage [26].

Elevated ANGPT2 levels have been found in patients with acute coronary syndrome [28,29], hypertension [30,31], congestive heart failure [32] and congenital heart failure [33]. ANGPT2 has been proposed as a prognostic biomarker of adverse cardiovascular events in myocardial infarction [34] and after percutaneous coronary intervention (PCI) [35,36]. In contrast, ANGPT1 plays a protective role in rodent models of vascular injuries [37,38].

The vascular endothelial growth factor (VEGF) family includes VEGF-A, VEGF-B, VEGF-C, and VEGF-D [39]. VEGFs and their receptors on blood and lymphatic endothelial cells play intricate roles in initiating and promoting inflammatory and tumor angiogenesis [40]. VEGF-A, the most potent proangiogenic factor [41], was first identified for its permeabilizing activity and named vascular permeability factor (VPF) [42]. VEGF-A and VEGF-B are key regulators of systemic and cardiac angiogenesis [39,43,44]. VEGF-C and VEGF-D are the most important modulators of inflammatory and tumor lymphangiogenesis [45,46]. Several studies have found elevated levels of circulating VEGF-A in patients with myocardial infarction [28,47–50]. By contrast, the roles of VEGF-A [32] VEGF-C and VEGF-D in HF remain unclear or totally unexplored.

Phospholipases A_2 (PLA_2) hydrolyze the fatty acids from membrane phospholipids releasing arachidonic acid and lysophospholipids [51–54]. Secreted or extracellular PLA_2 ($sPLA_2$) modulate vascular permeability [55] and activate inflammatory cells [53,56,57]. Circulating levels of $sPLA_2$ predict coronary events in patients with coronary artery disease [58] and in apparently healthy men and women [59]. Serum $sPLA_2$ levels also predict long-term mortality for HF after myocardial infarction [60]. Intima of coronary atherosclerotic lesions of patients with angina or myocardial infarction express $sPLA_2$ [61] and elevated serum levels of $sPLA_2$ increase the risk of early atherosclerosis [62].

While some studies are available on ANGPTs, VEGF isoforms, and $sPLA_2$ involvement in ischemic heart disease, very little is known in the clinical setting of IHF and, to the best of our knowledge, no data are available in NIHF. Thus, the aim of the present study is to evaluate the circulating levels of ANGPTs, VEGFs, and $sPLA_2$ activity in HF patients, particularly comparing the ischemic and non-ischemic etiologies.

2. Materials and Methods

2.1. Study Population

Patients with systolic HF were enrolled at the Department of Translational Medical Sciences of the University of Naples Federico II. Inclusion criteria were: age ≥ 18 years, diagnosis of HF from at least six months [2], left ventricular ejection fraction (LVEF) ≤ 45%, stable clinical condition during the month prior to inclusion, and an optimal guideline-based pharmacotherapy from at least three months, if not contraindicated. Exclusion criteria were represented by chronic obstructive pulmonary disease (COPD), diabetes mellitus (DM), immune disorders (rheumatoid arthritis, systemic lupus erythematosus, systemic sclerosis, Sjögren syndrome, vasculitis, psoriatic arthritis, dermatomyositis, ankylosing spondylitis), malignancies (also past), severe obesity as assessed through a body mass index (BMI) more than 32 kg/m^2, dialysis-dependent kidney failure, acute coronary syndromes and/or coronary revascularization in the previous 6 months, and an inability to provide informed consent. The control group was represented by subjects without HF and in accordance with the exclusion criteria. All patients underwent medical history evaluation and collection of demographic/clinical data, including age, gender, BMI, cardiovascular risk factors, and comorbidities. Clinical examination, transthoracic echocardiography, and serum BNP determination were performed at the time of the enrolment. The HF population was subsequently divided into two groups based on the HF etiology: ischemic HF (IHF) or non-ischemic HF (NIHF). Ischemic etiology was established based on either previous documented myocardial infarction and/or significant coronary artery disease with indication of cardiac revascularization. This study was approved by the Ethics Committee of the University of Naples Federico II (protocol number 124/17). All participants were carefully informed and signed a written consent to participate in the study.

2.2. Blood Sampling

Blood was collected during routine diagnostic procedures, scheduled in the course of hospital access for the determination of the main blood parameters (blood counts, biochemical. and coagulation profile), and the remaining plasma sample was labeled with a code that was documented into a data sheet. As mentioned above, blood samples were collected in patients under stable clinical conditions, strictly verifying all inclusion and exclusion criteria. The samples were collected by means of a clean venipuncture and minimal stasis using sodium citrate 3.2% as anticoagulant. After centrifugation (2000 g for 20 min at 22 °C), the plasma was divided into aliquots and stored at −80 °C until used. Technicians who performed the assays were blinded to the patients' history.

2.3. Assays of ANGPTs and VEGFs

Plasma levels of ANGPT1, ANGPT2, VEGF-A, VEGF-C, and VEGF-D were measured using commercially available ELISA kits (R&D System, Minneapolis, MN, USA) according to the manufacturer's instructions. The ELISA sensitivity was 156.25–10,000 pg/mL for ANGPT1, 31.1–4000 pg/mL for ANGPT2, 31.1–2000 pg/mL for VEGF-A, 62.5–4000 pg/mL for VEGF-C, and 31.3–2000 pg/mL for VEGF-D.

2.4. Assay of Phospholipase A_2 Activity

PLA_2 activity in the plasma of patients and healthy controls was measured by Life Technologies EnzChek (Milan, Italy) phospholipase A_2 assay. Briefly, a PLA_2 substrate cocktail consisting of 7-hydroxycoumarinyl-arachidonate (0.3 mM), 7-hydroxycoumarinyl-linolenate (0.3 mM), hydroxycoumarinyl 6-heptenoate (0.3 mM), dioleoylphosphatidylcholine (DOPC) (10 mM), and dioleoylphosphatidylglycerol (DOPG) (10 mM) was prepared in ethanol. Liposomes were formed by gradually adding 77 μL substrate/lipid cocktail to 10 mL of PLA_2 buffer (50 mM Tris–HCl, 100 mM NaCl, 1 mM $CaCl_2$) while stirring rapidly over 1 min using a magnetic stirrer. Fluorescence (excitation at 360 nm and emission at 460 nm) was measured and specific activity [relative fluorescent units (RFU)/mL] for each sample was calculated. Plasma (50 μL) was added to 96-well plates, and PLA_2 activity was evaluated by adding 50 μL of substrate cocktail.

2.5. Statistical Analysis

The sample size was determined by the primary outcome, which was defined through a comparison of ANGPT2 plasma levels between HF patients and healthy controls in a 1:1 ratio. Assuming an alpha error equal to 5% and a statistical power equal to 80%, considering the mean concentrations of ANGPT2 to be approximately 500 pg/mL in healthy individuals, according to previous evidence [32], a minimum of 70 patients (35 per group) are necessary to capture as significant a 40% difference in ANGPT2 plasma concentration between controls and HF patients. Data were analyzed with the GraphPad Prism 7 software package. Data were tested for normality using a D'Agostino-Pearson normality test. If normality was not rejected at the 0.05 significance level, we used parametric tests. Otherwise, for not-normally distributed data we used nonparametric tests. Statistical analysis was performed using a Student's *t*-test or one-way ANOVA and Bonferroni's multiple comparison test, as indicated in the figure legends. Correlations between two variables were assessed by Spearman's rank correlation analysis and reported as coefficients of correlation (*r*). Plasma concentrations of VEGFs and ANGPTs and activity of $sPLA_2$ are shown as the median (horizontal black line), the 25th and 75th percentiles (boxes), and the 5th and 95th percentiles (whiskers) of HF, NIHF, and IHF patients and controls. Statistically significant differences were accepted when the *p*-value was ≤ 0.05.

3. Results

3.1. Clinical and Demographic Characteristics of Overall Population

Table 1 summarizes the demographic and clinical characteristics of patients with IHF, NIHF, and matched healthy controls. The overall study population comprised 43 patients suffering from HF and 42 healthy donors, carefully selected according to inclusion/exclusion criteria. Patients with HF were divided into two groups based on HF etiology [3]: 19 with IHF and 25 with NIHF. Both HF groups were homogeneous in age, gender, BNP levels and LVEF. As expected, IHF and NIHF showed higher BNP levels and lower LVEFs compared to healthy controls (Table 1).

Table 1. Demographic and clinical characteristics of patients with ischemic heart failure (IHF) or non-ischemic heart failure (NIHF) and healthy controls.

Characteristics	Healthy Controls (*N* = 42)	IHF (*N* = 19)	NIHF (*N* = 25)
Age-median years (range)	75.5 (46–98)	77 (54–87)	65 (45–87)
Gender male-no. (%)	16 (38.1)	12 (63.1)	16 (64)
BMI (kg/m^2)	25.2 ± 4.1	25.4 ± 3.0	25.5 ± 4.2
Caucasian (%)	100	100	100
BNP (pg/mL)	50.6 ± 32.0	1025.8 ± 733.3 *	968.6 ± 802.2 *
Leukocytes (×10^3/mm^3)	7.2 ± 2.5	8.6 ± 4.1	7.9 ± 3.0
GFR (mL/min)	71.2 ± 23.3	48.5 ± 24.3	69.6 ± 32.4
LVEF (%)	61.6 ± 5.8	34.3 ± 6.9 *	34.6 ± 7.4 *

Data are expressed as the mean ± standard deviation of the mean (BMI, BNP, Leukocytes, GFR, LVEF) or median value (Age). IHF: ischemic heart failure; NIHF: non-ischemic heart failure; BNP: B-type natriuretic peptide; GFR: glomerular filtration rate (assessed through CKD-EPI equation); LVEF: left ventricular ejection fraction. * $p < 0.01$ when compared to healthy controls analyzed by one-way ANOVA and Bonferroni's multiple comparison test.

3.2. Plasma Concentrations of ANGPT1, ANGPT2, VEGF-A, VEGF-C, VEGF-D and PLA_2 Activity in Healthy Controls and HF Patients

As shown in Figure 1, lower concentrations of ANGPT1 and higher levels of ANGPT2 and ANGPT2/ANGPT1 ratios were detected in subjects suffering from HF compared to healthy controls. No differences were observed in plasma concentrations of VEGF-A and VEGF-C in the two groups (Figure 2). Otherwise, HF patients presented higher concentrations of VEGF-D compared to controls. Moreover, HF was associated with higher PLA_2 activity (Figure 3).

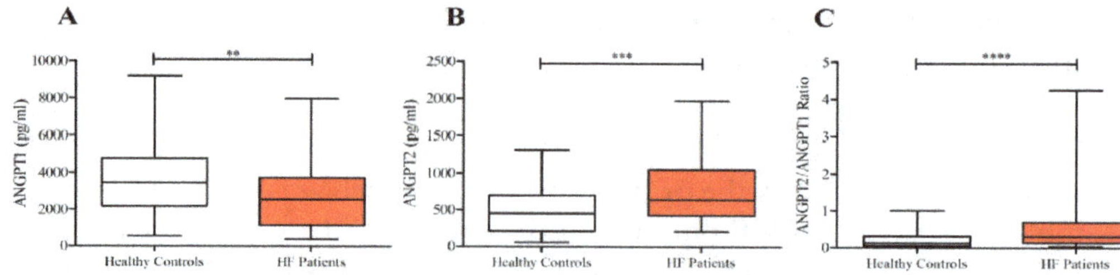

Figure 1. (**A**) Plasma concentrations of angiopoietin-1 (ANGPT1) in heart failure (HF) patients and in healthy controls; (**B**) Plasma concentrations of ANGPT2 in HF patients and in healthy controls; (**C**) ANGPT2/ANGPT1 ratio in HF patients and in healthy controls. Data are shown as the median (horizontal block line), the 25th and 75th percentiles (boxes), and the 5th and 95th percentiles (whiskers) (statistical analysis was performed by a Student's t-test). ** $p < 0.01$; *** $p < 0.001$; **** $p < 0.0001$.

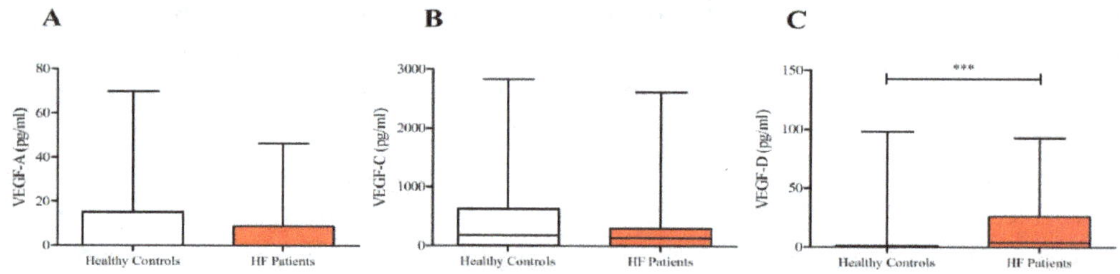

Figure 2. (**A**) Plasma concentrations ofvascular endothelial growth factor-A (VEGF-A) in heart failure (HF) patients and in healthy controls; (**B**) plasma concentrations of VEGF-C in HF patients and in healthy controls; (**C**) plasma concentrations of VEGF-D in HF patients and in healthy controls. Data are shown as the median (horizontal block line), the 25th and 75th percentiles (boxes), and the 5th and 95th percentiles (whiskers) (statistical analysis was performed by a Student's t-test). *** $p < 0.001$.

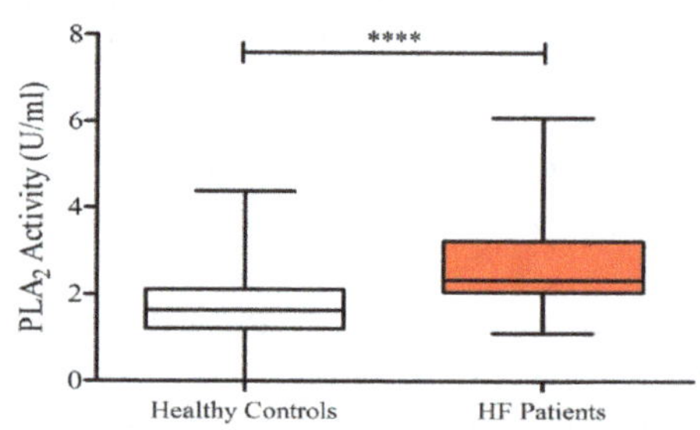

Figure 3. Plasma concentrations of $sPLA_2$ activity in HF patients and in healthy controls. Data are shown as the median (horizontal block line), the 25th and 75th percentiles (boxes), and the 5th and 95th percentiles (whiskers) (statistical analysis was performed by a Student's t-test). **** $p < 0.0001$.

3.3. Plasma Concentrations of ANGPT1, ANGPT2 and Their Ratio in Patients With IHF and NIHF

The concentrations of ANGPT1 were significantly reduced in NIHF compared to controls (Figure 4A). By contrast, the plasma concentrations of ANGPT2 were selectively increased only in NIHF compared to healthy donors (Figure 4B). Similarly, the ANGPT2/ANGPT1 ratio, a parameter of vascular permeability [63], was also increased only in NIHF patients compared to controls (Figure 4C). Importantly, no difference emerged between IHF group and healthy controls in the ANGPT2/ANGPT1 ratio, whereas there was a significant difference between the ANGPT2/ANGPT1 ratio in NIHF vs. IHF (Figure 4C). There were no differences in ANGPT1 or ANGPT2 between male and female values in both controls and patients. Moreover, the age of patients and the concentrations of the different mediators examined did not correlate.

3.4. Plasma Concentrations of VEGF-A, VEGF-C, and VEGF-C in Patients with IHF and NIHF

VEGF-A is a powerful permeability [42] and angiogenic mediator [41]. Elevated concentrations of VEGF-A have been found in patients with acute myocardial ischemia [28,47–50]. By contrast, the role of

VEGF-A in chronic heart failure remains unclear [32]. We found that the mean plasma concentrations of VEGF-A were essentially similar in patients with different types of HF and controls (Figure 5A).

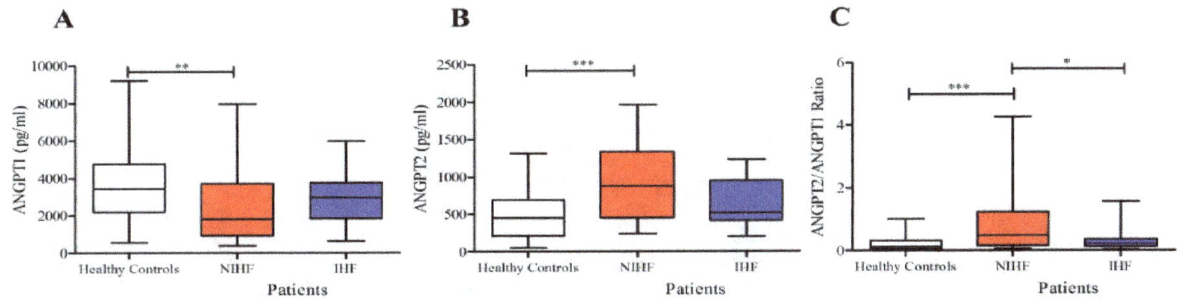

Figure 4. (**A**) Plasma concentrations of angiopoietin-1 (ANGPT1) in ischemic (IHF) and non-ischemic (NIHF) patients, and in healthy controls; (**B**) plasma concentrations of ANGPT2 in IHF and NIHF patients, and in healthy controls; (**C**) ANGPT2/ANGPT1 ratio in IHF and NIHF patients, and in healthy controls. Data are shown as the median (horizontal block line), the 25th and 75th percentiles (boxes), and the 5th and 95th percentiles (whiskers) (statistical analysis was performed by one-way ANOVA and Bonferroni's multiple comparison test). * $p < 0.05$; ** $p < 0.01$; *** $p < 0.001$.

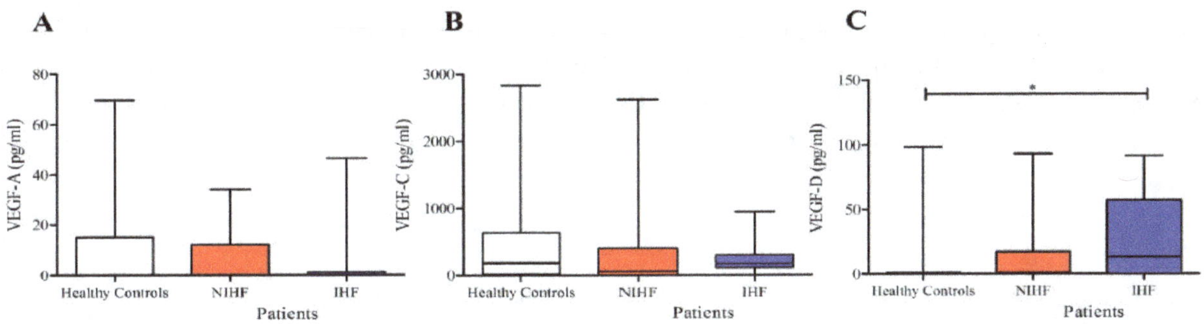

Figure 5. (**A**) Plasma concentrations of VEGF-A in IHF and NIHF patients and in healthy controls; (**B**) plasma concentrations of VEGF-C in IHF and NIHF patients and in healthy controls; (**C**) plasma concentrations of VEGF-D in IHF and NIHF patients and in healthy controls. Data are shown as the median (horizontal block line), the 25th and 75th percentiles (boxes), and the 5th and 95th percentiles (whiskers) (statistical analysis was performed by one-way ANOVA and Bonferroni's multiple comparison test). * $p < 0.05$

VEGF-C and VEGF-D are known to play a major role as lymphangiogenic factors acting on VEGF receptor 3 (VEGFR3) on lymphatic endothelial cells (LECs) [64,65]. More recently, it has been shown that these factors are produced by human cardiac mast cells [43] and, under certain circumstances, can exert a protective effect in cardiovascular disorders [66,67]. In addition, it has been demonstrated that VEGF-C and VEGF-D can exert different effects [45]. The mean plasma concentrations of VEGF-C did not differ in patients with different HF types and controls (Figure 5B). In contrast, the plasma concentrations of VEGF-D were increased in IHF patients compared to healthy controls (Figure 5C). There were no differences in VEGF-A, VEGF-C, and VEGF-D concentrations between male and female values in either controls and patients. Moreover, the age of patients and the concentrations of VEGFs examined did not correlate.

3.5. Plasma Concentrations of $sPLA_2$ Activity in Patients With IHF and NIHF

$sPLA_2$ modulates vascular permeability [55] and promotes inflammation [52,53,56]. Circulating $sPLA_2$ levels increase the risk of early atherosclerosis [62] and predict long-term mortality of HF after myocardial infarction [60]. Figure 6 shows that plasma activity of $sPLA_2$ activity was significantly increased in both groups of HF patients compared to healthy controls. There was no differences in

$sPLA_2$ activity between male and female values in both controls and patients. Moreover, the age of patients and the concentration of $sPLA_2$ activity did not correlate.

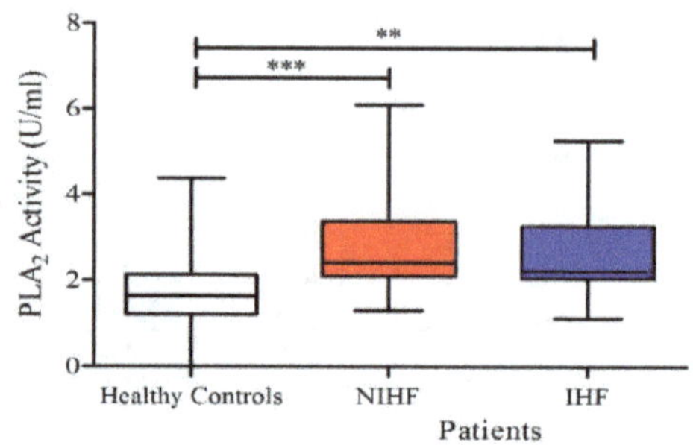

Figure 6. Plasma concentrations of $sPLA_2$ activity in IHF and NIHF patients and in healthy controls. Data are shown as the median (horizontal block line), the 25th and 75th percentiles (boxes), and the 5th and 95th percentiles (whiskers) (statistical analysis was performed by one-way ANOVA and Bonferroni's multiple comparison test). ** $p < 0.01$; *** $p < 0.001$.

3.6. Correlations between ANGPT1 or ANGPT2 Plasma Concentrations and $sPLA_2$ Activity in Patients with IHF and NIHF

As shown in Figure 7, there was an inverse correlation between plasma concentrations of ANGPT2 and ANGPT1 (Figure 7A) and $sPLA_2$ activity and ANGPT1 (Figure 7B) in NIHF patients. Furthermore, a positive correlation between PLA_2 activity and ANGPT2 was detected in NIHF (Figure 7C). No correlation was observed between $sPLA_2$ activity and the ANGPT2/ANGPT1 ratio in NIHF.

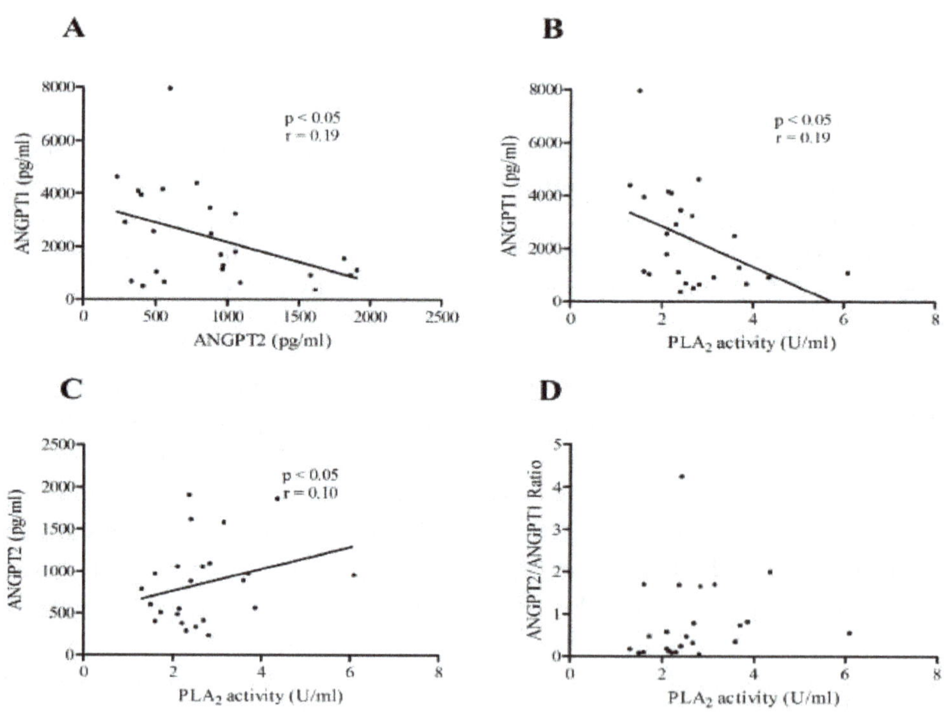

Figure 7. (**A**) Correlations between the plasma concentrations of ANGPT2 and ANGPT1 in NIHF patients; (**B**) correlation between circulating $sPLA_2$ activity and the concentration of ANGPT1 in NIHF patients; (**C**) correlation between the plasma concentration of $sPLA_2$ activity and ANGPT2 in NIHF patients; (**D**) correlation between the plasma concentration of $sPLA_2$ activity and the ANGPT2/ANGPT1 ratio in NIHF patients. Spearman's correlation coefficients (r) were calculated and are shown in the panels.

Contrariwise, no correlations were observed among the plasma concentrations of ANGPT1 and BNP, ANGPT2 and BNP, and $sPLA_2$ activity and BNP in NIHF patients. Similarly, no correlations were found between plasma concentrations of ANGPT1, ANGPT2, and $sPLA_2$ activity vs. LVEF in patients with IHF or NIHR.

4. Discussion

To the best of our knowledge, this is the first study reporting significant and distinct alterations of plasma concentrations from three different classes of proinflammatory mediators that are essential for vascular development, integrity and remodeling (i.e., angiopoietins, VEGFs, and secretory phospholipase A_2) in patients with two forms of HF (i.e., ischemic and non-ischemic).

ANGPTs bind to and activate the Tie2 receptor on endothelial cells [9,27]. ANGPT1, produced by periendothelial mural cells [16] acts as a vascular stabilizer by affecting the connections between endothelial cells and the cytoskeleton [68]. In contrast, ANGPT2, produced by blood endothelial cells [23], is rapidly released from Wiebel–Palade bodies in response to various stimuli [24]. ANGPT2 also binds to Tie2 [27] and antagonizes ANGPT1-mediated Tie2 phosphorylation, thereby inducing vascular instability and leakage [25,26,69]. In addition, ANGPT2 is an important permeability [63,70] and proinflammatory mediator [16].

Elevated circulating levels of ANGPT2 have been reported in acute coronary syndromes [28,29], and this mediator has been proposed as a negative prognostic marker after myocardial infarction [34] and PCI [35,36]. ANGPT2 is associated with a greater risk of cardiovascular mortality in the general population [71], as well as with higher mortality in patients suffering from myocardial infarction and cardiogenic shock [29,72]. A recent report demonstrates that ANGPT2 is highly expressed in endothelial cells at the border of the infarct area after ischemic injury in mice [15]. In the remodeling phase after myocardial infarction, endothelial- and macrophage-derived ANGPT2 promotes abnormal vascular remodeling and exacerbates inflammation. In contrast, ANGPT1 plays a protective role in preclinical models of vascular injury [37,38] and exerts anti-inflammatory effects [20].

Our study shows that HF is associated with reduced ANGPT1 plasma concentrations, increased ANGPT2 levels, and an increased ANGPT2/ANGPT1 ratio as compared with healthy controls. Of importance, different alterations of ANGPT1 and ANGPT2 expression have been detected in patients with IHF and NIHF. For instance, plasma levels of ANGPT1 are significantly decreased only in NIHF, but not in IHF patients compared to controls. Contrarywise, circulating levels of ANGPT2 are increased in NIHF, but not in IHF patients compared to healthy donors. Moreover, the ANGPT2/ANGPT1 ratio, an index of vascular permeability [63], was exclusively increased only in NIHF patients.

We did not find a correlation between plasma concentrations of ANGPT1 or ANGPT2 and BNP in either IHF or NIHF patients. In contrast, a recent study reported a significant correlation between serum concentrations of ANGPT2 and NT-proBNP in more than 200 patients that had undergone diagnostic cardiac catheterization [73]. Several explanations can justify these apparently different results. The latter study included patients with (54%) or without coronary artery disease, as well as with comorbidities (e.g., diabetes, hypertension) that may have influenced the results. In our study, the population of IHF and NIHF participants was selectively included, and patients with comorbidities were not selected. Although the two examined cohorts were rather small, the patients examined in our study were very homogeneous for the principal clinical and demographic features.

Our results may have clinical implications for patients suffering from HF. First, if confirmed in larger cohorts, the evaluation of plasma concentrations of ANGPT1, ANGPT2, and their ratio may be useful in the identification of different pathophysiological patterns underlying ischemic and non-ischemic HF. Second, the unique role of the ANGPTs/Tie2 signaling pathway in vascular stability suggests that it could serve as a target for therapeutic intervention in diseases whose pathophysiology comprises the alteration of vascular integrity [27], such as HF. Recently, it has been demonstrated that ANGPT2 inhibition, through an anti-ANGPT2 blocking antibody, substantially alleviated autoimmune inflammation [70]. Importantly, specific ANGPT2 deletion or the use of an anti-ANGPT2 antibody markedly reduced cardiac hypoxia, proinflammatory macrophage polarization, adverse vascular remodeling, and the consequent progression of HF after myocardial infarction in mice [15]. The results of the latter study contribute to elucidating the roles of ANGPT2 in the pathogenesis of post-ischemic cardiovascular remodeling. Finally, these fascinating experimental results designate ANGPT2 as a promising therapeutic target to prevent/ameliorate HF.

VEGF-A is a powerful permeability factor [42] and a potent proangiogenic and proinflammatory mediator [41,74]. Although several clinical studies have found elevated circulating levels of VEGF-A in myocardial infarction [28,47–50], the role of this mediator in HF still remains poorly elucidated. Our results show that, differently from acute vascular injuries, plasma levels of VEGF-A are not altered in the overall HF population or in either IHF or NIHF patients. Thus, our results suggest that this mediator could play different roles in an acute vs. chronic setting of myocardial ischemia.

VEGF-C and VEGF-D are major lymphangiogenic factors produced by human macrophages [52,75] and cardiac mast cells [43]. In a mouse model of HF, VEGF-C and VEGF-D were upregulated in the early stages of disease, with levels returning afterwards to baseline [76]. Levels of VEGF-C have been reported as elevated in patients with ischemic or non-ischemic cardiomyopathy [77]. An increased level of VEGF-D was found in an animal model of ischemic cardiomyopathy [78] as well as in human atherosclerotic lesions [79]. Recent evidence indicates that lymphangiogenesis [66] and VEGF-C improve cardiac functions after experimental myocardial infarction [80]. Our results indicate that the plasma concentrations of VEGF-C were similar in patients with HF (IHF and NIHF) and controls. Interestingly, the circulating concentrations of VEGF-D were increased in HF patients compared to controls, but significant differences were exclusively detected in IHF patients. The differential alterations of VEGF-C and VEGF-D in these patients is intriguing but not surprising. In fact, recent evidence demonstrates that VEGF-C and VEGF-D can differently modulate the immune system [45]. The possible role of VEGF-D in HF patients deserves further investigations.

PLA_2 activity was found increased in plasma from both groups of HF patients compared to healthy controls. PLA_2 modulates endothelial cell migration and vascular permeability in vitro and in humans [53,55–57,81]. Previous studies have demonstrated that circulating levels of $sPLA_2$ predict coronary events in patients with coronary artery disease [58], as well as in apparently healthy men and women [59]. Moreover, serum $sPLA_2$ levels also predicts readmission for HF after myocardial infarction [60]. More recently, elevated circulatory levels of $sPLA_2$ were associated with risk of early atherosclerosis [62]. Our study is, to our knowledge, the first to demonstrate that high plasma concentrations of PLA_2 activity can be found in HF patients, both with an ischemic and non-ischemic etiology.

Along with the epidemiologic transition of global population, the pathophysiology of HF has changed over time. According to the Framingham Heart Study, hypertension represented the most frequently associated condition in HF patients, irrespective of LVEF [82]. It is widely recognized that coronary heart disease represents the predominant cause of HFrEF [83]. Coronary stenosis-dependent cardiomyocyte hypoxia, through inadequate oxygen supply to metabolic needs and leading to ventricular dysfunction, may be the result of both acute and chronic cardiac ischemia. Indeed, in acute coronary syndromes, a sudden drop in myocardial perfusion rapidly determines cardiomyocyte injury. In the setting of chronic ischemia there is often an imbalance between coronary blood flow and augmented demand due to progressive atherosclerosis, especially under stress. This leads over time to hibernation, stunning, and secondary myocardial remodeling, resulting in reduced cardiac output [84].

NIHF pathophysiology is more heterogeneous due to several etiologic factors that are sometimes concurrent. The most relevant causes of NIHF are represented by primary valvular diseases, arterial hypertension, microbial cardiomyopathy, DM, toxic agents (drugs or alcohol), and genetic cardiomyopathies. Once all the listed factors have been excluded, idiopathic HF is the resulting diagnosis [85]. In NIHF there is a primary injury in the cardiomyocyte structure and function that manifests in cell apoptosis and a consequent substitution with fribotic tissue, without alteration in coronary flow.

However, independently from ischemic or non-ischemic etiology, all patients suffering from systolic HF present reduction of LVEF, maladaptive LV remodeling, and similar clinical presentations including dyspnea and hydro-saline retention. Our results identify an HF-dependent impact on the expression levels of several vascular permeability and inflammatory mediators, with different patterns in the clinical setting of NIHF and IHF that potentially reflect the above-mentioned pathophysiological differences.

Several immune cells produce $sPLA_2$ [86–88], ANGPTs [15,17,18,24,70,89], VEGF-A [43,52,74,90], and VEGF-C/VEGF-D [52,74,91]. In this study, we did not address the issue of the contribution of different cells to the increased plasma levels of these powerful inflammatory mediators observed in patients with IHF or NIHF. ANGPT2 appears to be a potential therapeutic option in experimental heart failure [15]. Future studies with the aim of identifying the cellular sources of these powerful mediators could lead to the identification of novel and selective therapeutic targets in IHF and NIHF patients.

The limited number of subjects enrolled represented the main limitation of the present investigation. However, it is important to point out that in order to identify specific differences between NIHF and IHF the study protocol included stringent exclusion criteria to reduce potential interference with the inflammatory and angiogenic patterns explored in the study. Indeed, very common comorbidities such as COPD, DM, immune disorders, malignancies, and severe obesity were excluded from the study. As a consequence, the patients examined were very homogeneous, but rather small. The results of this preliminary study will have to be extended in a future multicenter trial examining larger cohorts of IHF and NIHF patients.

5. Conclusions

In the present study we demonstrated that the ANGPT system is selectively modulated in NIHF patients, with an increased ANGPT2/ANGPT1 ratio compared to IHF and controls, whereas VEGF-D was exclusively augmented in IHF patients. In contrast, sPLA2 activity was increased in both IHF and NIHF patients compared to healthy controls. To the best of our knowledge this represents the first evidence reporting that several regulators of vascular permeability and inflammation is specifically altered in patients with IHF and NIHF, paving the way for the identification of new molecular mechanisms underlying HF pathophysiology and novel therapeutic targets.

Author Contributions: Conceptualization, G.V., S.L., G.M., and G.R.; methodology, S.L., L.B., G.G., and G.R.; software, S.L. and A.L.F.; validation, G.V., G.M., and G.R.; formal analysis, G.V., S.L., L.B., and A.L.F.; investigation, G.V., S.L., and A.L.F.; resources, G.M.; data curation, G.V., S.L., L.B., A.L.F., and G.R.; writing—original draft preparation, G.V., S.L., L.B., and G.M.; writing—review and editing, G.V., S.L., N.F., A.d.P., G.M., and G.R.; supervision, G.V., S.L., G.M., and G.R.; project administration, G.V., S.L., G.M., and G.R.; funding acquisition, G.M. All authors have read and agreed to the published version of the manuscript.

Acknowledgments: The authors apologize to the many researchers who contributed importantly to this field and whose works were not cited because of space and citation restrictions. Leonardo Bencivenga has been supported by a research grant provided by the Cardiopath PhD program. The authors thank Gjada Criscuolo for a critical reading of the manuscript.

Abbreviations

ACE	angiotensin-converting enzyme
ANGPT	angiopoietin
ARB	angiotensin receptor blocker
BMI	body mass index
BNP	B-type natriuretic peptide
COPD	chronic obstructive pulmonary disease
DM	diabetes mellitus

DOPC	dioleoylphosphatidylcholine
DOPG	dioleoyphosphatidylglycerol
EF	ejection fraction
GFR	glomerular filtration rate
HF	heart failure
IHF	ischemic heart failure
LVEF	left ventricular ejection fraction
NIHF	non-ischemic heart failure
PLA_2	phospholipase A_2
VEGF	vascular endothelial growth factor
VEGFR	vascular endothelial growth factor receptor

References

1. Hershberger, R.E.; Hedges, D.J.; Morales, A. Dilated cardiomyopathy: The complexity of a diverse genetic architecture. *Nat. Rev. Cardiol.* **2013**, *10*, 531–547. [CrossRef] [PubMed]
2. Ponikowski, P.; Voors, A.A.; Anker, S.D.; Bueno, H.; Cleland, J.G.F.; Coats, A.J.S.; Falk, V.; Gonzalez-Juanatey, J.R.; Harjola, V.P.; Jankowska, E.A.; et al. 2016 ESC Guidelines for the diagnosis and treatment of acute and chronic heart failure: The Task Force for the diagnosis and treatment of acute and chronic heart failure of the European Society of Cardiology (ESC) Developed with the special contribution of the Heart Failure Association (HFA) of the ESC. *Eur. Heart J.* **2016**, *37*, 2129–2200. [PubMed]
3. McNally, E.M.; Mestroni, L. Dilated cardiomyopathy: Genetic determinants and mechanisms. *Circ. Res.* **2017**, *121*, 731–748. [CrossRef] [PubMed]
4. Bozkurt, B.; Colvin, M.; Cook, J.; Cooper, L.T.; Deswal, A.; Fonarow, G.C.; Francis, G.S.; Lenihan, D.; Lewis, E.F.; McNamara, D.M.; et al. Current diagnostic and treatment strategies for specific dilated cardiomyopathies: A scientific statement from the american heart association. *Circulation* **2016**, *134*, e579–e646. [CrossRef] [PubMed]
5. Hartupee, J.; Mann, D.L. Neurohormonal activation in heart failure with reduced ejection fraction. *Nat. Rev. Cardiol.* **2017**, *14*, 30–38. [CrossRef]
6. Braunwald, E. Biomarkers in heart failure. *N. Engl. J. Med.* **2008**, *358*, 2148–2159. [CrossRef]
7. Wang, Q.; Zhao, Z.; Zhang, X.; Lu, C.; Ren, S.; Li, S.; Guo, J.; Liao, P.; Jiang, B.; Zheng, Y. Identifying microRNAs and their editing sites in Macaca mulatta. *Cells* **2019**, *8*, 682. [CrossRef]
8. Fiedler, U.; Augustin, H.G. Angiopoietins: A link between angiogenesis and inflammation. *Trends Immunol.* **2006**, *27*, 552–558. [CrossRef]
9. Akwii, R.G.; Sajib, M.S.; Zahra, F.T.; Mikelis, C.M. Role of Angiopoietin-2 in vascular physiology and pathophysiology. *Cells* **2019**, *8*, 471. [CrossRef]
10. Maisonpierre, P.C.; Suri, C.; Jones, P.F.; Bartunkova, S.; Wiegand, S.J.; Radziejewski, C.; Compton, D.; McClain, J.; Aldrich, T.H.; Papadopoulos, N.; et al. Angiopoietin-2, a natural antagonist for Tie2 that disrupts in vivo angiogenesis. *Science* **1997**, *277*, 55–60. [CrossRef]
11. Suri, C.; Jones, P.F.; Patan, S.; Bartunkova, S.; Maisonpierre, P.C.; Davis, S.; Sato, T.N.; Yancopoulos, G.D. Requisite role of angiopoietin-1, a ligand for the TIE2 receptor, during embryonic angiogenesis. *Cell* **1996**, *87*, 1171–1180. [CrossRef]
12. Fagiani, E.; Lorentz, P.; Kopfstein, L.; Christofori, G. Angiopoietin-1 and -2 exert antagonistic functions in tumor angiogenesis, yet both induce lymphangiogenesis. *Cancer Res.* **2011**, *71*, 5717–5727. [CrossRef] [PubMed]
13. Schulz, P.; Fischer, C.; Detjen, K.M.; Rieke, S.; Hilfenhaus, G.; von Marschall, Z.; Bohmig, M.; Koch, I.; Kehrberger, J.; Hauff, P.; et al. Angiopoietin-2 drives lymphatic metastasis of pancreatic cancer. *FASEB J.* **2011**, *25*, 3325–3335. [CrossRef] [PubMed]
14. Eklund, L.; Kangas, J.; Saharinen, P. Angiopoietin-Tie signalling in the cardiovascular and lymphatic systems. *Clin. Sci. (Lond.)* **2017**, *131*, 87–103. [CrossRef] [PubMed]
15. Lee, S.J.; Lee, C.K.; Kang, S.; Park, I.; Kim, Y.H.; Kim, S.K.; Hong, S.P.; Bae, H.; He, Y.; Kubota, Y.; et al. Angiopoietin-2 exacerbates cardiac hypoxia and inflammation after myocardial infarction. *J. Clin. Investig.* **2018**, *128*, 5018–5033. [CrossRef]
16. Daneman, R.; Zhou, L.; Kebede, A.A.; Barres, B.A. Pericytes are required for blood-brain barrier integrity during embryogenesis. *Nature* **2010**, *468*, 562–566. [CrossRef]

17. Prevete, N.; Staiano, R.I.; Granata, F.; Detoraki, A.; Necchi, V.; Ricci, V.; Triggiani, M.; De Paulis, A.; Marone, G.; Genovese, A. Expression and function of Angiopoietins and their tie receptors in human basophils and mast cells. *J. Biol. Regul. Homeost. Agents* **2013**, *27*, 827–839.
18. Fang, H.Y.; Hughes, R.; Murdoch, C.; Coffelt, S.B.; Biswas, S.K.; Harris, A.L.; Johnson, R.S.; Imityaz, H.Z.; Simon, M.C.; Fredlund, E.; et al. Hypoxia-inducible factors 1 and 2 are important transcriptional effectors in primary macrophages experiencing hypoxia. *Blood* **2009**, *114*, 844–859. [CrossRef]
19. Davis, S.; Aldrich, T.H.; Jones, P.F.; Acheson, A.; Compton, D.L.; Jain, V.; Ryan, T.E.; Bruno, J.; Radziejewski, C.; Maisonpierre, P.C.; et al. Isolation of angiopoietin-1, a ligand for the TIE2 receptor, by secretion-trap expression cloning. *Cell* **1996**, *87*, 1161–1169. [CrossRef]
20. Gamble, J.R.; Drew, J.; Trezise, L.; Underwood, A.; Parsons, M.; Kasminkas, L.; Rudge, J.; Yancopoulos, G.; Vadas, M.A. Angiopoietin-1 is an antipermeability and anti-inflammatory agent in vitro and targets cell junctions. *Circ. Res.* **2000**, *87*, 603–607. [CrossRef]
21. Jeansson, M.; Gawlik, A.; Anderson, G.; Li, C.; Kerjaschki, D.; Henkelman, M.; Quaggin, S.E. Angiopoietin-1 is essential in mouse vasculature during development and in response to injury. *J. Clin. Investig.* **2011**, *121*, 2278–2289. [CrossRef] [PubMed]
22. Thurston, G.; Rudge, J.S.; Ioffe, E.; Zhou, H.; Ross, L.; Croll, S.D.; Glazer, N.; Holash, J.; McDonald, D.M.; Yancopoulos, G.D. Angiopoietin-1 protects the adult vasculature against plasma leakage. *Nat. Med.* **2000**, *6*, 460–463. [CrossRef]
23. Gehling, U.M.; Ergun, S.; Schumacher, U.; Wagener, C.; Pantel, K.; Otte, M.; Schuch, G.; Schafhausen, P.; Mende, T.; Kilic, N.; et al. In vitro differentiation of endothelial cells from AC133-positive progenitor cells. *Blood* **2000**, *95*, 3106–3112. [CrossRef] [PubMed]
24. Fiedler, U.; Scharpfenecker, M.; Koidl, S.; Hegen, A.; Grunow, V.; Schmidt, J.M.; Kriz, W.; Thurston, G.; Augustin, H.G. The Tie-2 ligand angiopoietin-2 is stored in and rapidly released upon stimulation from endothelial cell Weibel-Palade bodies. *Blood* **2004**, *103*, 4150–4156. [CrossRef] [PubMed]
25. Fiedler, U.; Reiss, Y.; Scharpfenecker, M.; Grunow, V.; Koidl, S.; Thurston, G.; Gale, N.W.; Witzenrath, M.; Rosseau, S.; Suttorp, N.; et al. Angiopoietin-2 sensitizes endothelial cells to TNF-alpha and has a crucial role in the induction of inflammation. *Nat. Med.* **2006**, *12*, 235–239. [CrossRef]
26. Roviezzo, F.; Tsigkos, S.; Kotanidou, A.; Bucci, M.; Brancaleone, V.; Cirino, G.; Papapetropoulos, A. Angiopoietin-2 causes inflammation in vivo by promoting vascular leakage. *J. Pharmacol. Exp. Ther.* **2005**, *314*, 738–744. [CrossRef]
27. Saharinen, P.; Eklund, L.; Alitalo, K. Therapeutic targeting of the angiopoietin-TIE pathway. *Nat. Rev. Drug Discov.* **2017**, *16*, 635–661. [CrossRef]
28. Lee, K.W.; Lip, G.Y.; Blann, A.D. Plasma angiopoietin-1, angiopoietin-2, angiopoietin receptor tie-2, and vascular endothelial growth factor levels in acute coronary syndromes. *Circulation* **2004**, *110*, 2355–2360. [CrossRef]
29. Poss, J.; Fuernau, G.; Denks, D.; Desch, S.; Eitel, I.; de Waha, S.; Link, A.; Schuler, G.; Adams, V.; Bohm, M.; et al. Angiopoietin-2 in acute myocardial infarction complicated by cardiogenic shock—A biomarker substudy of the IABP-SHOCK II-Trial. *Eur. J. Heart Fail.* **2015**, *17*, 1152–1160. [CrossRef]
30. Patel, J.V.; Lim, H.S.; Varughese, G.I.; Hughes, E.A.; Lip, G.Y. Angiopoietin-2 levels as a biomarker of cardiovascular risk in patients with hypertension. *Ann. Med.* **2008**, *40*, 215–222. [CrossRef]
31. David, S.; Kumpers, P.; Lukasz, A.; Kielstein, J.T.; Haller, H.; Fliser, D. Circulating angiopoietin-2 in essential hypertension: Relation to atherosclerosis, vascular inflammation, and treatment with olmesartan/pravastatin. *J. Hypertens.* **2009**, *27*, 1641–1647. [CrossRef] [PubMed]
32. Chong, A.Y.; Caine, G.J.; Freestone, B.; Blann, A.D.; Lip, G.Y. Plasma angiopoietin-1, angiopoietin-2, and angiopoietin receptor tie-2 levels in congestive heart failure. *J. Am. Coll. Cardiol.* **2004**, *43*, 423–428. [CrossRef] [PubMed]
33. Lukasz, A.; Beutel, G.; Kumpers, P.; Denecke, A.; Westhoff-Bleck, M.; Schieffer, B.; Bauersachs, J.; Kielstein, J.T.; Tutarel, O. Angiopoietin-2 in adults with congenital heart disease and heart failure. *PLoS ONE* **2013**, *8*, e66861. [CrossRef] [PubMed]
34. Iribarren, C.; Phelps, B.H.; Darbinian, J.A.; McCluskey, E.R.; Quesenberry, C.P.; Hytopoulos, E.; Vogelman, J.H.; Orentreich, N. Circulating angiopoietins-1 and -2, angiopoietin receptor Tie-2 and vascular endothelial growth factor-A as biomarkers of acute myocardial infarction: A prospective nested case-control study. *BMC Cardiovasc. Disord.* **2011**, *11*, 31. [CrossRef] [PubMed]

35. Jian, W.; Li, L.; Wei, X.M.; Wu, C.Q.; Gui, C. Prognostic value of angiopoietin-2 for patients with coronary heart disease after elective PCI. *Medicine (Baltimore)* **2019**, *98*, e14216. [CrossRef]
36. Zeng, Z.Y.; Gui, C.; Li, L.; Wei, X.M. Effects of percutaneous coronary intervention on serum Angiopoietin-2 in patients with coronary heart disease. *Chin. Med. J. (Engl.)* **2016**, *129*, 631–635. [CrossRef]
37. Moxon, J.V.; Trollope, A.F.; Dewdney, B.; de Hollander, C.; Nastasi, D.R.; Maguire, J.M.; Golledge, J. The effect of angiopoietin-1 upregulation on the outcome of acute ischaemic stroke in rodent models: A meta-analysis. *J. Cereb. Blood Flow Metab.* **2019**, *39*, 2343–2354. [CrossRef]
38. Chiang, W.C.; Huang, Y.C.; Fu, T.I.; Chen, P.M.; Chang, F.C.; Lai, C.F.; Wu, V.C.; Lin, S.L.; Chen, Y.M. Angiopoietin 1 influences ischemic reperfusion renal injury via modulating endothelium survival and regeneration. *Mol. Med.* **2019**, *25*, 5. [CrossRef]
39. Varricchi, G.; Loffredo, S.; Galdiero, M.R.; Marone, G.; Cristinziano, L.; Granata, F.; Marone, G. Innate effector cells in angiogenesis and lymphangiogenesis. *Curr. Opin. Immunol.* **2018**, *53*, 152–160. [CrossRef]
40. Varricchi, G.; de Paulis, A.; Marone, G.; Galli, S.J. Future Needs in Mast Cell Biology. *Int. J. Mol. Sci.* **2019**, *20*, 4397. [CrossRef]
41. Sammarco, G.; Varricchi, G.; Ferraro, V.; Ammendola, M.; De Fazio, M.; Altomare, D.F.; Luposella, M.; Maltese, L.; Curro, G.; Marone, G.; et al. Mast cells, angiogenesis and lymphangiogenesis in human gastric cancer. *Int. J. Mol. Sci.* **2019**, *20*, 2106. [CrossRef] [PubMed]
42. Senger, D.R.; Galli, S.J.; Dvorak, A.M.; Perruzzi, C.A.; Harvey, V.S.; Dvorak, H.F. Tumor cells secrete a vascular permeability factor that promotes accumulation of ascites fluid. *Science* **1983**, *219*, 983–985. [CrossRef] [PubMed]
43. Varricchi, G.; Loffredo, S.; Borriello, F.; Pecoraro, A.; Rivellese, F.; Genovese, A.; Spadaro, G.; Marone, G. Superantigenic activation of human cardiac mast cells. *Int. J. Mol. Sci.* **2019**, *20*, 1828. [CrossRef] [PubMed]
44. Varricchi, G.; Pecoraro, A.; Marone, G.; Criscuolo, G.; Spadaro, G.; Genovese, A.; Marone, G. Thymic stromal lymphopoietin isoforms, inflammatory disorders, and cancer. *Front. Immunol.* **2018**, *9*, 1595. [CrossRef] [PubMed]
45. Fankhauser, M.; Broggi, M.A.S.; Potin, L.; Bordry, N.; Jeanbart, L.; Lund, A.W.; Da Costa, E.; Hauert, S.; Rincon-Restrepo, M.; Tremblay, C.; et al. Tumor lymphangiogenesis promotes T cell infiltration and potentiates immunotherapy in melanoma. *Sci. Transl. Med.* **2017**, *9*, eaal4712. [CrossRef] [PubMed]
46. Stacker, S.A.; Williams, S.P.; Karnezis, T.; Shayan, R.; Fox, S.B.; Achen, M.G. Lymphangiogenesis and lymphatic vessel remodelling in cancer. *Nat. Rev. Cancer* **2014**, *14*, 159–172. [CrossRef]
47. Heeschen, C.; Dimmeler, S.; Hamm, C.W.; Boersma, E.; Zeiher, A.M.; Simoons, M.L.; Investigators, C. Prognostic significance of angiogenic growth factor serum levels in patients with acute coronary syndromes. *Circulation* **2003**, *107*, 524–530. [CrossRef]
48. Hojo, Y.; Ikeda, U.; Zhu, Y.; Okada, M.; Ueno, S.; Arakawa, H.; Fujikawa, H.; Katsuki, T.; Shimada, K. Expression of vascular endothelial growth factor in patients with acute myocardial infarction. *J. Am. Coll. Cardiol.* **2000**, *35*, 968–973. [CrossRef]
49. Kawamoto, A.; Kawata, H.; Akai, Y.; Katsuyama, Y.; Takase, E.; Sasaki, Y.; Tsujimura, S.; Sakaguchi, Y.; Iwano, M.; Fujimoto, S.; et al. Serum levels of VEGF and basic FGF in the subacute phase of myocardial infarction. *Int. J. Cardiol.* **1998**, *67*, 47–54. [CrossRef]
50. Kranz, A.; Rau, C.; Kochs, M.; Waltenberger, J. Elevation of vascular endothelial growth factor-A serum levels following acute myocardial infarction. Evidence for its origin and functional significance. *J. Mol. Cell. Cardiol.* **2000**, *32*, 65–72. [CrossRef] [PubMed]
51. Dennis, E.A.; Cao, J.; Hsu, Y.H.; Magrioti, V.; Kokotos, G. Phospholipase A2 enzymes: Physical structure, biological function, disease implication, chemical inhibition, and therapeutic intervention. *Chem. Rev.* **2011**, *111*, 6130–6185. [CrossRef] [PubMed]
52. Granata, F.; Staiano, R.I.; Loffredo, S.; Petraroli, A.; Genovese, A.; Marone, G.; Triggiani, M. The role of mast cell-derived secreted phospholipases A2 in respiratory allergy. *Biochimie* **2010**, *92*, 588–593. [CrossRef] [PubMed]
53. Loffredo, S.; Ferrara, A.L.; Bova, M.; Borriello, F.; Suffritti, C.; Veszeli, N.; Petraroli, A.; Galdiero, M.R.; Varricchi, G.; Granata, F.; et al. Secreted phospholipases A2 in hereditary angioedema with C1-inhibitor deficiency. *Front. Immunol.* **2018**, *9*, 1721. [CrossRef] [PubMed]
54. Murakami, M.; Lambeau, G. Emerging roles of secreted phospholipase A(2) enzymes: An update. *Biochimie* **2013**, *95*, 43–50. [CrossRef] [PubMed]

55. Rizzo, M.T.; Nguyen, E.; Aldo-Benson, M.; Lambeau, G. Secreted phospholipase A(2) induces vascular endothelial cell migration. *Blood* **2000**, *96*, 3809–3815. [CrossRef]
56. Loffredo, S.; Marone, G. Hereditary angioedema: The plasma contact system out of control: Comment. *J. Thromb. Haemost.* **2018**, *16*, 2347–2348. [CrossRef] [PubMed]
57. Lambeau, G.; Gelb, M.H. Biochemistry and physiology of mammalian secreted phospholipases A2. *Ann. Rev. Biochem.* **2008**, *77*, 495–520. [CrossRef] [PubMed]
58. Kugiyama, K.; Ota, Y.; Takazoe, K.; Moriyama, Y.; Kawano, H.; Miyao, Y.; Sakamoto, T.; Soejima, H.; Ogawa, H.; Doi, H.; et al. Circulating levels of secretory type II phospholipase A(2) predict coronary events in patients with coronary artery disease. *Circulation* **1999**, *100*, 1280–1284. [CrossRef] [PubMed]
59. Boekholdt, S.M.; Keller, T.T.; Wareham, N.J.; Luben, R.; Bingham, S.A.; Day, N.E.; Sandhu, M.S.; Jukema, J.W.; Kastelein, J.J.; Hack, C.E.; et al. Serum levels of type II secretory phospholipase A2 and the risk of future coronary artery disease in apparently healthy men and women: The EPIC-Norfolk prospective population study. *Arterioscler. Thromb. Vasc. Biol.* **2005**, *25*, 839–846. [CrossRef]
60. Xin, H.; Chen, Z.Y.; Lv, X.B.; Liu, S.; Lian, Z.X.; Cai, S.L. Serum secretory phospholipase A2-IIa (sPLA2-IIA) levels in patients surviving acute myocardial infarction. *Eur. Rev. Med. Pharmacol. Sci.* **2013**, *17*, 999–1004.
61. Nijmeijer, R.; Meuwissen, M.; Krijnen, P.A.; van der Wal, A.; Piek, J.J.; Visser, C.A.; Hack, C.E.; Niessen, H.W. Secretory type II phospholipase A2 in culprit coronary lesions is associated with myocardial infarction. *Eur. J. Clin. Investig.* **2008**, *38*, 205–210. [CrossRef]
62. Sun, C.Q.; Zhong, C.Y.; Sun, W.W.; Xiao, H.; Zhu, P.; Lin, Y.Z.; Zhang, C.L.; Gao, H.; Song, Z.Y. Elevated Type II secretory phospholipase A2 increases the risk of early atherosclerosis in patients with newly diagnosed metabolic syndrome. *Sci. Rep.* **2016**, *6*, 34929. [CrossRef]
63. Loffredo, S.; Bova, M.; Suffritti, C.; Borriello, F.; Zanichelli, A.; Petraroli, A.; Varricchi, G.; Triggiani, M.; Cicardi, M.; Marone, G. Elevated plasma levels of vascular permeability factors in C1 inhibitor-deficient hereditary angioedema. *Allergy* **2016**, *71*, 989–996. [CrossRef]
64. Randolph, G.J.; Ivanov, S.; Zinselmeyer, B.H.; Scallan, J.P. The lymphatic system: Integral roles in immunity. *Ann. Rev. Immunol.* **2017**, *35*, 31–52. [CrossRef] [PubMed]
65. Zheng, W.; Aspelund, A.; Alitalo, K. Lymphangiogenic factors, mechanisms, and applications. *J. Clin. Investig.* **2014**, *124*, 878–887. [CrossRef] [PubMed]
66. Henri, O.; Pouehe, C.; Houssari, M.; Galas, L.; Nicol, L.; Edwards-Levy, F.; Henry, J.P.; Dumesnil, A.; Boukhalfa, I.; Banquet, S.; et al. Selective stimulation of cardiac lymphangiogenesis reduces myocardial edema and fibrosis leading to improved cardiac function following myocardial infarction. *Circulation* **2016**, *133*, 1484–1497. [CrossRef] [PubMed]
67. Shimizu, Y.; Polavarapu, R.; Eskla, K.L.; Pantner, Y.; Nicholson, C.K.; Ishii, M.; Brunnhoelzl, D.; Mauria, R.; Husain, A.; Naqvi, N.; et al. Impact of Lymphangiogenesis on cardiac remodeling after ischemia and reperfusion injury. *J. Am. Heart Assoc.* **2018**, *7*, e009565. [CrossRef]
68. Karaman, S.; Leppanen, V.M.; Alitalo, K. Vascular endothelial growth factor signaling in development and disease. *Development* **2018**, *145*, dev.151019. [CrossRef]
69. Park, J.S.; Kim, I.K.; Han, S.; Park, I.; Kim, C.; Bae, J.; Oh, S.J.; Lee, S.; Kim, J.H.; Woo, D.C.; et al. Normalization of tumor vessels by Tie2 activation and Ang2 inhibition enhances drug delivery and produces a favorable tumor microenvironment. *Cancer Cell* **2016**, *30*, 953–967. [CrossRef]
70. Li, Z.; Korhonen, E.A.; Merlini, A.; Strauss, J.; Wihuri, E.; Nurmi, H.; Antila, S.; Paech, J.; Deutsch, U.; Engelhardt, B.; et al. Angiopoietin-2 blockade ameliorates autoimmune neuroinflammation by inhibiting leukocyte recruitment into the CNS. *J. Clin. Investig.* **2020**, *130*, 1977–1990. [CrossRef]
71. Lorbeer, R.; Baumeister, S.E.; Dorr, M.; Nauck, M.; Grotevendt, A.; Volzke, H.; Vasan, R.S.; Wallaschofski, H.; Lieb, W. Circulating angiopoietin-2, its soluble receptor Tie-2, and mortality in the general population. *Eur. J. Heart Fail.* **2013**, *15*, 1327–1334. [CrossRef] [PubMed]
72. Link, A.; Poss, J.; Rbah, R.; Barth, C.; Feth, L.; Selejan, S.; Bohm, M. Circulating angiopoietins and cardiovascular mortality in cardiogenic shock. *Eur. Heart J.* **2013**, *34*, 1651–1662. [CrossRef] [PubMed]
73. Jian, W.; Mo, C.H.; Yang, G.L.; Li, L.; Gui, C. Angiopoietin-2 provides no incremental predictive value for the presence of obstructive coronary artery disease over N-terminal pro-brain natriuretic peptide. *J. Clin. Lab. Anal.* **2019**, *33*, e22972. [CrossRef] [PubMed]

74. Detoraki, A.; Staiano, R.I.; Granata, F.; Giannattasio, G.; Prevete, N.; de Paulis, A.; Ribatti, D.; Genovese, A.; Triggiani, M.; Marone, G. Vascular endothelial growth factors synthesized by human lung mast cells exert angiogenic effects. *J. Allergy Clin. Immunol.* **2009**, *123*, 1142–1149.e5. [CrossRef]
75. Staiano, R.I.; Loffredo, S.; Borriello, F.; Iannotti, F.A.; Piscitelli, F.; Orlando, P.; Secondo, A.; Granata, F.; Lepore, M.T.; Fiorelli, A.; et al. Human lung-resident macrophages express CB1 and CB2 receptors whose activation inhibits the release of angiogenic and lymphangiogenic factors. *J. Leukoc. Biol.* **2016**, *99*, 531–540. [CrossRef]
76. Huusko, J.; Lottonen, L.; Merentie, M.; Gurzeler, E.; Anisimov, A.; Miyanohara, A.; Alitalo, K.; Tavi, P.; Yla-Herttuala, S. AAV9-mediated VEGF-B gene transfer improves systolic function in progressive left ventricular hypertrophy. *Mol. Ther.* **2012**, *20*, 2212–2221. [CrossRef]
77. Abraham, D.; Hofbauer, R.; Schafer, R.; Blumer, R.; Paulus, P.; Miksovsky, A.; Traxler, H.; Kocher, A.; Aharinejad, S. Selective downregulation of VEGF-A(165), VEGF-R(1), and decreased capillary density in patients with dilative but not ischemic cardiomyopathy. *Circ. Res.* **2000**, *87*, 644–647. [CrossRef]
78. Park, J.H.; Yoon, J.Y.; Ko, S.M.; Jin, S.A.; Kim, J.H.; Cho, C.H.; Kim, J.M.; Lee, J.H.; Choi, S.W.; Seong, I.W.; et al. Endothelial progenitor cell transplantation decreases lymphangiogenesis and adverse myocardial remodeling in a mouse model of acute myocardial infarction. *Exp. Mol. Med.* **2011**, *43*, 479–485. [CrossRef]
79. Rutanen, J.; Leppanen, P.; Tuomisto, T.T.; Rissanen, T.T.; Hiltunen, M.O.; Vajanto, I.; Niemi, M.; Hakkinen, T.; Karkola, K.; Stacker, S.A.; et al. Vascular endothelial growth factor-D expression in human atherosclerotic lesions. *Cardiovasc. Res.* **2003**, *59*, 971–979. [CrossRef]
80. Klotz, L.; Norman, S.; Vieira, J.M.; Masters, M.; Rohling, M.; Dube, K.N.; Bollini, S.; Matsuzaki, F.; Carr, C.A.; Riley, P.R. Cardiac lymphatics are heterogeneous in origin and respond to injury. *Nature* **2015**, *522*, 62–67. [CrossRef]
81. David, S.; Kumpers, P.; Hellpap, J.; Horn, R.; Leitolf, H.; Haller, H.; Kielstein, J.T. Angiopoietin 2 and cardiovascular disease in dialysis and kidney transplantation. *Am. J. Kidney Dis.* **2009**, *53*, 770–778. [CrossRef] [PubMed]
82. McKee, P.A.; Castelli, W.P.; McNamara, P.M.; Kannel, W.B. The natural history of congestive heart failure: The Framingham study. *N. Engl. J. Med.* **1971**, *285*, 1441–1446. [CrossRef] [PubMed]
83. Sacks, D.; Baxter, B.; Campbell, B.C.V.; Carpenter, J.S.; Cognard, C.; Dippel, D.; Eesa, M.; Fischer, U.; Hausegger, K.; Hirsch, J.A.; et al. Multisociety consensus quality improvement revised consensus statement for endovascular therapy of acute ischemic stroke. *Int. J. Stroke* **2018**, *13*, 612–632. [CrossRef] [PubMed]
84. Albakri, A. Clinical and Medical Investigations Ischemic heart failure: A review of clinical status and meta-analysis of diagnosis and clinical management methods. *Clin. Med. Investig.* **2018**, *3*, 2–15.
85. Balmforth, C.; Simpson, J.; Shen, L.; Jhund, P.S.; Lefkowitz, M.; Rizkala, A.R.; Rouleau, J.L.; Shi, V.; Solomon, S.D.; Swedberg, K.; et al. Outcomes and effect of treatment according to etiology in HFrEF: An analysis of PARADIGM-HF. *JACC Heart Fail.* **2019**, *7*, 457–465. [CrossRef] [PubMed]
86. Hallstrand, T.S.; Lai, Y.; Hooper, K.A.; Oslund, R.C.; Altemeier, W.A.; Matute-Bello, G.; Gelb, M.H. Endogenous secreted phospholipase A2 group X regulates cysteinyl leukotrienes synthesis by human eosinophils. *J. Allergy Clin. Immunol.* **2016**, *137*, 268–277.e8. [CrossRef]
87. Murakami, M.; Yamamoto, K.; Miki, Y.; Murase, R.; Sato, H.; Taketomi, Y. The roles of the secreted phospholipase A2 gene family in immunology. *Adv. Immunol.* **2016**, *132*, 91–134.
88. Triggiani, M.; Giannattasio, G.; Calabrese, C.; Loffredo, S.; Granata, F.; Fiorello, A.; Santini, M.; Gelb, M.H.; Marone, G. Lung mast cells are a source of secreted phospholipases A2. *J. Allergy Clin. Immunol.* **2009**, *124*, 558–565.e1–3. [CrossRef]
89. Marone, G.; Borriello, F.; Varricchi, G.; Genovese, A.; Granata, F. Basophils: Historical reflections and perspectives. *Chem. Immunol. Allergy* **2014**, *100*, 172–192.
90. Loffredo, S.; Staiano, R.I.; Granata, F.; Genovese, A.; Marone, G. Immune cells as a source and target of angiogenic and lymphangiogenic factors. *Chem. Immunol. Allergy* **2014**, *99*, 15–36.
91. Varricchi, G.; Marone, G. Mast cells: Fascinating but still elusive after 140 years from their discovery. *Int. J. Mol. Sci.* **2020**, *21*, 464. [CrossRef]

9

Risk Stratification in Hypertrophic Cardiomyopathy: Insights from Genetic Analysis and Cardiopulmonary Exercise Testing

Damiano Magrì [1,*,†], Vittoria Mastromarino [1,2], Giovanna Gallo [1], Elisabetta Zachara [3], Federica Re [3], Piergiuseppe Agostoni [4,5], Dario Giordano [1], Speranza Rubattu [1,6,*], Maurizio Forte [6], Maria Cotugno [6], Maria Rosaria Torrisi [1,7], Simona Petrucci [1,7], Aldo Germani [1,7], Camilla Savio [7], Antonello Maruotti [8,9,10], Massimo Volpe [1,6], Camillo Autore [1], Maria Piane [1,7,†] and Beatrice Musumeci [1]

1 Department of Clinical and Molecular Medicine, Sapienza University, 00100 Rome, Italy; vittoriamastromarino@libero.it (V.M.); giovanna.gallo@uniroma1.it (G.G.); dariogiordano@outlook.com (D.G.); mara.torrisi@uniroma1.it (M.R.T.); simona.petrucci@uniroma1.it (S.P.); aldo.germani@uniroma1.it (A.G.); massimo.volpe@uniroma1.it (M.V.); camillo.autore@uniroma1.it (C.A.); maria.piane@uniroma1.it (M.P.); beatrice.musumeci@uniroma1.it (B.M.)

2 Unit of Pediatric Cardiology and Cardiac Surgery, Sant'Orsola Hospital, 40100 Bologna, Italy

3 Cardiac Arrhythmia Center and Cardiomyopathies Unit, San Camillo—Forlanini Hospital, 00100 Rome, Italy; elisabettazachara@gmail.com (E.Z.); re.federica77@gmail.com (F.R.)

4 Centro Cardiologico Monzino, IRCCS, 20100 Milan, Italy; piergiuseppe.agostoni@unimi.it

5 Department of Clinical Sciences and Community Health, University of Milan, 20100 Milan, Italy

6 IRCCS Neuromed, 86077 Pozzilli (IS), Italy; maurizio.forte@neuromed.it (M.F.); maria.cotugno@neuromed.it (M.C.)

7 UOC Medical Genetics and Advanced Cell Diagnostics, S. Andrea University Hospital, 00100 Rome, Italy; camilla.savio@ospedalesantandrea.it

8 Department of Scienze Economiche, Politiche e delle Lingue Moderne—Libera Università SS Maria Assunta, 00100 Rome, Italy; a.maruotti@lumsa.it

9 Department of Mathematics, University of Bergen, 5052 Bergen, Norway

10 School of Computing, University of Portsmouth, Portsmouth PO1, UK

* Correspondence: damiano.magri@uniroma1.it (D.M.); rubattu.speranza@neuromed.it (S.R.)

† These authors contributed equally.

Abstract: The role of genetic testing over the clinical and functional variables, including data from the cardiopulmonary exercise test (CPET), in the hypertrophic cardiomyopathy (HCM) risk stratification remains unclear. A retrospective genotype–phenotype correlation was performed to analyze possible differences between patients with and without likely pathogenic/pathogenic (LP/P) variants. A total of 371 HCM patients were screened at least for the main sarcomeric genes *MYBPC3* (myosin binding protein C), *MYH7* (β-myosin heavy chain), *TNNI3* (cardiac troponin I) and *TNNT2* (cardiac troponin T): 203 patients had at least an LP/P variant, 23 patients had a unique variant of uncertain significance (VUS) and 145 did not show any LP/P variant or VUS. During a median 5.4 years follow-up, 51 and 14 patients developed heart failure (HF) and sudden cardiac death (SCD) or SCD-equivalents events, respectively. The LP/P variant was associated with a more aggressive HCM phenotype. However, left atrial diameter (LAd), circulatory power (peak oxygen uptake*peak systolic blood pressure, CP%) and ventilatory efficiency (C-index = 0.839) were the only independent predictors of HF whereas only LAd and CP% were predictors of the SCD end-point (C-index = 0.738). The present study reaffirms the pivotal role of the clinical variables and, particularly of those CPET-derived, in the HCM risk stratification.

Keywords: hypertrophic cardiomyopathy; cardiopulmonary exercise test; genetic testing

1. Introduction

Hypertrophic cardiomyopathy (HCM), the most common genetic heart disease, inherited with an autosomal dominant pattern, incomplete penetrance and variable expressivity, is characterized by markedly different instrumental and clinical spectra [1–3]. Accordingly, there is always great interest in investigating approaches potentially able to identify early those HCM patients at high risk of cardiovascular events both in terms of sudden cardiac death (SCD) and heart failure (HF). Indeed, albeit the SCD is a devastating but relatively rare event, HF development and its related complications still represent an incoming concern in HCM patients [4–6].

In such a context, due to its genetic nature, many researchers attempted not only an HCM genotype–phenotype correlation but also a possible genotype-based risk stratification. Indeed, HCM is predominantly a sarcomeric disease and variants in *MYH7* and *MYBPC3* genes, encoding for the cardiac thick myofilament proteins β-myosin heavy chain and myosin binding protein C, respectively, together account about 50% of the HCM families. Conversely, likely pathogenic/pathogenic (LP/P) variants in thin filament protein genes, such as *TNNT2*, *TNNI3* and *TPM1* encoding for cardiac troponin T, troponin I and alpha-tropomyosin, account for less than 10% [6–9]. Several studies have demonstrated that being carriers of sarcomeric variants might exert a negative prognostic impact on outcome, as well as multiple simultaneous variants, such as the so-called "gene dosage effect" [8–13]. What remains unclear, up to now, is whether the genetic profile of the single HCM patient might provide a real significant incremental risk prediction beyond the clinical risk factors, including those derived from a maximal cardiopulmonary exercise test (CPET) [2,3]. Indeed, growing evidence suggests that a CPET assessment, combined with other clinical and instrumental variables, represents a useful tool in stratifying both the SCD and the HF-related events' risk in HCM patients [14–18].

Therefore, the current multicenter retrospective study investigates a possible adjunctive role of genetic testing analysis in the HCM patients' management over the main clinical and functional parameters. Particularly, a genotype–phenotype correlation was performed to analyze possible differences between HCM patients with and without LP/P variants with respect to their main clinical and functional features and, mainly, their SCD and HF-related events' rate.

2. Methods

2.1. Study Sample

Data from a total of 665 consecutive outpatients with HCM were analyzed. All patients were part of a cohort recruited and prospectively followed in three HCM Italian centers between September 2007 and December 2019: Azienda Ospedaliera Universitaria Sant'Andrea, "Sapienza" University, Rome (n = 437); Azienda Ospedaliera San Camillo Forlanini, Rome (n = 189); Centro Cardiologico Monzino, University of Milan, Milan (n = 39). The diagnosis of HCM was based on maximal wall thickness (MWT) ≥ 15 mm unexplained by abnormal loading conditions or in accordance with published criteria for the diagnosis of disease in relatives of patients with unequivocal disease [2,3]. Patients with known metabolic diseases or syndromic causes of HCM were excluded from the present study.

The study complied with the ethical standards of the Declaration of Helsinki and was reviewed and approved by the institutional ethics committees. Written informed consent was obtained from all participants. The authors from each participating center guarantee the integrity of data from their institution and have agreed to the article as written.

2.2. Patients Clinical and Functional Assessment

Data were independently collected at each participating center using a uniform methodology. Each HCM patient underwent a clinical assessment, including history with pedigree analysis and the New York Heart Association (NYHA) classification, 24 h ECG Holter monitoring, transthoracic Doppler echocardiography and maximal CPET. The usual five SCD risk factors were also collected [2,3]: (a) FH-SCD (history of HCM-related SCD in at least one first-degree or other relatives younger than 50 years old); (b) massive left ventricular (LV) hypertrophy (maximal wall thickness, MWT, ≥30 mm); (c) at least one run of nonsustained ventricular tachycardia (NSVT, ≥3 consecutive ventricular beats at a rate of ≥120 beats per minute and <30 s in duration on 24 h ECG Holter monitoring); (d) unexplained syncope judged inconsistent with neurocardiogenic origin; (e) abnormal blood pressure response to exercise (ABPRE, failure to increase systolic blood pressure, SBP, by at least 20 mmHg from rest to peak exercise or a fall of ≥20 mmHg from SBP).

The following echocardiographic measurements, obtained according to the international guidelines [19], were considered: LV end-diastolic diameter (LVEDd, parasternal long axis), the greatest LV thickness (MWT, measured at any LV site), left atrial diameter (LAd, parasternal long axis), the highest maximal LV outflow tract gradient among those measured at rest, in orthostatic position and after Valsalva maneuver (LVOTGmax, apical four-chamber view) [20] and LV ejection fraction with Simpson's biplane methods (LVEF, apical four-chamber view).

All CPETs were performed using an electronically braked cycle ergometer. A personalized ramp exercise protocol was performed, aiming at a test duration of 10 ± 2 min [21]. The exercise was preceded by a few minutes of resting breath-by-breath gas exchange monitoring and by an unloaded warm-up. In the absence of clinical events, CPET was interrupted when patients stated that they had reached maximal effort. A 12-lead ECG, diastolic and systolic blood pressure were recorded during CPET, in order to obtain the following parameters: rest heart rate (HR), peak HR, %pHR ((peak HR/(220 − age)) × 100), and ΔSBP (peak SBP − rest SBP) [22]. A breath-by-breath analysis of expiratory gases and ventilation (VE) has been performed, and peak values were obtained in the last 20 s of exercise. The predicted peak VO_2 was determined by using the gender-, age- and weight-adjusted formula. Circulatory power (CP = peak VO_2 × SBP) was obtained considering peak VO_2 value as a percentage of predicted (CP%) [19,23]. Anaerobic threshold (AT) was measured by V-slope analysis of VO_2 and VCO_2, and it was confirmed by ventilator equivalents and end-tidal pressures of CO_2 and O_2 [24]. The end of the isocapnic buffering period was identified when VE/VCO_2 increased and the end-tidal pressure of CO_2 decreased. VE/VCO_2 slope was calculated as the slope of the linear relationship between VE and VCO_2 from the 1st minute after the beginning of the loaded exercise and the end of the isocapnic buffering period [24].

2.3. Genetic Testing

All patients included in the study received genetic counseling and underwent genetic testing for HCM, performed by Sanger sequencing (from 2007 to 2010) or NGS (next-generation sequencing, from 2011 to 2019). The genes analyzed in the participating laboratories from the HCM centers had changed and/or added over time. In this retrospective study, we report the genotype–phenotype correlation analysis only for those patients screened at least for the sarcomeric genes *MYBPC3* (myosin binding protein C, cardiac) *MYH7* (β-myosin heavy chain, cardiac), *TNNI3* (troponin I, cardiac) and *TNNT2* (troponin T type 2, cardiac). All coding regions and boundaries of flanking introns ±25 were analyzed for all genes considered in this study. In addition, all variants reported in this paper, identified by NGS technology, were validated by Sanger sequencing. Patients with variants located in nonsarcomeric genes were also excluded.

All the identified variants were re-evaluated based on new evidence from the scientific literature and classified according to the criteria of the American College of Medical Genetics and Genomics (ACMG) [25,26]. Only the genetic variants predicted to alter the protein and with a minor allele frequency (MAF) ≤0.2% (considering the prevalence of HCM disease in the general population), were considered. For this evaluation, we used MAF data derived from GnomAD (Genome Aggregation Database https://gnomad.broadinstitute.org/). The clinical classification of variants was carried out according to the 5-class system: benign (B), likely benign (LB), likely pathogenic (LP), pathogenic (P) and variants of uncertain significance (VUS). Genetic results were considered informative for LP or P variants, noninformative for B, LB or VUS variants. Variants are reported using the Human Genome Variation Society nomenclature guidelines (https://varnomen.hgvs.org/).

2.4. Clinical Outcomes

All patients had planned clinical reviews every 6–12 months or earlier according to the clinical status. Follow-up duration was defined as the time interval between the clinical examination and either the first event or the last visit/telephone interview in case of no events.

The HF end-point was represented by the following events: death due to HF, cardiac transplantation, progression to a stable NYHA class III–IV due to an end-stage phase with or without LVEF < 50% (hypokinetic dilated phase or restrictive phenotype evolution), severe functional deterioration leading to hospitalization for septal reduction, hospitalization due to HF symptoms or signs development. The SCD end-point was also tested, which included SCD or an equivalent event. SCD was defined as witnessing sudden death with or without documented ventricular fibrillation or death within 1 h of new symptoms or nocturnal deaths with no antecedent history of worsening symptoms. Aborted SCD during follow-up and appropriate ICD therapies (defined as intervention triggered by ventricular fibrillation or rapid ventricular tachycardia at >180 bpm) were considered equivalent to SCD in accordance with previous studies [17,18,27,28].

The causes of death, as well as the other events, were ascertained by experienced cardiologists at each center using hospital and primary health care records, death certificates, post-mortem reports, and interviews with relatives and/or physicians. To avoid a composite cardiovascular end-point including also cerebrovascular events, due to the small number of such events and in accordance with other studies by our research group [17,18,22], death due to ischemic or hemorrhagic stroke (n. 2 events) and nonfatal cerebrovascular (n. 5 events), as well as death due to noncardiovascular causes (n. 2 events), were excluded from the survival analysis.

2.5. Statistical Analysis

All data are expressed as mean ± standard deviation or as absolute number (percentage). Preliminarily, an extension of the Shapiro–Wilk test of normality was performed. Categorical variables were compared with a difference between proportion tests whereas a two-sample *t*-test was used to compare the continuous data between the two study groups (no variants and VUS Versus LP/P variants). In comparing the two populations, the variance was estimated separately for both groups and the Welch–Satterthwaite modification to the degrees of freedom was used.

We, therefore, focused on the distribution of survival times by adopting the Cox proportional hazards regression model. We performed a backward selection of the predictors to be included in the model. A 5% significance level was used in the backward elimination procedure to select covariates for the final multivariate model for the combined as well as the HF end-point while, due to the low events' number, a 15% significance level was adopted for the SCD one. To avoid the inclusion of collinear variables in the multivariate Cox analysis, we built several models in which VO_2-derived variables, known to be collinear, were added to the prognostic model one at a time. We retain the model with the best trade-off between model complexity and model fit judged by the log-likelihood. We also performed a calibration analysis. We computed the average calibration error for both approaches and tested the observed versus average predicted probabilities for each class of risk. The Brier quadratic error score and a χ^2 test of goodness of fit based on the Brier score were also checked. We did not find any clear indication of overfitting from the post hoc analysis and, consequently, in the present paper we simply reported results based on the backward elimination procedure only. Discrimination of variables included in the final multivariate model specification was performed by Harrell's C-index.

Therefore, we investigated the proportional hazards assumption by tests and graphical diagnostics based on scaled Schoenfeld residuals. Test of proportional hazards assumption for each covariate was obtained by correlating the corresponding set of scaled Schoenfeld residuals with the Kaplan–Meier estimate of the survival distribution. To check for the presence of influential observations, we produced a matrix of estimated changes in the regression coefficients upon deleting each observation in turn and comparing the magnitudes of the largest values to the regression coefficients.

Statistical analysis was performed using R (R Development Core Team, 2014). A p-value lower than or equal to 0.05 was generally considered as statistically significant.

3. Results

From an initial study sample of 665 consecutive HCM outpatients, a total of 294 patients (44%) were excluded because they did not undergo genetic testing ($n = 197$), because they were lost at follow-up ($n = 39$), because of the presence of nonsarcomeric variants ($n = 22$) or, eventually, because the genetic analysis was not performed according to the previously described inclusion criteria ($n = 36$). Thus, a total of 371 HCM patients were effectively enrolled and analyzed in the present study. The diagram displayed in Figure 1 resumes the step-by-step classification of the study population.

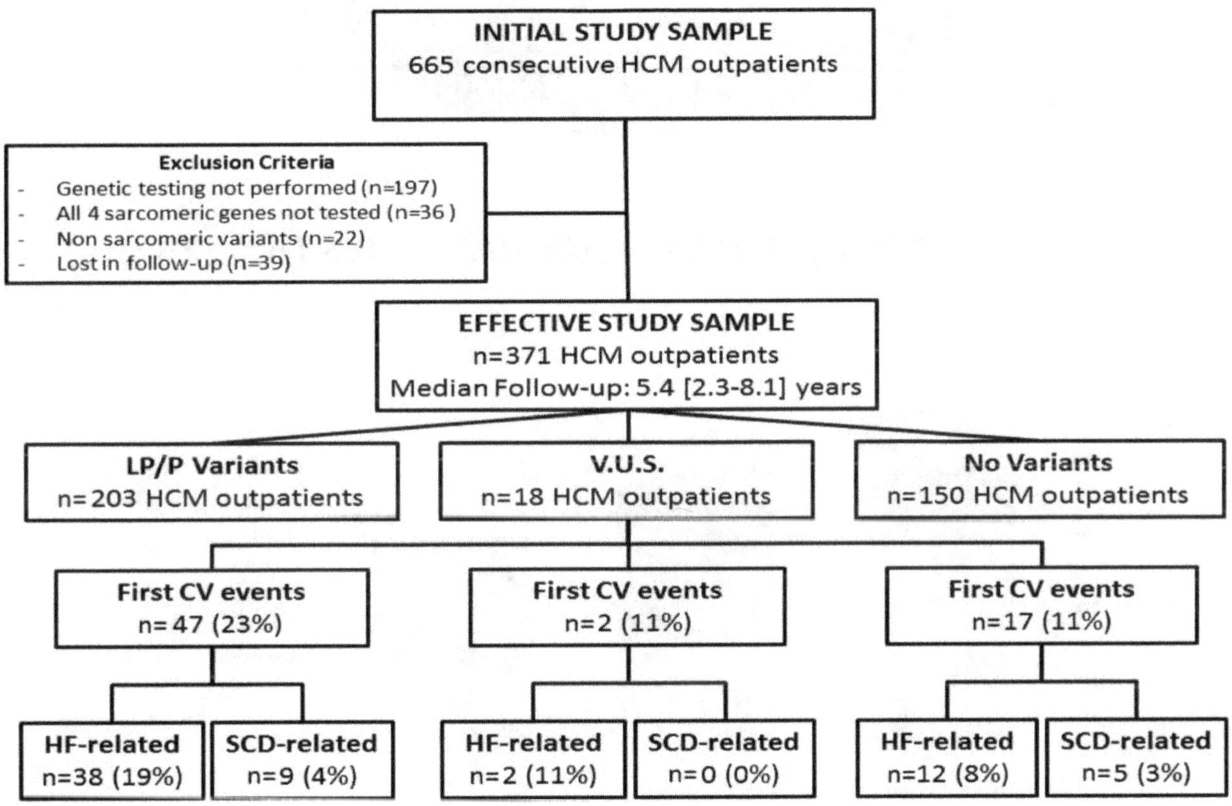

Figure 1. Diagram showing the step-by-step classification of the hypertrophic cardiomyopathy (HCM) population considered in our study. LP/P: likely pathogenic/pathogenic sarcomeric variants; V.U.S.: variant of uncertain significance; CV: cardiac events; HF: heart failure; SCD: sudden cardiac death.

3.1. Genetic Results

Two hundred and three (55%) genetic tests were informative as they detected at least an LP/P variant, whereas the percentage of patients with VUS was 6% ($n = 23$ patients); 39% ($n = 145$ patients) did not show any P/LP variant or VUS (Figure 2). Excluding the B/LB variants, 124 unique variants were identified and detailed extensively in the Supplementary files (Tables S1 and S2). These variants included 91 (73%) missense, 2 (2%) intronic, 10 (8%) frameshift, 8 (6%) splicing, 11 (9%) nonsense, 1 (1%) inframe variants (Figure S1). According to ACMG criteria, 94 variants were classified as LP/P and 30 of them as VUS. *MYBPC3* and *MYH7* resulted in the most mutated genes with 88 LP/P variants (75%, Figure 2). Twenty-four patients resulted to be carriers of multiple variants, considering those with at least one P/LP variant and other P/LP or VUS variants (Table S3). Among these, 14 patients were double heterozygous with one variant in two different genes while the remaining 10 had multiple variants in the same gene. It was not possible to determinate the phase of these variants, since segregation studies among relatives could not be performed.

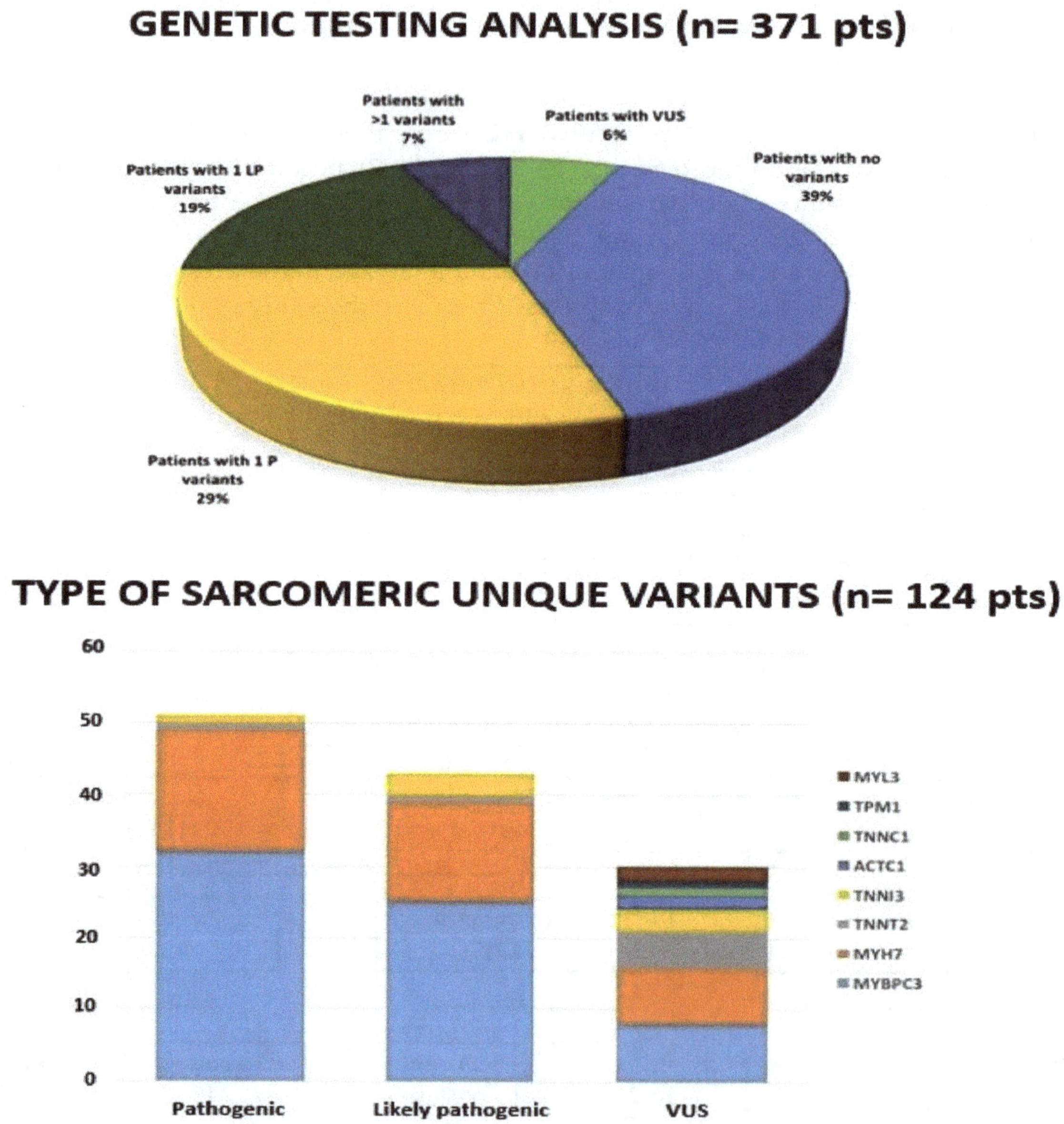

Figure 2. (**Top panel**): results of genetic testing analysis in the overall study sample. (**Bottom panel**): type and distribution of likely pathogenic/pathogenic (LP/P) variants and variants of uncertain significance (VUS). *MYL3*: myosin light chain 3; *TPM1*: tropomyosin 1; *TNNC1*: troponin C1; *ACTC1*: actin alpha cardiac muscle 1; *TNNI3*: cardiac troponin I; *TNNT2*: cardiac troponin T; *MYH7*: β-myosin heavy chain; *MYBPC3*: myosin binding protein C.

3.2. Clinical and Functional Characteristics

The demographic and clinical data of the entire cohort are reported in Table 1. The population mainly consisted of middle-aged predominantly male (64%) patients with a quite preserved NYHA class (NYHA I–II 94%). At the study run-in, echocardiographic evidence of the end-stage phase was present in 4%, atrial fibrillation in 3% and a septal myectomy had been performed in 11% patients.

Documented cardiovascular comorbidities included systemic hypertension (27%), diabetes (6%) and coronary artery disease (4%).

Table 1. Main clinical variables of the entire study sample at the study run-in (n = 371 patients).

General Data	
Age, years	49 ± 16
Male, n (%)	238 (64)
Age at diagnosis, years	40 ± 19
NYHA III–IV, n (%)	24 (6)
ICD, n (%)	43 (12)
Previous myectomy, n (%)	20 (5)
SCD risk factors	
NSVT, n (%)	121 (32)
FH-SCD, n (%)	48 (13)
MWT > 30 mm, n (%)	26 (7)
Unexplained syncope, n (%)	56 (15)
ABPRE, n (%)	45 (16)
Echocardiographic data	
LVEDd, mm	45 ± 5
LAd, mm	43 ± 7
MWT, mm	20 ± 5
LVOT obstruction, n (%)	125 (33)
$LVOTG_{max}$, mmHg	11 (6–39)
LVEF, %	62 ± 7
CPET data	
Peak HR, % of predicted	79 ± 13
Peak VO_2, mL/kg/min	23 ± 7
Peak VO_2, % of predicted	77 ± 18
Peak SBP, mmHg	164 ± 27
CP%, % of predicted * mmHg	12,937 ± 4300
VE/VCO_2 slope	28.4 ± 5.5
Medical treatment	
β-blocker, n (%)	228 (61)
Nondihydropyridine CCB, n (%)	31 (8)
ACE-I/ARB, n (%)	107 (29)
Diuretics, n (%)	78 (21)
Amiodaron, n (%)	33 (9)

Data are expressed as mean ± SD, as an absolute number of patients (% on total sample) or as median (25th–75th percentile). VUS: variant of uncertain significance; LP: likely pathogenic; P: pathogenic; NYHA: New York Heart Association; ICD: implantable cardioverter defibrillator; SCD: sudden cardiac death; NSVT: nonsustained ventricular tachycardia; FH: family history; ABPRE: abnormal blood pressure response at exercise; LVEDd: left ventricular end-diastolic diameter; LAd: left atrial diameter; MWT: maximum wall thickness; $LVOTG_{max}$: maximal LV outflow tract gradient; LVEF: LV ejection fraction; SBP: peak systolic blood pressure; HR: heart rate; VO_2: oxygen uptake; CP: circulatory power; VE/VCO_2 slope: relation between ventilation versus carbon dioxide production; CCB: calcium channel blocker; ACE-I/ARB: angiotensin-converting enzyme inhibitors/angiotensin receptor blocker.

Table 2 shows the comparison of clinical features between patients with and without LP/P variants. The LP/P variants group showed a younger age, a slightly higher prevalence of FH-SCD and ABPRE and a worse functional capacity in terms of pVO_2, CP% and VE/VCO_2 slope. With respect to the other clinical features, at the study run-in, the LP/P variants group had a greater prevalence of patients with end-stage phase (6% vs. 2%, $p = 0.011$) and atrial fibrillation (3% vs. 1%, $p = 0.032$), whereas no difference in the prevalence of previous myectomy was found (5% for both groups). Concerning the documented cardiovascular comorbidities, no difference was found in coronary artery disease (3% vs. 5%), whereas the LP/P variants group showed a lower prevalence of systemic hypertension (15% vs. 31%, $p < 0.001$) and diabetes (3% vs. 8%, $p = 0.007$).

Table 2. Main clinical variables of the study sample at the study run-in according to genetic testing results.

General Data	No Variants and VUS (n = 168)	LP/P Variants (n = 203)	p-Values
Age, years	53 ± 18	45 ± 16	<0.001
Male, n (%)	112 (67)	124(61)	NS
Age at diagnosis, years	47 ± 20	35 ± 17	<0.001
NYHA III-IV, n (%)	10 (6)	14 (7)	NS
ICD, n (%)	11 (6)	32 (16)	0.019
Previous myectomy, n (%)	9 (5)	11 (5)	NS
SCD risk factors			
NSVT, n (%)	48 (28)	73 (36)	NS
FH-SCD, n (%)	16 (9)	32 (16)	0.049
MWT > 30 mm, n (%)	10 (6)	16 (8)	NS
Unexplained syncope, n (%)	29 (17)	26 (13)	NS
ABPRE, n (%)	11 (7)	34 (17)	0.003
Echocardiographic data			
LVEDd, mm	46 ± 4	45 ± 6	NS
LAd, mm	43 ± 7	43 ± 7	NS
MWT, mm	20 ± 5	20 ± 5	NS
LVOT obstruction, n (%)	79 (47)	45 (22)	<0.001
$LVOTG_{max}$, mmHg	16 (9–39)	10 (5–33)	0.023
LVEF, %	63 ± 4	61 ± 6	<0.001
CPET data			
Peak HR, % of predicted	78 ± 12	79 ± 13	NS
Peak VO_2, mL/kg/min	23 ± 7	23 ± 7	NS
Peak VO_2, % of predicted	79 ± 18	75 ± 18	0.032
Peak SBP, mmHg	175 ± 26	157 ± 26	<0.001
CP%, % of predicted * mmHg	14,070 ± 4269	12,015 ± 4020	<0.001
VE/VCO_2 slope	27.5 ± 4.9	29.1 ± 6.0	0.019
Medical treatment			
β-blocker, n (%)	105 (62)	122 (60)	NS
Non dihydropyridine CCB, n (%)	11 (7)	20 (10)	NS
ACE-I/ARB, n (%)	58 (34)	48 (24)	0.014
Diuretics, n (%)	37 (22)	41 (21)	NS
Amiodaron, n (%)	16 (9)	17 (8)	NS

Data are expressed as mean ± SD, as the absolute number of patients (% on total sample) or as median (25th–75th percentile). NS: not significant. See Table 1 for other abbreviations.

3.3. End-Point Analysis

Median follow-up was 5.4 years (25th–75th centile: 2.3 to 8.1 years) with a total of 2271 patients-year. During the entire follow-up, a total of 129 (35%) patients experienced at least one of the pre-specified events. In patients who developed multiple events, time to the first was used as an event time cutoff and, accordingly, SCD or HF-related events at five-years' cumulative hazard equal to 0.369 was estimated. Patients who completed the follow-up period before the tenth year were censored at the time of the last clinical evaluation.

A total of 14 SCD or SCD-equivalents were analyzed. Specifically, SCD occurred in three patients; four patients experienced a resuscitated SCD and seven patients had an appropriate ICD intervention. A total of 52 HF-related events were analyzed. Specifically, HF-related death occurred in two patients, seven patients underwent cardiac transplantation, 20 patients were hospitalized due to HF signs/symptoms, 12 patients were hospitalized for septal reduction procedure due to significant HF signs/symptoms development and 11 patients evolved to end-stage or restrictive phenotype evolution. Table 3 reports the detailed Cox proportional univariate survival analysis for both the study end-points. Most of the single variables were significantly associated with the HF end-point whereas few of them to the SCD end-point. Particularly, besides a number of clinical variables, the LP/P variant presence was significantly associated with the HF but not to the SCD end-point (Figure 3). Instead, at multivariate analysis, covariates showing significant effects for the primary HF-related end-point were the following: LAd, CP% and VE/VCO_2 slope (C-index 0.839, $p < 0.001$) while LAd and the CP% remained independently associated with the SCD end-point (C-index 0.738, Table 4).

Table 3. Main significant univariate Cox proportional survival analysis according to the clinical variables for the two main study end-points.

	HF Endpoint ($n = 52$)			SCD Endpoint ($n = 14$)		
	H.R. (95% C.I.)	*p*-Values	C-Index	H.R. (95% C.I.)	*p*-Values	C-Index
Age at CPET	–	NS	–	0.964 (0.934–0.996)	0.038	0.613
Male sex	–	NS	–	–	NS	–
Age at diagnosis	–	NS	–	0.944 (0.906–0.983)	0.006	0.729
FH-SCD	1.869 (1.010–3.460)	0.046	0.522	2.830 (0.892–8.979)	0.077	0.607
Unexplained Syncope	–	NS	–	–	NS	–
NSVT	1.917 (1.102–3.333)	0.021	0.548	–	NS	–
ABPRE	3.418 (1.769–6.605)	<0.001	0.641	–	NS	–
MWT > 30 mm	–	NS	–	3.956 (1.210–12.940)	0.023	0.569
MWT	–	NS	–	1.100 (1.012–1.195)	0.025	0.593
LVOTO	2.110 (1.215–3.664)	<0.01	0.641	–	NS	–
LAd	1.077 (1.039–1.116)	<0.001	0.704	1.054 (0.984–1.129)	0.112	0.660
$LVOTG_{max}$	1.016 (1.008–1.024)	<0.001	0.672	0.971 (0.937–1.007)	0.123	0.577
LVEF	0.929 (0.899–0.959)	<0.001	0.587	–	NS	–
pVO_2, mL/kg/min	0.851 (0.799–0.905)	<0.001	0.739	–	NS	–
pVO_2, % of predicted	0.851 (0.799–0.905)	<0.001	0.749	–	NS	–
VE/VCO_2 slope	1.017 (1.069–1.146)	<0.001	0.724	–	NS	–
CP%	0.998 (0.997–0.999)	<0.001	0.778	0.998 (0.997–1.000)	0.052	0.705
LP or P variants	2.395 (1.171–4.856)	0.013	0.609	–	NS	–

H.R.: hazard ratio; C.I.: confidence interval. See Table 1 for other abbreviations.

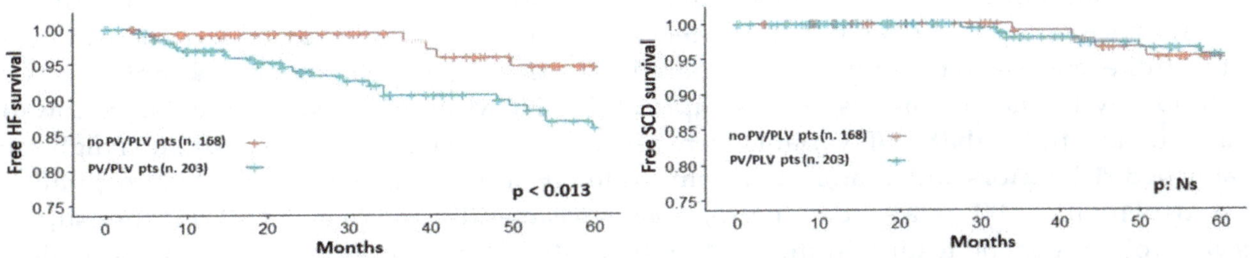

Figure 3. Kaplan–Meier estimator of survival free from heart failure (HF, **left panel**) and sudden cardiac death (SCD, **right panel**) related events according to the presence of likely pathogenic/pathogenic sarcomeric variants (PLV/PV).

Table 4. Significant multivariate Cox proportional survival analysis and test for proportional hazards assumption for the two study end-points.

	Multivariate Cox Proportional Survival Analysis					
	HF Endpoint			SCD Endpoint		
	H.R. (95% C.I.)	*p*-Values	C-Index	H.R. (95% C.I.)	*p*-Values	C-Index
LAd	1.083 (1.039–1.130)	<0.001	0.839	1.078 (1.005–1.163)	0.0485	0.738
CP%	0.998 (0.997–0.999)	<0.001		0.998 (0.9996–1.000)	0.0488	
VE/VCO$_2$ slope	1.044 (0.999–1.090)	0.05				

See Tables 1 and 2 for other abbreviations.

4. Discussion

The present multicenter retrospective study, conducted on a suitable cohort of consecutive HCM outpatients regularly followed at three Italian tertiary HCM centers, shows that HCM patients with LP/P sarcomeric variants tend to present a more aggressive form of disease with an earlier onset, a worse functional status and a greater risk of HF development and HF-related complications, compared to HCM patients with VUS or any variants. However, contextually, our data do not support a strict role of genetic testing over HCM patients' comprehensive clinical assessment. Indeed, the LP/P variants presence does not emerge at multivariate analysis as an independent risk factor, being other instrumental variables (i.e., LAd, CP% and VE/VCO$_2$ slope) much stronger outcome predictors.

Over the last decades a number of clinical features were investigated in order to identify those HCM patients at high risk of adverse events, both arrhythmic and HF-related. Indeed, albeit most of the cases show a benign course with a life expectancy equal to the general population [1], the SCD remains a rare but devastating event which is still the leading cause of death in the young population and athletes [2,3,6]. Furthermore, proper due to the improvement in the HCM management, both pharmacological and nonpharmacological (i.e., ICD, myectomy, LVAD/heart transplantation), there is a growing percentage of HCM patients who develop HF as well as HF-related complications [1,5,29]. The present study, as an ancillary result, confirms the abovementioned concern by showing a significant rate of HF-related events ($n = 114$ events) with a relatively low number of SCD and SCD-equivalent ($n = 14$ events) at a midterm follow-up.

Given the wide HCM clinical spectrum, its genetic nature and the need for targeted prevention strategies, previous studies sought to investigate and weigh the influence of sarcomere variants on the HCM clinical phenotype and outcome [7–13,16]. Indeed, HCM represents a sarcomeric disease with LP/P variants in *MYBPC3* and *MYH7* genes (thick filaments) together accounting for about 50% of the HCM families whereas LP/P variants in *TNNT2*, *TNNI3* (thin filaments) accounting for less than 10% [1,6]. In such a context, an old study by Olivotto and colleagues, conducted in the pre-NGS scenario on a cohort of 203 HCM patients with a median follow-up of 4.5 years, suggested that HCM patients with sarcomere variants had a greater probability of a worse outcome (i.e., cardiac death, nonfatal stroke, end-stage progression) compared to those with nonsarcomeric variants [8]. A more recent study by Li and colleagues, on a sample of 558 HCM patients with a median follow-up of 4.5 years, demonstrated that LP/P variants were associated to an early disease onset, to a high burden of established risk factors and, mainly, to a composite HF end-points (i.e., HF-related hospitalization, heart transplantation, HF-related death, progression to an end-stage phase) [10]. Further support to a possible role of genetic testing in the HCM risk stratification comes from Velzen and colleagues that, on a population of 626 HCM patients with a long-term follow-up (>10 years), confirmed that patients with LP/P variants had a more aggressive phenotype (i.e., young age, high prevalence of SCD risk factors) and found an independent association with all-cause mortality, HF-related and SCD mortality [12]. Eventually, the recent SHARE study, conducted on a large cohort of 2763 HCM patients followed-up for a median of 2.9 years, confirmed that patients carrying sarcomeric LP/P variants had an earlier disease onset and a greater risk of developing the overall composite outcome (SCD or SCD-equivalent, LVAD/cardiac transplantation, progression to an end-stage phase, all-cause mortality, atrial fibrillation and stroke) [13]. The present study confirms that HCM patients carrying LP/P variants have a worse clinical feature in terms of disease onset as well as of historical risk factors [29]. However, we proved just a univariate association between the HCM-mutated status and a composite HF end-point. Although a close comparison with the abovementioned studies remains difficult because of different methodological approaches (i.e., number of genes screened, variants classification, end-points' construction), the most likely reason underlying this negative datum could be the optimal clinical and functional characterization of our study cohort. Indeed, we specifically challenged the prognostic impact of LP/P variants not only with the historical variables but also, and specifically, with the CPET-derived parameters. Thus, we showed originally that patients with LP/P variants, although younger than the counterpart, exhibited also a more severe functional limitation both in terms of pVO_2 and ventilatory efficiency values. Furthermore, due to a concomitant blunted increase of SBP during exercise, HCM patients with LP/P variants showed significantly lower values of CP%. Each of the three abovementioned CPET-derived variables has a specific pathophysiological meaning in the HCM patients' context [30,31] and a possible capability as an outcome predictor. Particularly, the pVO_2 is a multidimensional parameter dependent on cardiac output (heart rate * stroke volume) and artero-venous O_2 extraction [24,32] and it has been extensively shown to be a strong predictor of poor outcome in HCM [14–18] as well as in HF patients [33,34]. The CP%, according to its formula [23,24], magnifies the prognostic power of the pVO_2 through the ABPRE [17,18] which, in turn, depends on the intrinsic myocardial function/geometry as well on abnormal peripheral autonomic reflexes [35,36]. Eventually, the ventilatory efficiency (i.e., VE/VCO_2 slope) has been shown to correlate with pulmonary capillary wedge pressure and left ventricular diastolic properties in HCM [37]. Although usually preserved in HCM patients, the VE/VCO_2 slope tends to worsen significantly only in the late systolic dysfunction phase but it is conceivable that it could mirror also an early exercise-induced left ventricular diastolic functional derangement [16,31,37–39].

5. Limitations

The relatively small number of patients enrolled, together with the low number of hard events, represents a certain limitation that does not allow us to define the true weight of the genetic analysis results in terms of HCM risk prediction when compared to a full clinical assessment. However, it should be noted that our data do not argue against the overall importance of genetic testing in HCM management. Indeed, the identification of unaffected mutated relatives can be possible only after the detection of P/LP variants in affected HCM probands by gene sequencing [40]. Furthermore, molecular analysis of HCM genes remains one of the pivotal approaches in distinguishing the so-called HCM phenocopies where early diagnosis is crucial to managing it optimally [2,3]. On the other hand, whenever a P/LP variant is not found in HCM patients, the HCM diagnosis should be carefully re-evaluated. Again, concerning risk stratification, a comprehensive clinical assessment might be essential.

Another limitation that needs to be acknowledged is that, apart from the main four genes (*MYBPC3, MYH7, TNNI3, TNNT2*) that were tested in all patients, other genes known to be HCM-related (i.e., *ACTC1, TPM1, TNNC1*, or *MYL2* and *MYL3*) were tested in most but not all patients. However, it should be remarked that these variants are rarely detected in HCM patients [6,7]. Moreover, given the few numbers of patients carrying variants in thin filaments genes (<15%) as well patients with multiple variants (6%) in our study sample, our survival analysis considered the overall impact of the LP/P sarcomeric variants without distinguishing the type of compromised filaments or a possible "gene dosage effect". Similarly, growing data report possible relationships between specific variants location in functional domains of sarcomeric proteins and prognostic implications. Particularly, pathogenic missense variants located in the converter domain of the *MYH7* gene were found associated with a worse outcome [41,42]. Furthermore, Garcia-Giustiniani and colleagues found a significant association between p.(Gly716Arg), p.(Arg719Trp) and p.(Arg719Gln) variants with a high risk of events (i.e., 50-year survival of only 20% of carriers) [43]. In the present study cohort, although six different pathogenic missense variants falling within the converter domain (p.(Gly716Arg), p.(Arg719Trp), p.(Arg719Gln), p.(Ile736Thr), p.(Gly741Arg) and p.(Arg723Cys)) were found, the small number of patients carrying these variants as well as their relatively young age unable us to support their specific prognostic power. For the same underlying reasons (i.e., small number of patients carrying VUS only), we cannot speculate about an intermediate prognosis in this subset of patients as hypothesized in the SHARE study [13]. Eventually, we found multiple variants in the same gene in 10 patients and in this specific setting, we cannot determinate whether the genetic alterations were on the same chromosome (heterozygous state) or not (compound heterozygous state).

Finally, besides the genetic profile per se, we examined the prognostic effect of several clinical and instrumental variables at a single time point. Accordingly, we cannot exclude that changes in some variables, as for instance an upgrading of treatment during follow-up or upcoming risk factors, altered our survival analysis. However, it is reasonable that seriate clinical and functional evaluations in HCM patients at the highest risk could further magnify our findings rather than rebut them.

6. Conclusions

Our data underline the importance of a multidimensional clinical assessment over the genetic testing analysis in the HCM risk stratification. This unexpected finding, different from other literature reports, might be likely explained by the limited size of the sample cohort. The LP/P variants were anyway associated with a more aggressive HCM phenotype in terms of early disease onset, high burden of historical risk factor and, for the first time, poor functional status. Of note, within a number of clinical and instrumental variables, the present study reaffirms the pivotal role of the variables derived from a CPET assessment.

Author Contributions: Conceptualization, D.M., M.P., S.R., C.A. and B.M.; methodology, M.P., A.M., M.R.T., C.S., S.P., A.G., M.F. and M.C.; formal analysis, D.M., V.M., G.G., M.P., S.R. and A.M.; investigation, D.M., V.M., G.G., D.G., E.Z., F.R., C.A., B.M., S.R., M.P., C.S., A.G. and S.P.; resources, D.M., S.R., C.A. and M.V.; data curation, D.M.,V.M., G.G, M.P. and S.R.; writing—original draft preparation, D.M., V.M. and G.G; writing—review and editing, D.M., S.R., E.Z., F.R., C.A., M.V. and P.A.; visualization, D.M., V.M. and G.G.; supervision, C.A., S.R. and M.V.; project administration, D.M., C.A., B.M., S.R., E.Z. and F.R.; funding acquisition, D.M., S.R., C.A. and M.V. All authors have read and agreed to the published version of the manuscript.

References

1. Maron, B.J.; Maron, M.S. Hypertrophic cardiomyopathy. *Lancet* **2013**, *381*, 242–255. [CrossRef]
2. Gersh, B.J.; Maron, B.J.; Bonow, R.O.; Dearani, J.A.; Fifer, M.A.; Link, M.S.; Naidu, S.S.; Nishimura, R.A.; Ommen, S.R.; Rakowski, H.; et al. 2011 ACCF/AHA Guideline for the Diagnosis and Treatment of Hypertrophic Cardiomyopathy: Executive Summary: A Report of the American College of Cardiology Foundation/American Heart Association Task Force on Practice Guidelines. *Circulation* **2011**, *124*, 2761–2796. [CrossRef]
3. Elliott, P.M.; Anastasakis, A.; Borger, M.A.; Borggrefe, M.; Cecchi, F.; Charron, P.; Hagege, A.A.; Lafont, A.; Limongelli, G.; Mahrholdt, H.; et al. 2014 ESC Guidelines on diagnosis and management of hypertrophic cardiomyopathy: The Task Force for the Diagnosis and Management of Hypertrophic Cardiomyopathy of the European Society of Cardiology (ESC). *Eur. Heart J.* **2014**, *35*, 2733–2779. [CrossRef]

4. Maron, B.J.; Ommen, S.R.; Semsarian, C.; Spirito, P.; Olivotto, I.; Maron, M.S. Hypertrophic cardiomyopathy: Present and future, with translation into contemporary cardiovascular medicine. *J. Am. Coll. Cardiol.* **2014**, *64*, 83–99. [CrossRef]
5. Musumeci, M.B.; Russo, D.; Limite, L.R.; Canepa, M.; Tini, G.; Casenghi, M.; Francia, P.; Adduci, C.; Pagannone, E.; Magrì, D.; et al. Long-Term Left Ventricular Remodeling of Patients with Hypertrophic Cardiomyopathy. *Am. J. Cardiol.* **2018**, *122*, 1924–1931. [CrossRef]
6. Marian, A.J.; Braunwald, E. Hypertrophic Cardiomyopathy: Genetics, Pathogenesis, Clinical Manifestations, Diagnosis, and Therapy. *Circ. Res.* **2017**, *121*, 749–770. [CrossRef]
7. Rubattu, S.; Bozzao, C.; Pennacchini, E.; Pagannone, E.; Musumeci, M.B.; Piane, M.; Germani, A.; Savio, C.; Francia, P.; Volpe, M.; et al. A Next-Generation Sequencing Approach to Identify Gene Mutations in Early- and Late-Onset Hypertrophic Cardiomyopathy Patients of an Italian Cohort. *Int. J. Mol. Sci.* **2016**, *17*, 1239. [CrossRef]
8. Olivotto, I.; Girolami, F.; Ackerman, M.J.; Nistri, S.; Bos, J.M.; Zachara, E.; Ommen, S.R.; Theis, J.L.; Vaubel, R.A.; Re, F.; et al. Myofilament protein gene mutation screening and outcome of patients with hypertrophic cardiomyopathy. *Mayo Clin. Proc.* **2008**, *83*, 630–638. [CrossRef]
9. Selvi Rani, D.; Nallari, P.; Dhandapany, P.S.; Rani, J.; Meraj, K.; Ganesan, M.; Narasimhan, C.; Thangaraj, K. Coexistence of Digenic Mutations in Both Thin (TPM1) and Thick (MYH7) Filaments of Sarcomeric Genes Leads to Severe Hypertrophic Cardiomyopathy in a South Indian FHCM. *DNA Cell Biol.* **2015**, *34*, 350–359. [CrossRef]
10. Li, Q.; Gruner, C.; Chan, R.H.; Care, M.; Siminovitch, K.; Williams, L.; Woo, A.; Rakowski, H. Genotype-positive status in patients with hypertrophic cardiomyopathy is associated with higher rates of heart failure events. *Circ. Cardiovasc. Genet.* **2014**, *7*, 416–422. [CrossRef]
11. Lopes, L.R.; Syrris, P.; Guttmann, O.P.; O'Mahony, C.; Tang, H.C.; Dalageorgou, C.; Jenkins, S.; Hubank, M.; Monserrat, L.; McKenna, W.J.; et al. Novel genotype-phenotype associations demonstrated by high-throughput sequencing in patients with hypertrophic cardiomyopathy. *Heart* **2015**, *101*, 294–301. [CrossRef]
12. Van Velzen, H.G.; Vriesendorp, P.A.; Oldenburg, R.A.; van Slegtenhorst, M.A.; van der Velden, J.; Schinkel, A.F.L.; Michels, M. Value of Genetic Testing for the Prediction of Long-Term Outcome in Patients with Hypertrophic Cardiomyopathy. *Am. J. Cardiol.* **2016**, *118*, 881–887. [CrossRef]
13. Ho, C.Y.; Day, S.M.; Ashley, E.A.; Michel, M.; Pereira, A.C.; Jacoby, D.; Cirino, A.L.; Fox, J.C.; Lakdawala, N.K.; Ware, J.S.; et al. Genotype and Lifetime Burden of Disease in Hypertrophic Cardiomyopathy: Insights from the Sarcomeric Human Cardiomyopathy Registry (SHaRe). *Circulation* **2018**, *138*, 1387–1398. [CrossRef]
14. Masri, A.; Pierson, L.M.; Smedira, N.G.; Agarwal, S.; Lytle, B.W.; Naji, P.; Thamilarasan, M.; Lever, H.M.; Cho, L.S.; Desai, M.Y. Predictors of longterm outcomes in patients with hypertrophic cardiomyopathy undergoing cardiopulmonary stress testing and echocardiography. *Am. Heart J.* **2015**, *169*, 684–692. [CrossRef]
15. Coats, C.J.; Rantell, K.; Bartnik, A.; Patel, A.; Mist, B.; McKenna, W.J.; Elliott, P.M. Cardiopulmonary exercise testing and prognosis in hypertrophic cardiomyopathy. *Circ. Heart Fail.* **2015**, *8*, 1022–1031. [CrossRef]
16. Finocchiaro, G.; Haddad, F.; Knowles, J.W.; Caleshu, C.; Pavlovic, A.; Homburger, J.; Shmargad, Y.; Sinagra, G.; Magavern, E.; Wong, M.; et al. Cardiopulmonary responses and prognosis in hypertrophic cardiomyopathy: A potential role for comprehensive noninvasive hemodynamic assessment. *JACC Heart Fail.* **2015**, *3*, 408–418. [CrossRef]
17. Magrì, D.; Re, F.; Limongelli, G.; Agostoni, P.; Zachara, E.; Correale, M.; Mastromarino, V.; Santolamazza, C.; Casenghi, M.; Pacileo, G.; et al. Heart Failure Progression in Hypertrophic Cardiomyopathy—Possible Insights From Cardiopulmonary Exercise Testing. *Circ. J.* **2016**, *80*, 2204–2211. [CrossRef]
18. Magrì, D.; Limongelli, G.; Re, F.; Agostoni, P.; Zachara, E.; Correale, M.; Mastromarino, V.; Santolamazza, C.; Casenghi, M.; Pacileo, G.; et al. Cardiopulmonary exercise test and sudden cardiac death risk in hypertrophic cardiomyopathy. *Heart* **2016**, *102*, 602–609. [CrossRef]
19. Lang, R.M.; Badano, L.P.; Mor-Avi, V.; Afilalo, J.; Armstrong, A.; Ernande, L.; Flachskampf, F.A.; Foster, E.; Goldstein, S.A.; Kuznetsova, T.; et al. Recommendations for cardiac chamber quantification by echocardiography in adults: An update from the American Society of Echocardiography and the European Association of Cardiovascular Imaging. *J. Am. Soc. Echocardiogr.* **2015**, *28*, 1–39. [CrossRef]

20. Autore, C.; Bernabò, P.; Barillà, C.S.; Bruzzi, P.; Spirito, P. The prognostic importance of left ventricular outflow obstruction in hypertrophic cardiomyopathy varies in relation to the severity of symptoms. *J. Am. Coll. Cardiol.* **2005**, *45*, 1076–1080. [CrossRef]
21. Agostoni, P.; Bianchi, M.; Moraschi, A.; Palermo, P.; Cattadori, G.; La Gioia, R.; Bussotti, M.; Wasserman, K. Work-rate affects cardiopulmonary exercise test results in heart failure. *Eur. J. Heart Fail.* **2005**, *7*, 498–504. [CrossRef]
22. Magrì, D.; Agostoni, P.; Sinagra, G.; Re, F.; Correale, M.; Limongelli, G.; Zachara, E.; Mastromarino, V.; Santolamazza, C.; Casenghi, M.; et al. Clinical and prognostic impact of chronotropic incompetence in patients with hypertrophic cardiomyopathy. *Int. J. Cardiol.* **2018**, *271*, 125–131. [CrossRef]
23. Corrà, U.; Mezzani, A.; Giordano, A.; Bosimini, E.; Giannuzzi, P. Exercise haemodynamic variables rather than ventilatory efficiency indexes contribute to risk assessment in chronic heart failure patients treated with carvedilol. *Eur. Heart J.* **2009**, *30*, 3000–3006. [CrossRef]
24. Wasserman, K.; Hansen, J.E.; Sue, D.Y.; Stringer, W.; Whipp, B.J. Normal Values. In *Principles of Exercise Testing and Interpretation*, 4th ed.; Weinberg, R., Ed.; Lippincott Williams and Wilkins: Philadelphia, PA, USA, 2005; pp. 160–182.
25. Richards, S.; Aziz, N.; Bale, S.; Bick, D.; Das, S.; Gastier-Foster, J.; Grody, W.W.; Hegde, M.; Lyon, E.; Spector, E.; et al. Standards and guidelines for the interpretation of sequence variants: A joint consensus recommendation of the American College of Medical Genetics and Genomics and the Association for Molecular Pathology. *Genet. Med.* **2015**, *17*, 405–424. [CrossRef]
26. Hershberger, R.E.; Givertz, M.M.; Ho, C.Y.; Judge, D.P.; Kantor, P.; McBride, K.L.; Morales, A.; Taylor, M.R.G.; Vatta, M.; Ware, S.M.; et al. Genetic evaluation of cardiomyopathy: A clinical practice resource of the American College of Medical Genetics and Genomics (ACMG). *Genet. Med.* **2018**, *20*, 899–909. [CrossRef]
27. O'Mahony, C.; Jichi, F.; Pavlou, M.; Monserrat, L.; Anastasakis, A.; Rapezzi, C.; Biagini, E.; Gimeno, J.R.; Limongelli, G.; McKenna, W.J.; et al. A novel clinical risk prediction model for sudden cardiac death in hypertrophic cardiomyopathy (HCM Risk-SCD). *Eur. Heart J.* **2014**, *35*, 2010–2020. [CrossRef]
28. O'Mahony, C.; Akhtar, M.M.; Anastasiou, Z.; Guttmann, O.P.; Vriesendorp, P.A.; Michels, M.; Magrì, D.; Autore, C.; Fernández, A.; Ochoa, J.P.; et al. Effectiveness of the 2014 European Society of Cardiology guideline on sudden cardiac death in hypertrophic cardiomyopathy: A systematic review and meta-analysis. *Heart* **2019**, *105*, 623–631. [CrossRef]
29. Biagini, E.; Olivotto, I.; Iascone, M.; Parodi, M.I.; Girolami, F.; Frisso, G.; Autore, C.; Limongelli, G.; Cecconi, M.; Maron, B.J.; et al. Significance of sarcomere gene mutations analysis in the end-stage phase of hypertrophic cardiomyopathy. *Am. J. Cardiol.* **2014**, *114*, 769–776. [CrossRef]
30. Magrì, D.; Santolamazza, C. Cardiopulmonary Exercise Test in Hypertrophic Cardiomyopathy. *Ann. Am. Thorac. Soc.* **2017**, *14* (Suppl. 1), 102–109. [CrossRef]
31. Magrì, D.; Agostoni, P.; Cauti, F.M.; Musumeci, B.; Egidy Assenza, G.; De Cecco, C.N.; Muscogiuri, G.; Maruotti, A.; Ricotta, A.; Pagannone, E.; et al. Determinants of peak oxygen uptake in patients with hypertrophic cardiomyopathy: A single-center study. *Intern. Emerg. Med.* **2014**, *9*, 293–302. [CrossRef]
32. Magrì, D. Peak oxygen uptake in heart failure: Look behind the number! *Eur. J. Prev. Cardiol.* **2018**, *25*, 1934–1936. [CrossRef]
33. Agostoni, P.; Corrà, U.; Cattadori, G.; Veglia, F.; La Gioia, R.; Scardovi, A.B.; Emdin, M.; Metra, M.; Sinagra, G.; Limongelli, G.; et al. Metabolic exercise test data combined with cardiac and kidney indexes, the MECKI score: A multiparametric approach to heart failure prognosis. *Int. J. Cardiol.* **2013**, *167*, 2710–2718. [CrossRef]
34. Paolillo, S.; Veglia, F.; Salvioni, E.; Corrà, U.; Piepoli, M.; Lagioia, R.; Limongelli, G.; Sinagra, G.; Cattadori, G.; Scardovi, A.B.; et al. Heart failure prognosis over time: How the prognostic role of oxygen consumption and ventilatory efficiency during exercise has changed in the last 20 years. *Eur. J. Heart Fail.* **2019**, *21*, 208–217. [CrossRef]
35. Ciampi, Q.; Betocchi, S.; Lombardi, R.; Manganelli, F.; Storto, G.; Losi, M.A.; Pezzella, E.; Finizio, F.; Cuocolo, A.; Chiariello, M. Hemodynamic determinants of exercise-induced abnormal blood pressure response in hypertrophic cardiomyopathy. *J. Am. Coll. Cardiol.* **2002**, *40*, 278–284. [CrossRef]
36. Kawasaki, T.; Azuma, A.; Kuribayashi, T.; Akakabe, Y.; Yamano, M.; Miki, S.; Sawada, T.; Kamitani, T.; Matsubara, H.; Sugihara, H. Vagal enhancement due to subendocardial ischemia as a cause of abnormal blood pressure response in hypertrophic cardiomyopathy. *Int. J. Cardiol.* **2008**, *129*, 59–64. [CrossRef]

37. Arena, R.; Owens, D.S.; Arevalo, J.; Smith, K.; Mohiddin, S.A.; McAreavey, D.; Ulisney, K.L.; Tripodi, D.; Fananapazir, L.; Plehn, J.F. Ventilatory efficiency and resting hemodynamics in hypertrophic cardiomyopathy. *Med. Sci. Sports Exerc.* **2008**, *40*, 799–805. [CrossRef]
38. Salvioni, E.; Corrà, U.; Piepoli, M.; Rovai, S.; Correale, M.; Paolillo, S.; Pasquali, M.; Magrì, D.; Vitale, G.; Fusini, L.; et al. Gender and age normalization and ventilation efficiency during exercise in heart failure with reduced ejection fraction. *ESC Heart Fail.* **2020**, *7*, 371–380. [CrossRef]
39. Musumeci, M.B.; Mastromarino, V.; Casenghi, M.; Tini, G.; Francia, P.; Maruotti, A.; Romaniello, A.; Magrì, D.; Lillo, R.; Adduci, C.; et al. Pulmonary hypertension and clinical correlates in hypertrophic cardiomyopathy. *Int. J. Cardiol.* **2017**, *248*, 326–332. [CrossRef]
40. Maron, B.J.; Maron, M.S.; Semsarian, C. Genetics of hypertrophic cardiomyopathy after 20 years: Clinical perspectives. *J. Am. Coll. Cardiol.* **2012**, *60*, 705–715. [CrossRef]
41. Homburger, J.R.; Green, E.M.; Caleshu, C.; Sunitha, M.S.; Taylor, R.E.; Ruppel, K.M.; Prasad Rao Metpally, R.; Colan, S.D.; Michels, M.; Day, S.M.; et al. Multidimensional Structure-Function Relationships in Human β-Cardiac Myosin from Population-Scale Genetic Variation. *Proc. Natl. Acad. Sci. USA* **2016**, *113*, 6701–6706. [CrossRef]
42. Alamo, L.; Ware, J.S.; Pinto, A.; Gillilan, R.E.; Seidman, J.G.; Seidman, C.E.; Padrón, R. Effects of Myosin Variants on Interacting-Heads Motif Explain Distinct Hypertrophic and Dilated Cardiomyopathy Phenotypes. *eLife* **2017**, *6*, e24634. [CrossRef]
43. García-Giustiniani, D.; Arad, M.; Ortíz-Genga, M.; Barriales-Villa, R.; Fernández, X.; Rodríguez-García, I.; Mazzanti, A.; Veira, E.; Maneiro, E.; Rebolo, P.; et al. Phenotype and Prognostic Correlations of the Converter Region Mutations Affecting the β Myosin Heavy Chain. *Heart* **2015**, *101*, 1047–1053. [CrossRef]

10

Levosimendan Improves Oxidative Balance in Cardiogenic Shock/Low Cardiac Output Patients

Elena Grossini [1,*], Serena Farruggio [1], Daniele Pierelli [2], Virginia Bolzani [3], Lidia Rossi [3], Piero Pollesello [4] and Carolina Monaco [2]

1. Laboratory of Physiology, Department of Translational Medicine, UPO, 28100 Novara, Italy; serefar@live.it
2. Cardiothoracic Intensive Care Unit, AOU, 28100 Novara, Italy; daniele.pierelli@gmail.com (D.P.); carolina.monaco@maggioreosp.novara.it (C.M.)
3. Cardiology Division, AOU, 28100 Novara, Italy; virgi.bolzani@gmail.com (V.B.); rossilidia7@gmail.com (L.R.)
4. Critical Care, OrionPharma, 02101 Espoo, Finland; piero.pollesello@orionpharma.com

* Correspondence: elena.grossini@med.uniupo.it

Abstract: The beneficial effects exerted by levosimendan against cardiac failure could be related to the modulation of oxidative balance. We aimed to examine the effects of levosimendan in patients with cardiogenic shock or low cardiac output on cardiac systo-diastolic function and plasma oxidants/antioxidants (glutathione, GSH; thiobarbituric acid reactive substances, TBARS). In four patients undergoing coronary artery bypass grafting or angioplasty, cardiovascular parameters and plasma GSH and TBARS were measured at T0 (before levosimendan infusion), T1 (1 h after the achievement of the therapeutic dosage of levosimendan), T2 (end of levosimendan infusion), T3 (72 h after the end of levosimendan infusion), and T4 (end of cardiogenic shock). We found an improvement in the indices of systolic (ejection fraction, cardiac output, cardiac index) and diastolic (E to early diastolic mitral annular tissue velocity, E/'; early to late diastolic transmitral flow velocity, EA) cardiac function at early T2. A reduction of central venous pressure and pulmonary wedge pressure was also observed. Plasma levels of GSH and TBARS were restored by levosimendan at T1, as well. The results obtained indicate that levosimendan administration can regulate oxidant/antioxidant balance as an early effect in cardiogenic shock/low cardiac output patients. Modulation of oxidative status on a mitochondrial level could thus play a role in exerting the cardio-protection exerted by levosimendan in these patients.

Keywords: antioxidants; calcium sensitizer; heart failure; mitochondria function; peroxidation

1. Introduction

Levosimendan is an inotrope used for the treatment of acutely decompensated heart failure patients with low cardiac output or cardiogenic shock [1–4].

Among its mechanisms of action, the sensitization of cardiac troponin C to calcium in cardiac muscle [5–7] and the opening adenosine triphosphate-sensitive potassium (K_{ATP}) channels in vascular smooth muscle cells [8,9] have been described. Due to these pharmacological actions, levosimendan improves atrio-ventricular coupling and cardiac mechanical efficiency without increasing myocardial oxygen consumption [10–13]. Moreover, levosimendan has been shown to have a direct effect on mitochondria [14–19].

Preliminary data obtained in vitro, ex vivo, and in vivo in animal models have shown that levosimendan could improve endothelial and mitochondrial function, and protect against peroxidation, as well. In anesthetized pigs subjected to renal ischemia/reperfusion, the intrarenal levosimendan administration was able to increase renal function and keep the oxidant balance, as shown by the increased plasma levels of glutathione (GSH) and the reduced release of peroxidation markers, like thiobarbituric acid reactive substances (TBARS) [20]. Similar nominally beneficial effects against peroxidation were observed in anesthetized rats subjected to hepatic ischemia/reperfusion and treated with levosimendan [21].

TBARS, which reflect the release of malon(MDA) generated through the peroxidation of polyunsaturated fatty acids, have been widely adopted as indicators of oxidative stress in various cardiovascular diseases [22]. GSH plays an important role in the maintenance of the thiol-redox status of the cell, and for this reason could act as antioxidant. GSH deficiency might manifest itself through an increased susceptibility to oxidative stress and to the augmented onset and progression of many diseases, including the cardiovascular diseases [23].)

Similar beneficial effects against peroxidation, as were observed in the renal model of ischemia/reperfusion, have been observed in anesthetized rats subjected to hepatic ischemia/reperfusion and treated with levosimendan [21]. Finally, in rat hepatocytes, the administration of levosimendan dose-dependently counteracted the injuries caused by oxidative stress, as evidenced by the keeping GSH content and the reduction of TBARS release [24]. In all the above conditions, endothelial and mitochondrial function were found to be ameliorated by levosimendan, which prevented the fall of mitochondrial membrane potential and restored nitric oxide (NO) release.

The beneficial effects elicited by levosimendan against oxidative stress could represent a further mechanism of protection in heart failure (HF) patients. The implication of oxidative stress in the pathophysiology of HF is well established. Oxidative stress may impair cardiac functions through damage to the cellular proteins and membranes by initiation of lipid peroxidation, thereby inducing cellular death and apoptosis. Moreover, it could exert direct negative inotropic effects through the reduction of cytosolic intracellular free calcium [25]. Thus, there is strong circumstantial evidence that oxidative stress is a prognostic factor in HF patients. Keith et al. showed that circulating MDA, a marker of lipid peroxidation, was significantly different between control subjects and patients with HF [26]. In addition, MDA plasma levels have been positively correlated not only with the presence of HF, but also with New York Heart Association (NYHA) functional class [27].

It is worth noting that levosimendan administration to decompensated HF subjects was able to improve oxidative damage, as shown by the TBARS measurement, by five days [28]. To date, however, the information available about the effects of levosimendan on oxidative stress and cardiac systo-diastolic function in cardiogenic shock/low cardiac output patients for ischemic disease, is scarce.

For this reason, in the present study, we aimed to examine, at the same time, the effects of intravenous levosimendan treatment on (1) systolic and diastolic functions, (2) hemodynamic variables, and (3) oxidant/antioxidant systems, in patients admitted to the cardiothoracic intensive care unit (ICU) for cardiogenic shock or decompensated heart failure after coronary artery bypass grafting (CABG) or percutaneous transluminal coronary angioplasty (PTCA). To our knowledge, this is the first time these parallel assessments have been performed in a clinical setting.

2. Materials and Methods

This was a prospective, longitudinal study approved by the Ethical Committee of Azienda Ospedaliero Universitaria (AOU) Maggiore della Carità of Novara (655/CE; Studio n. CE 107/17; approval date 16/06/2017). All procedures were compliant with the ethical standards of the Helsinki Declaration and conformed to standards currently applied in Italy. Patients' informed written consent was collected before starting the study.

In this pilot study, 4 adult patients admitted to the cardiothoracic ICU of AOU Maggiore della Carità of Novara were enrolled.

Inclusion criteria were: Aged over 18 years, reduced systolic function (ejection fraction, EF, < 30%) due to cardiogenic shock post-CABG or decompensated heart failure after PTCA.

Exclusion criteria: Acute renal or liver failure, septic condition.

Two male patients underwent CABG for three vessel-diseases. In PTCA patients (one male and one female), three arterial grafts were positioned on the left anterior descending coronary artery, and intra-aortic balloon pumps (IABP) were used. Demographic data are reported in Table 1.

Table 1. Demographic data of patients.

Males/Females	**3/1**
Age (years)	63 ± 13.5
BMI (body mass index)	26.63 ± 1.2
Diabetes	1/4
Hypertension	0
Smoker (>1 cigarette)	0
Dyslipidemia	0

Hemodynamic variables were monitored by means of a Swan–Ganz pulmonary artery catheter in all patients [29,30].

The central venous pressure (CVP), mean pulmonary arterial pressure (PAP), cardiac output (CO), cardiac index (CI), systemic vascular resistance index (SVRI), pulmonary vascular resistance index (PVRI), and the pulmonary capillary wedge pressure (PCWP) were continuously measured. Heart rate (HR), and systolic (SAP) and diastolic (DAP) arterial blood pressure were also recorded. Arterial and venous oxygen partial pressure (pO_2), and arterial and venous oxygen saturation (SO_2) were examined by hemogasanalyis (Radiometer ABL 90 Flex).

In all patients, systo-diastolic cardiac function was examined by an expert cardiologist through echocardiography (GE Vivid-i), following the time-course reported below, and as recommended by international guidelines [31–33].

After baseline data evaluation, levosimendan was administered intravenously at the dose of 0.1 μg/kg/min without a loading dose, which is adopted in the ICU for the treatment of cardiogenic shock or low cardiac output patients [34,35]. In all patients, vasopressor support was implemented by epinephrine (0.01–0.1 μg/kg/min) and in one patient with dopamine (2 μg/kg/min), as well. Mechanically assisted ventilation was provided to CABG patients.

Venous samples were taken for GSH and TBARS measurements, following the time-course reported below.

2.1. *Collection of Samples*

For the determination of GSH and TBARS, 10 mL of blood samples were taken from each donor using BD Vacutainer tubes (sodium heparin as anticoagulant). Each sample was immediately centrifuged by a refrigerated centrifuge (Eppendorf, mod. 5702 with rotor A-4-38) for 10 min, at a speed of 3100 g at 4 °C. The plasma obtained was divided into 5 tubes that were stored at −20 °C at the Physiology laboratory of the University of Eastern Piedmont of Novara.

2.2. *GSH Quantification*

GSH measurement was performed by using the Glutathione Assay Kit (Cayman Chemical, Ann Arbor, MI, USA), as previously described [36,37]. Each plasma sample was deproteinated by adding an equal volume of MPA solution to the sample which was then centrifuged at 2000 g for 2 min. The supernatant was collected, and 50 μL/mL of TEAM reagent was added to each sample in order to increase the pH. Fifty microliters of the samples were transferred to a 96-well plate where GSH was detected following the manufacturer's instructions through a spectrophotometer (VICTOR™ X Multilabel Plate Reader), at excitation/emission wavelengths of 405–414 nm. Glutathione was expressed as μM. The measurements were performed in triplicate.

2.3. *TBARS Quantification*

TBARS were determined as MDA release. The MDA measurement was performed by using the TBARS assay Kit (Cayman Chemical), as previously [36,38]. For the assays, 100 μL of each plasma sample was added to 100 μL of sodium dodecyl sulfate (SDS) solution and 2 mL of the Color Reagent, following the manufacturer's instructions. Each sample was boiled for 1 h and then transferred to ice for 10 min in order to stop the reaction. Each sample was centrifuged for 10 min at 1600 g at 4 °C and 150 μL was transferred to a 96-well plate where MDA was detected following the manufacturer's instructions through a spectrophotometer (VICTOR™ X Multilabel Plate Reader), at excitation/emission wavelengths of 530–540 nm. MDA production was expressed in μM. The measurements were performed in triplicate.

2.4. *Time-Course of Measurements*

T0, before the beginning of levosimendan administration: Hemodynamic variable measurements and cardiac systo-diastolic evaluation, GSH and TBARS sampling.

T1, at the end of 0.1 μg/kg/min levosimendan infusion (duration 24 h): Hemodynamic variable measurements and cardiac systo-diastolic evaluation, GSH and TBARS sampling.

T2, 24 h after the end of levosimendan infusion: Hemodynamic variable measurements and cardiac systo-diastolic evaluation, GSH and TBARS sampling.

T3, at 72 h after the end of levosimendan administration: Hemodynamic variable measurements and cardiac systo-diastolic evaluation, GSH and TBARS sampling.

T4, at the end of inotropic support: Hemodynamic variable measurements and cardiac systo-diastolic evaluation, GSH and TBARS sampling.

2.5. *Statistical Analysis*

All data were recorded using the Institution's database. Statistical analysis was performed by using GraphPad Prism 6.0. Non-nominal variables were checked for normality before statistical analysis. ANOVA for repeated measurements was used to compare results obtained in each patient at various timings. All non-nominal data were expressed as means ± standard deviation (SD). A p value lower than 0.05 was taken for statistical significance.

3. Results

The patients were overweight, and one patient was diabetic, but major cardiovascular risk factors like hypertension, smoking, or dyslipidemia were not identified (Table 1). At T0, mean EF amounted to 25%. In the two patients who underwent cardiothoracic surgery, extracorporeal circulation lasted 145 ± 21 min.

Improvements were recorded in CO, CI, and SAP, as shown in Figures 1 and 2A,B.

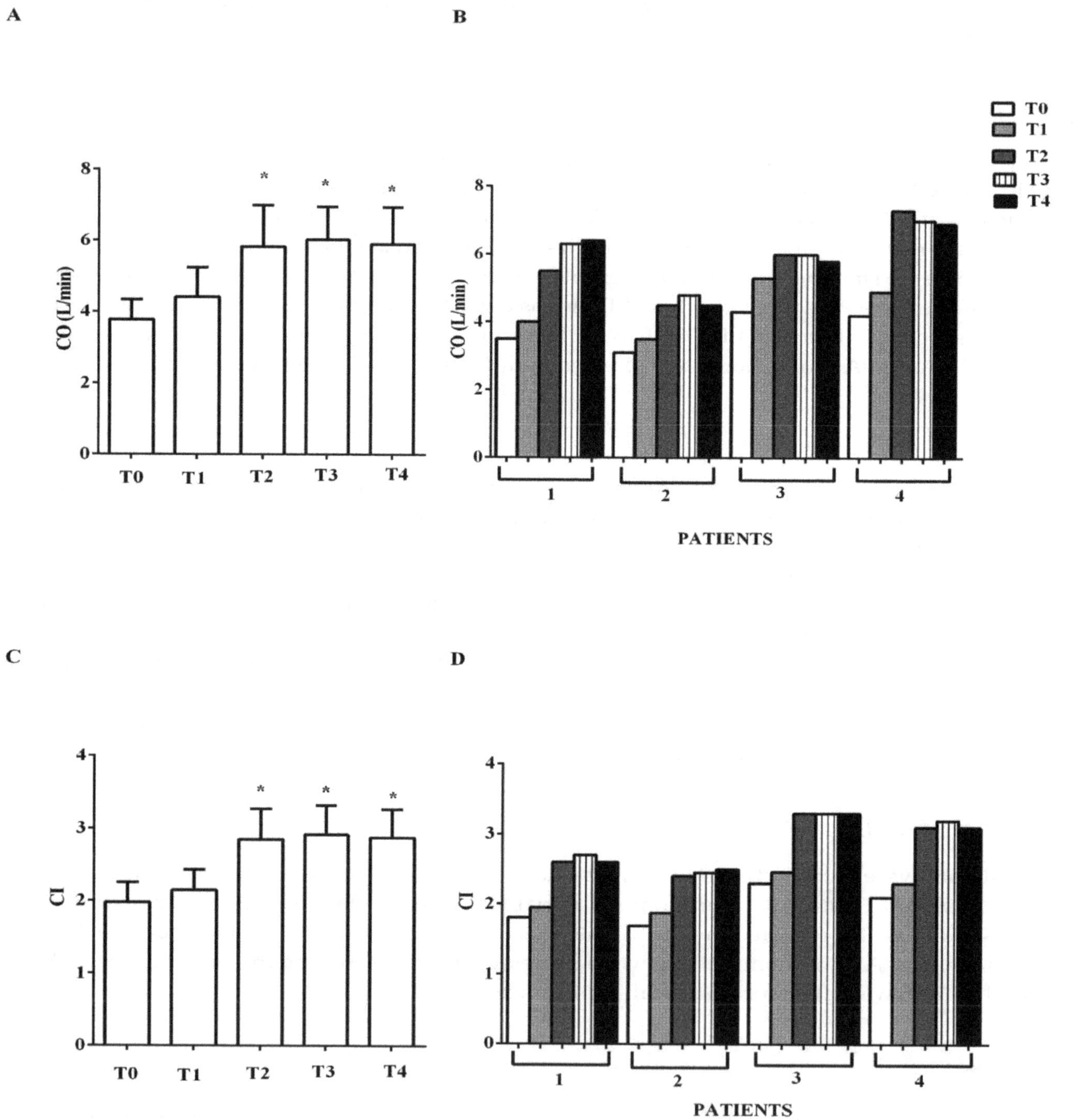

Figure 1. In (**A**,**B**), effects of levosimendan on cardiac output (CO) and in (**C**,**D**), on cardiac index (CI). In A and C, values are means ± SD. In B and D, columns represent single patients. * $p < 0.05$ vs. T0.

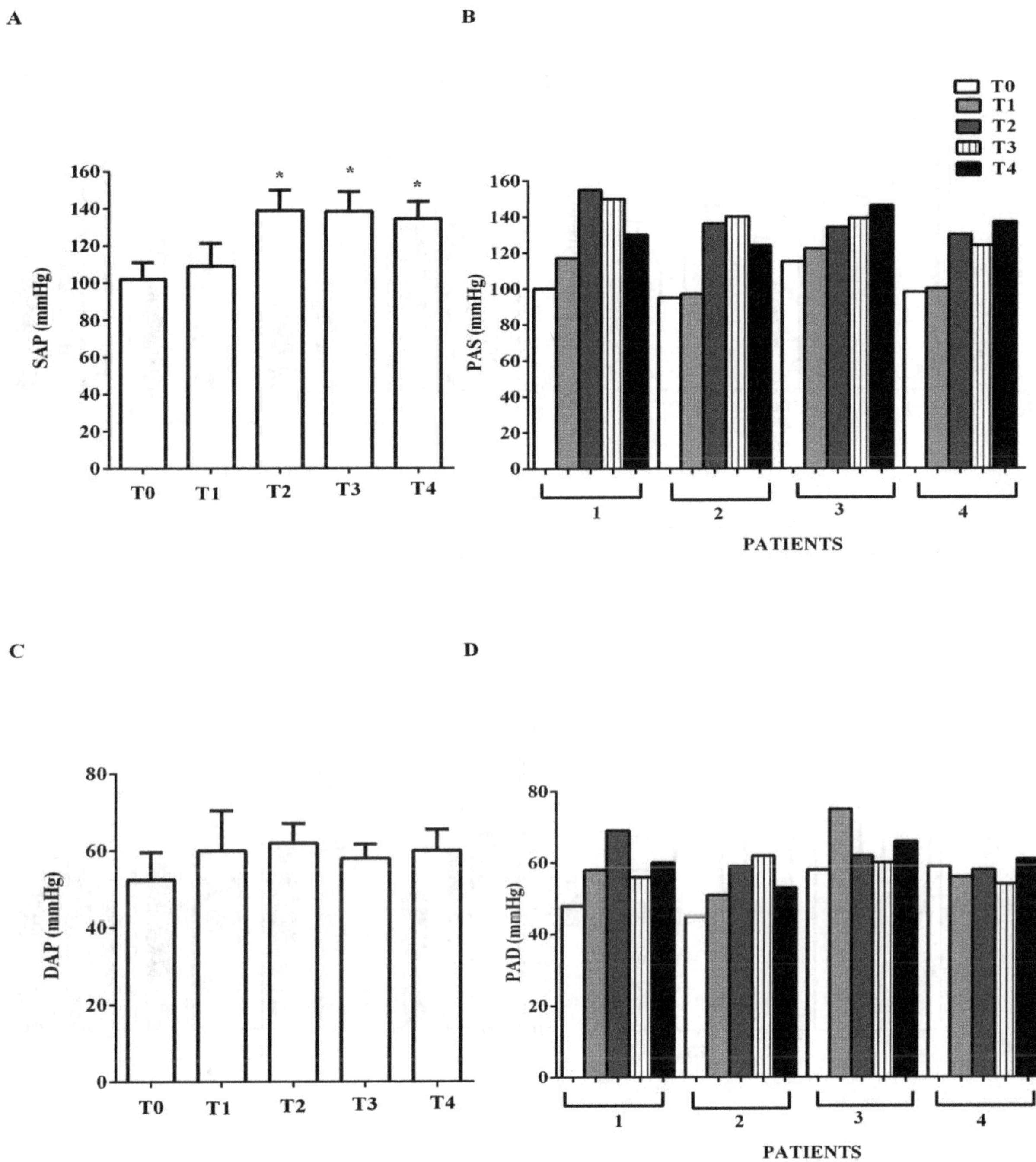

Figure 2. In (**A**,**B**), effects of levosimendan on systolic (SAP) and in (**C**,**D**), diastolic (DAP) arterial blood pressure. In A and C, values are means ± SD. In B and D, columns represent single patients. * $p < 0.05$ vs. T0.

EF increased from mean 26.25% ± 2.2 to 43.7% ± 2.9 at early T2, and to 48% ± 1.4 at T4 ($p < 0.05$). A reduction of CVP, pulmonary capillary wedge pressure (wedge), and PVRI was also observed (Figure 3A,B and Figure 4B,D). PAP at T4 was lower than PAP at T0 (Figure 3C,D).

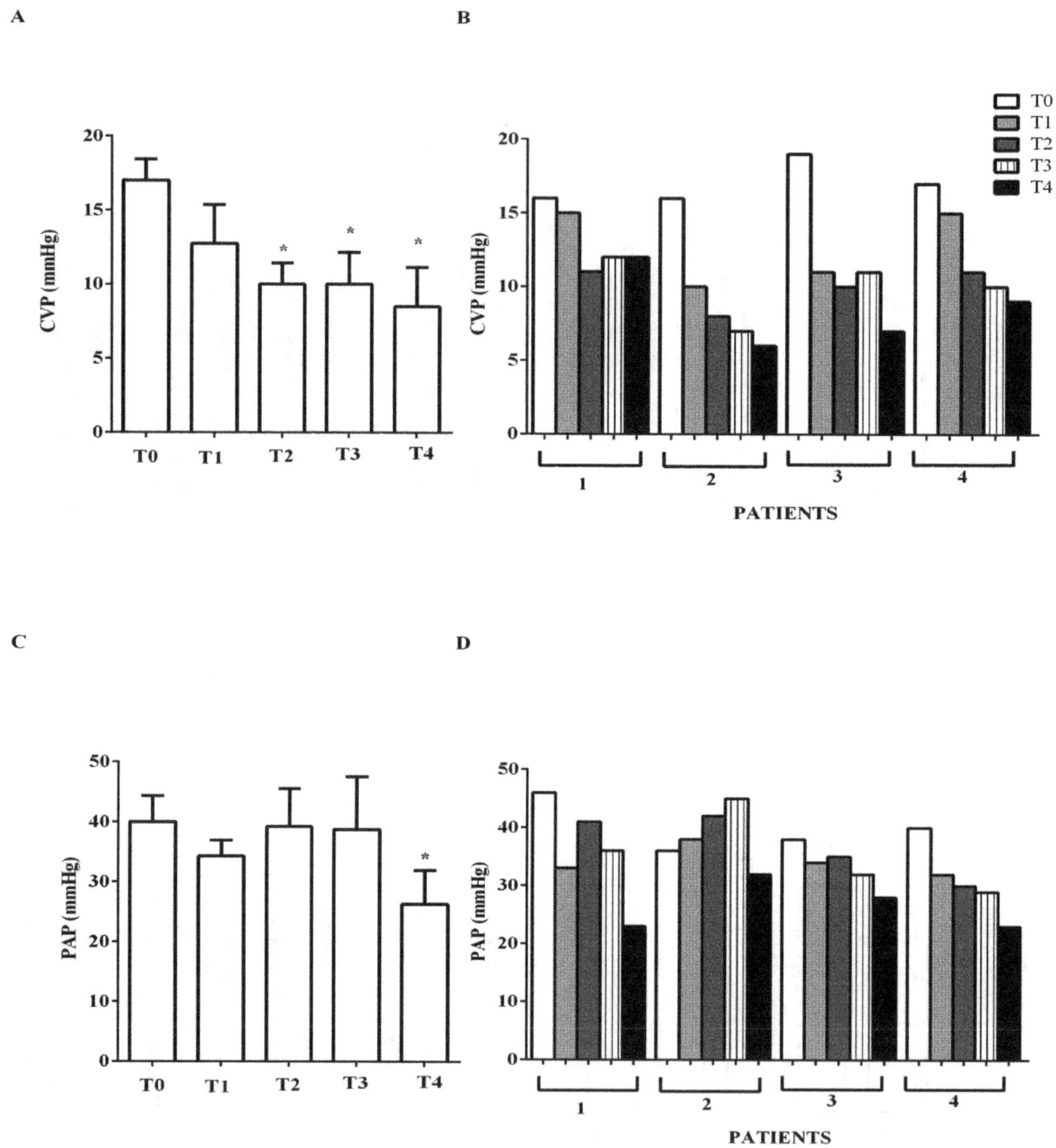

Figure 3. In (**A**,**B**), effects of levosimendan on central venous pressure (CVP) and in (**C**,**D**) on mean pulmonary arterial pressure (PAP). In A and C, values are means ± SD. In B and D, columns represent single patients. * $p < 0.05$ vs. T0.

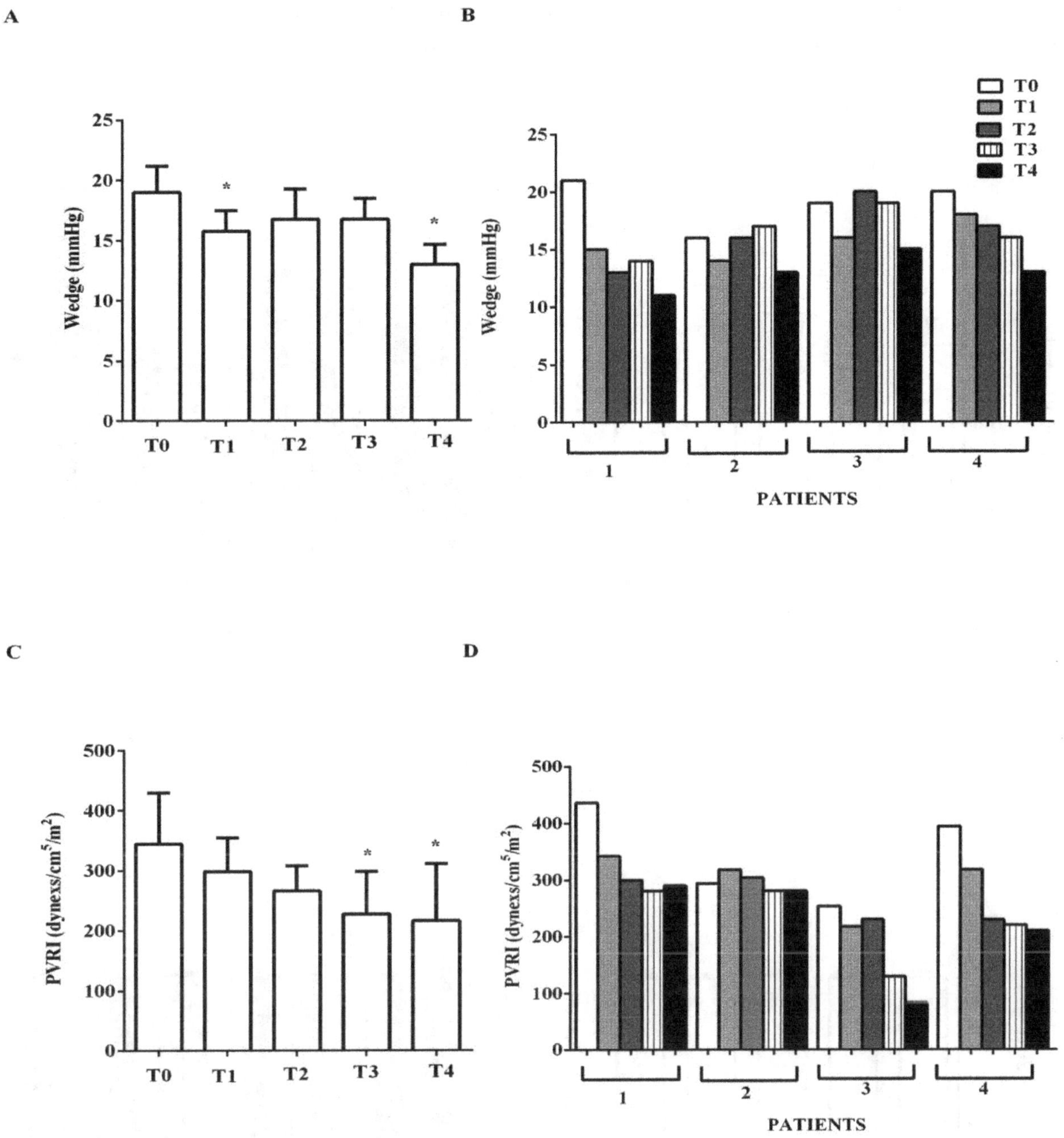

Figure 4. In (**A**,**B**), effects of levosimendan on pulmonary capillary wedge pressure (wedge) and in (**C**,**D**), on pulmonary vascular resistance index (PVRI). In A and C, values are means ± SD. In B and D, columns represent single patients. * $p < 0.05$ vs. T0.

Indices of diastolic function (E/E′, E/A) were improved by levosimendan administration (E to early diastolic mitral annular tissue velocity, E/, from mean 14.5 ± 1.3 at T0, to mean 11 ± 1.4 at T2, to mean 6.7 ± 1.7 at T4; early to late diastolic transmitral flow velocity, E/A, from >1 at T0 to <1 at T4; $p < 0.05$). No significant changes of HR were observed (mean values at T0 to T4, respectively: 96.75, 90.75, 95.75, 88, 91 beats/min), nor in DAP (Figure 2C,D). In the two PTCA patients, IABP was removed at T2 and mechanical ventilation was suspended after 1 and 3 days, respectively. In all patients, epinephrine was reduced from mean 0.06 ± 0.04 μg/kg/min at T0, to 0.04 ± 0.02 μg/kg/min at T2, to 0.001 ± 0.009 μg/kg/min at T3; at T4 it was suspended. Dopamine was reduced from 2 μg/kg/min at T0, to 1 μg/kg/min at T2; at T4 it was suspended.

Arterial oxygen saturation and oxygen partial pressure amounted to about 98% and 96 mmHg at T0 and did not vary significantly throughout the time-course (Figure 5).

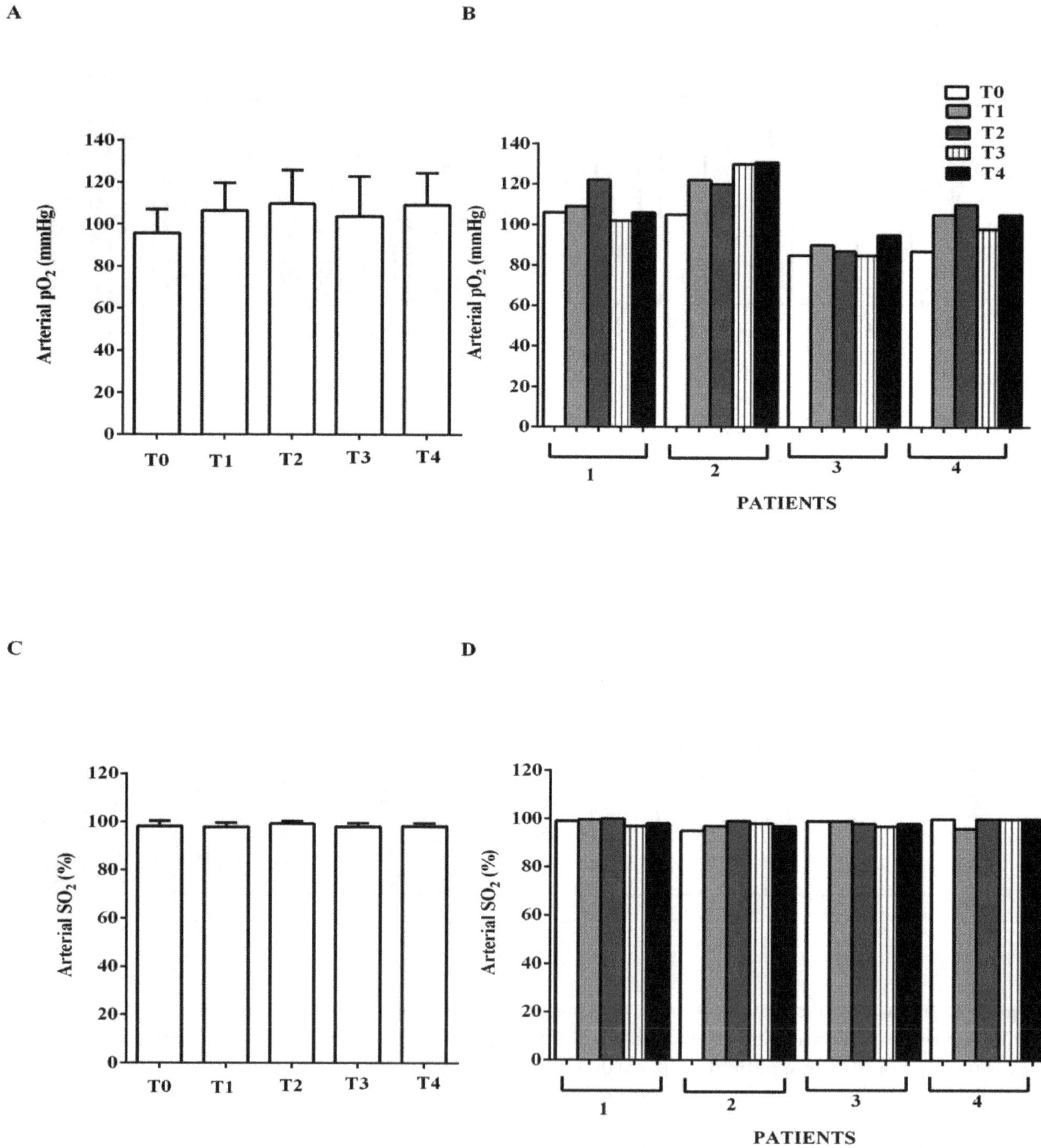

Figure 5. In (**A**,**B**), effects of levosimendan on arterial partial pressure (pO_2) and in (**C**,**D**), on arterial oxygen saturation (SO_2). In A and C, values are means ± SD. In B and D, columns represent single patients.

ygen venous partial pressure and venous oxygen saturation amounted to about 37 mmHg and 63% at T0 and did not show any changes (Figure 6).

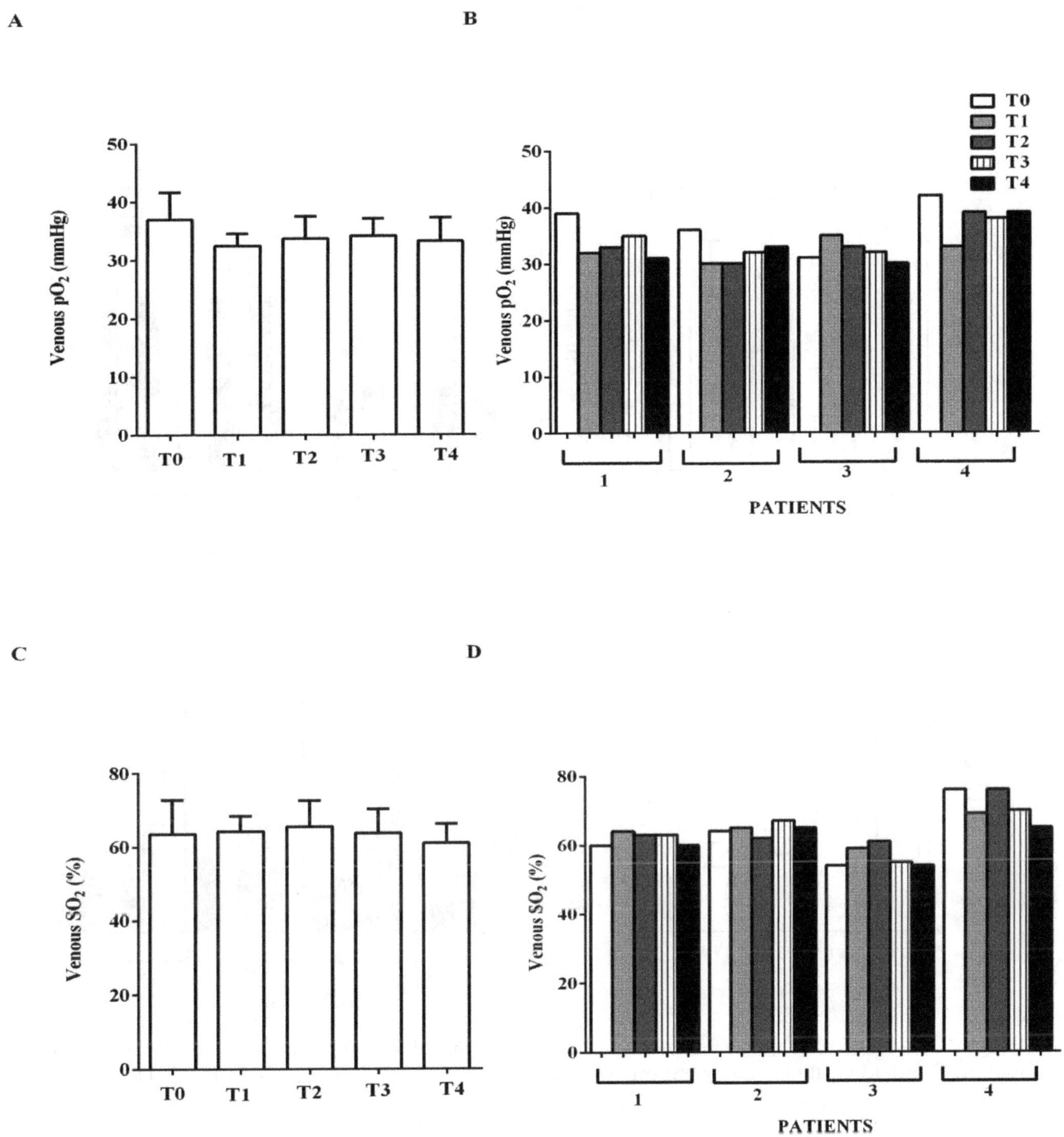

Figure 6. In (**A**,**B**), effects of levosimendan on venous oxygen partial pressure (pO_2) and in (**C**,**D**), on venous oxygen saturation (SO_2). In A and C, values are means ± SD. In B and D, columns represent single patients.

As depicted in Figure 7, at T0, the levels of GSH and MDA were 0.21 ± 0.16 μM and 7.1 ± 1.9 μM, respectively. Immediately after levosimendan administration, an improvement of the above parameters was observed. GSH at T1 rose to 1.16 ± 0.5 μM, whereas MDA declined to 4.3 ± 1.1 μM (both $p < 0.05$ vs. T0). At T2, T3, and T4, the levels of GSH increased (3.1 ± 1.3; 3.8 ± 1.2; 2.8 ± 1.2 μM, respectively; all $p < 0.05$ vs. T0) and those of MDA decreased progressively (2.5 ± 0.9; 2.4 ± 0.9; 2.1 ± 0.8 μM; all $p < 0.05$ vs. T0).

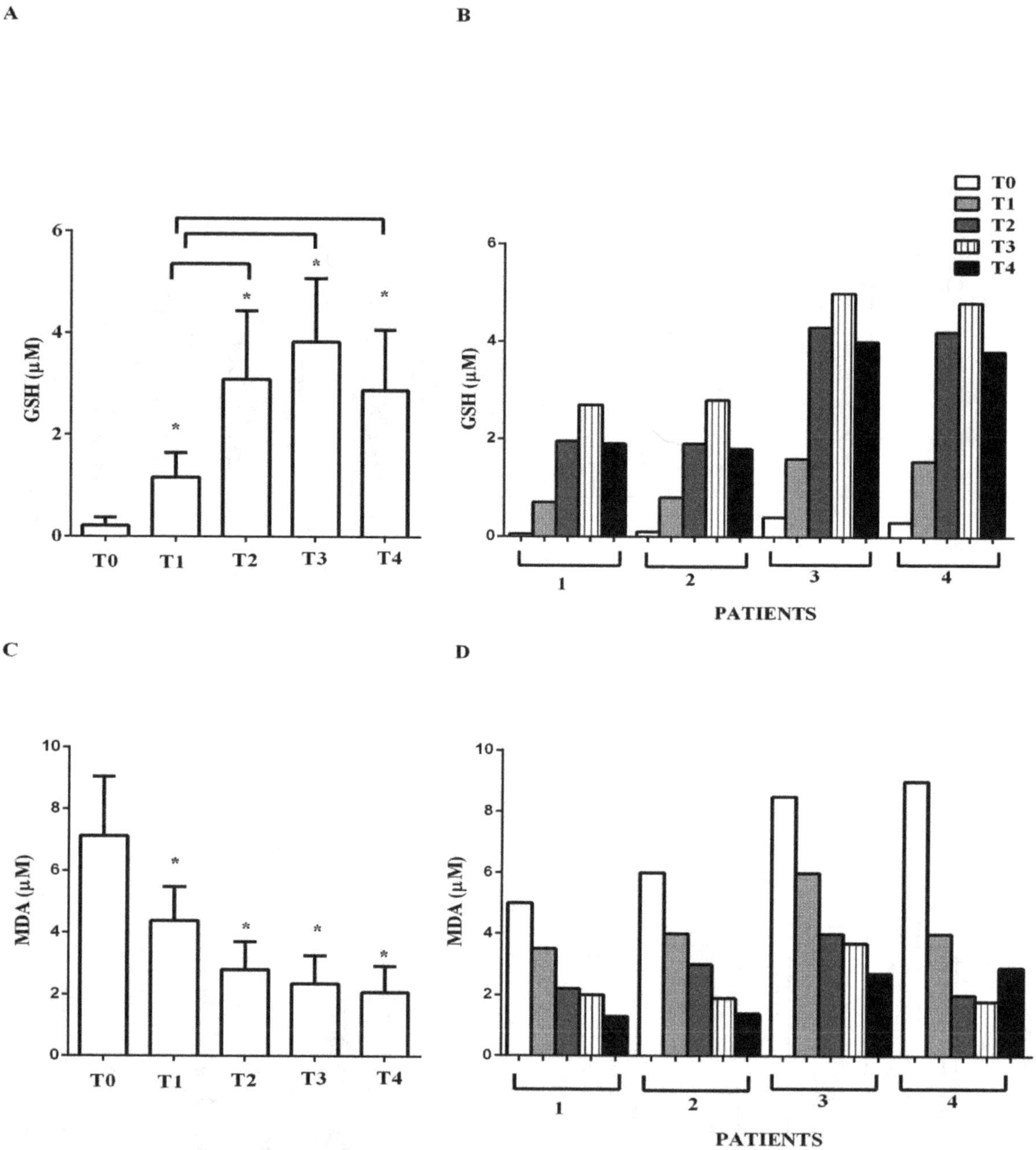

Figure 7. In (**A**,**B**), effects of levosimendan on plasma glutathione (GSH) and in (**C**,**D**), on plasma malonyldialdeide (MDA) concentration. In A and C, values are means ± SD. In B and D, columns represent single patients. * $p < 0.05$ vs. T0.

4. Discussion

The results obtained in the present study show protective effects elicited by levosimendan administration in cardiogenic shock or low cardiac output patients post-CABG or PTCA, through the modulation of oxidant/antioxidant balance.

The balance between ROS production and their removal by antioxidant systems is described as the "redox state". Oxidative stress arises any time the production of ROS exceeds the levels of antioxidants. In HF, an increased production of ROS, originating mainly by mitochondria from failing hearts, has been widely evidenced [39]. Chronic increases in ROS production may lead to a cycle of mitochondrial DNA damage, leading to a functional decline, further ROS generation, and cellular injury. ROS can directly impair contractile function by modifying proteins central to excitation–contraction coupling, ion transporters, and Ca^{2+} cycling, as well [40].

It is noteworthy that cardiac oxidative stress has been associated with diastolic dysfunction, as well [41], via changes in Ca^{2+} handling. Hence, increased ROS production can impair the activity of Ca^{2+}/calmodulin kinase (CaMK) II or SERCA2, or affect Ca^{2+} sensitivity of myofilaments. As a result, a diastolic SR Ca^{2+} leak and a reduction of relaxation stiffness of cardiomyocytes would happen [42].

In addition, changes of mitochondrial function could lead to increased intracellular Ca^{2+}, resulting in cardiomyocyte super-contracture, disruption of plasmalemma and therefore necrotic cell death. Although it was not clearly shown, at the basis of the above effects there could be the increased mitochondrial ROS generation [43].

Furthermore, KA_{TP} channels could represent a target for ROS in HF [44]. It has been shown that ROS-dependent modification of mitochondrial K_{ATP} channels, in particular, could represent a feedback mechanism for the regulation of mitochondrial K_{ATP} channel activity itself. Moreover, K_{ATP} channels have been widely shown to play important roles in protection of the heart from ischemic injury [45]. The opening of K_{ATP} channels could contribute to the regulation of cardiac mitochondrial function [46] and cardioprotection induced by ischemic preconditioning, as well.

For this reason, any factor able to affect K_{ATP} channel activity could represent a rescue method against cardiac damage.

The mechanisms of action of levosimendan are mainly related to the increase of Ca^{2+} sensitivity of troponin C and the opening of K_{ATP} channels in myocardium and vessels. Being a calcium sensitizer and not a calcium mobilizer, levosimendan does not increase myocardial oxygen consumption nor prevent myocardial apoptosis and remodeling [1].

For those reasons, levosimendan is widely used for the treatment of low cardiac output conditions for its effects on systemic and pulmonary hemodynamics and for the relief of symptoms of HF [47].

Recent evidence indicates that levosimendan could reduce oxidative markers and increase the antioxidant system. In decompensated HF patients, a reduction of TBARS levels was observed after 5 days from the start of levosimendan administration [28], while, in the animal model of renal and liver ischemia/reperfusion plasma, TBARS and GSH concentration was restored by levosimendan infusion [20,21]. A role for the modulation of the "redox state", as a possible mechanism of action of levosimendan in the protection against HF, might therefore be hypothesized.

In our study, the infusion of levosimendan in cardiogenic shock or low cardiac output patients post-CABG or PTCA improved GSH and reduced TBARS early at the achievement of the therapeutic levosimendan dosage. Those effects preceded those on hemodynamics and cardiac systo-diastolic function, which were evidenced by the improvement of EF, CO, CI, E/E', and E/A.

Our data confirm previous data about the protective effects exerted by levosimendan against peroxidation, and highlight their potential as further mechanisms through which levosimendan could exert its action on cardiac function. Although it was not examined, the maintenance of mitochondria function by levosimendan could be presumed to play a role in its antioxidant effects.

Hence, mitochondria have emerged as a central factor in the pathogenesis and progression of HF. It is widely accepted that mitochondrial dysfunction can contribute to impaired myocardial energetics and increased oxidative stress in cardiomyopathies, cardiac ischemic damage, and HF. Mitochondrial permeability transition pore opening has been shown to act as a critical trigger of myocyte death and myocardial remodeling. Increased mitochondrial permeabilization is a mechanistic pathway at the basis of myocardial apoptosis [48].

Previous findings have evidenced that levosimendan is able to prevent the fall of mitochondrial membrane potential and transition pore opening in cardiomyocytes [49]. In this way, it could modulate ROS release and apoptotic signaling. Thus, it could be hypothesized that the keeping mitochondrial function by levosimendan could represent the starting mechanism for the reduction of ROS release and the restoration of myocardial energetics and cell viability. These events would be followed by the improvement of cardiac systole and diastole and hemodynamics.

In conclusion, the results obtained have shown that levosimendan improved GSH and reduced TBARS early before the onset of the cardiovascular effects.

The main limitation of this study is the low number of patients and the different etiologies. However, the aim of this pilot study was to evaluate if levosimendan could exert its protective effects in patients with cardiac low output syndrome or cardiogenic shock on cardiovascular function and hemodynamics as a result of its ability to prevent the GSH reduction and TBARS increase, regardless of the etiology. Moreover, no comparison was performed with a "control" group. However, in this study, all patients were in control of themselves and we analyzed, at different time points, the concomitant changes of hemodynamic variables and cardiac systo-diastolic function, as well as the changes in the levels of oxidants and antioxidants. The results obtained have shown that levosimendan improved GSH and reduced TBARS early before the onset of the cardiovascular effects. Thus, in spite of the low number of cases, levosimendan infusion was able to significantly exert beneficial effects on both the oxidant and antioxidant system, hemodynamics, and cardiac function in cardiogenic shock/low cardiac output patients. A larger number of cases will be necessary to perform a more detailed analysis of the protective effects of levosimendan and evaluation of any differences among various patients.

Overall, the results obtained in this pilot study set the rationale for a clinical trial in a larger population, whose number will be established through a power calculation, and stratified for age, sex, BMI, comorbidities, and etiologies. In this regard, the role of IABP as a modulator of oxidative stress could be further analyzed. In addition, it would be interesting to collect more data about the "redox state" and inflammation and compare the effects of levosimendan with those of other inotropes.

Finally, it seems important to follow the putative anti-inflammatory effects of this drug, not only in cardiac patients, but also in patients with conditions such as pulmonary hypertension or amyotrophic lateral sclerosis, in which levosimendan is currently being clinically evaluated [50,51].

Author Contributions: Author Contributions: Conception and design: E.G., C.M. and P.P.; patient data and samples: D.P., L.R. and V.B.; experiments, collection and assembly of data: S.F., C.M., D.P., L.R. and V.B.; data analysis and interpretation: E.G. and P.P.; manuscript writing and editing: e.g., S.F., C.M., D.P., L.R., V.B. and P.P. All authors have read and agreed to the published version of the manuscript.

Acknowledgments: We thank Azienda Ospedaliera Universitaria AOU Maggiore della Carità for its help. We thank Hughes Associated, Oxford, for the language check of the document

References

1. Farmakis, D.; Alvarez, J.; Gal, T.B.; Brito, D.; Fedele, F.; Fonseca, C.; Gordon, A.C.; Gotsman, I.; Grossini, E.; Guarracino, F.; et al. Levosimendan beyond inotropy and acute heart failure: Evidence of pleiotropic effects on the heart and other organs: An expert panel position paper. *Int. J. Cardiol.* **2016**, *222*, 303–312. [CrossRef] [PubMed]
2. Follath, F.; Cleland, J.G.; Just, H.; Papp, J.G.; Scholz, H.; Peuhkurinen, K.; Harjola, V.P.; Mitrovic, V.; Abdalla, M.; Sandell, E.P.; et al. Steering Committee and Investigators of the Levosimendan Infusion versus Dobutamine (LIDO) Study. Efficacy and safety of intravenous levosimendan compared with dobutamine in severe low-output heart failure (the LIDO study): A randomised double-blind trial. *Lancet* **2002**, *360*, 196–202. [CrossRef]
3. Moiseyev, V.S.; Põder, P.; Andrejevs, N.; Ruda, M.Y.; Golikov, A.P.; Lazebnik, L.B.; Kobalava, Z.D.; Lehtonen, L.A.; Laine, T.; et al. Nieminen MSRUSSLAN Study Investigators. Safety and efficacy of a novel calcium sensitizer, levosimendan, in patients with left ventricular failure due to an acute myocardial infarction. A randomized, placebo-controlled, double-blind study (RUSSLAN). *Eur. Heart J.* **2002**, *23*, 1422–1432. [CrossRef] [PubMed]
4. Herpain, A.; Bouchez, S.; Girardis, M.; Guarracino, F.; Knotzer, J.; Levy, B.; Liebregts, T.; Pollesello, P.; Ricksten, S.E.; Riha, H.; et al. Use of Levosimendan in Intensive Care Unit Settings: An Opinion Paper. *J. Cardiovasc. Pharmacol.* **2019**, *73*, 3–14. [CrossRef]

5. Pollesello, P.; Ovaska, M.; Kaivola, J.; Tilgmann, C.; Lundström, K.; Kalkkinen, N.; Ulmanen, I.; Nissinen, E.; Taskinen, J. Binding of a new Ca^{2+} sensitizer, levosimendan, to recombinant human cardiac troponin C. A molecular modelling, fluorescence probe, and proton nuclear magnetic resonance study. *J. Biol. Chem.* **1994**, *269*, 28584–28590.
6. Pääkkönen, K.; Annila, A.; Sorsa, T.; Pollesello, P.; Tilgmann, C.; Kilpeläinen, I.; Karisola, P.; Ulmanen, I.; Drakenberg, T. Solution structure and main chain dynamics of the regulatory domain (Residues 1-91) of human cardiac troponin C. *J. Biol. Chem.* **1998**, *273*, 15633–15638. [CrossRef]
7. Sorsa, T.; Heikkinen, S.; Abbott, M.B.; Abusamhadneh, E.; Laakso, T.; Tilgmann, C.; Serimaa, R.; Annila, A.; Rosevear, P.R.; Drakenberg, T. Binding of levosimendan, a calcium sensitizer, to cardiac troponin C. *J. Biol. Chem.* **2001**, *276*, 9337–9343. [CrossRef]
8. Yokoshiki, H.; Katsube, Y.; Sunagawa, M.; Sperelakis, N. The novel calcium sensitizer levosimendan activates the ATP-sensitive K+ channel in rat ventricular cells. *J. Pharmacol. Exp. Ther.* **1997**, *283*, 375–383.
9. Pataricza, J.; Krassói, I.; Höhn, J.; Kun, A.; Papp, J.G. Functional role of potassium channels in the vasodilating mechanism of levosimendan in porcine isolated coronary artery. *Cardiovasc. Drugs Ther.* **2003**, *17*, 115–121. [CrossRef]
10. Kaheinen, P.; Pollesello, P.; Levijoki, J.; Haikala, H. Effects of levosimendan and milrinone on oxygen consumption in isolated guinea-pig heart. *J. Cardiovasc. Pharmacol.* **2004**, *43*, 555–561. [CrossRef]
11. Eriksson, O.; Pollesello, P.; Haikala, H. Effect of levosimendan on balance between ATP production and consumption in isolated perfused guinea-pig heart before ischemia or after reperfusion. *J. Cardiovasc. Pharmacol.* **2004**, *44*, 316–321. [CrossRef] [PubMed]
12. Ukkonen, H.; Saraste, M.; Akkila, J.; Knuuti, M.J.; Lehikoinen, P.; Någren, K.; Lehtonen, L.; Voipio-Pulkki, L.M. Myocardial efficiency during calcium sensitization with levosimendan: A noninvasive study with positron emission tomography and echocardiography in healthy volunteers. *Clin. Pharmacol. Ther.* **1997**, *61*, 596–607. [CrossRef]
13. Ukkonen, H.; Saraste, M.; Akkila, J.; Knuuti, J.; Karanko, M.; Iida, H.; Lehikoinen, P.; Någren, K.; Lehtonen, L.; Voipio-Pulkki, L.M. Myocardial efficiency during levosimendan infusion in congestive heart failure. *Clin. Pharmacol. Ther.* **2000**, *68*, 522–531. [CrossRef] [PubMed]
14. Kopustinskiene, D.M.; Pollesello, P.; Saris, N.E. Levosimendan is a mitochondrial K(ATP) channel opener. *Eur. J. Pharmacol.* **2001**, *428*, 311–314. [CrossRef]
15. Kopustinskiene, D.M.; Pollesello, P.; Saris, N.E. Potassium-specific effects of levosimendan on heart mitochondria. *Biochem. Pharmacol.* **2004**, *68*, 807–812. [CrossRef]
16. Soeding, P.F.; Crack, P.J.; Wright, C.E.; Angus, J.A.; Royse, C.F. Levosimendan preserves the contractile responsiveness of hypoxic human myocardium via mitochondrial K(ATP) channel and potential pERK 1/2 activation. *Eur. J. Pharmacol.* **2011**, *655*, 59–66. [CrossRef]
17. Torraco, A.; Carrozzo, R.; Piemonte, F.; Pastore, A.; Tozzi, G.; Verrigni, D.; Assenza, M.; Orecchioni, A.; D'Egidio, A.; Marraffa, E.; et al. Effects of levosimendan on mitochondrial function in patients with septic shock: A randomized trial. *Biochimie* **2014**, *102*, 166–173. [CrossRef]
18. Sommer, S.; Leistner, M.; Aleksic, I.; Schimmer, C.; Alhussini, K.; Kanofsky, P.; Leyh, R.G.; Sommer, S.P. Impact of levosimendan and ischaemia-reperfusion injury on myocardial subsarcolemmal mitochondrial respiratory chain, mitochondrial membrane potential, Ca^{2+} cycling and ATP synthesis. *Eur. J. Cardiothorac. Surg.* **2016**, *49*, 54–62. [CrossRef]
19. Bunte, S.; Behmenburg, F.; Bongartz, A.; Stroethoff, M.; Raupach, A.; Heinen, A.; Minol, J.P.; Hollmann, M.W.; Huhn, R.; Sixt, S.U. Preconditioning by Levosimendan is Mediated by Activation of Mitochondrial Ca^{2+}-Sensitive Potassium (mBKCa) Channels. *Cardiovasc. Drugs Ther.* **2018**, *32*, 427–434. [CrossRef]
20. Grossini, E.; Molinari, C.; Pollesello, P.; Bellomo, G.; Valente, G.; Mary, D.; Vacca, G.; Caimmi, P. Levosimendan protection against kidney ischemia/reperfusion injuries in anesthetized pigs. *J. Pharmacol. Exp. Ther.* **2012**, *342*, 376–388. [CrossRef]
21. Grossini, E.; Pollesello, P.; Bellofatto, K.; Sigaudo, L.; Farruggio, S.; Origlia, V.; Mombello, C.; Mary, D.A.; Valente, G.; Vacca, G. Protective effects elicited by levosimendan against liver ischemia/reperfusion injury in anesthetized rats. *Liver Transpl.* **2014**, *20*, 361–375. [CrossRef]
22. Ho, E.; Karimi Galougahi, K.; Liu, C.C.; Bhindi, R.; Figtree, G.A. Biological markers of oxidative stress: Applications to cardiovascular research and practice. *Redox Biol.* **2013**, *1*, 483–491. [CrossRef]

23. Ballatori, N.; Krance, S.M.; Notenboom, S.; Shi, S.; Tieu, K.; Hammond, C.L. Glutathione dysregulation and the etiology and progression of human diseases. *Biol. Chem.* **2009**, *390*, 191–214. [CrossRef] [PubMed]
24. Grossini, E.; Bellofatto, K.; Farruggio, S.; Sigaudo, L.; Marotta, P.; Raina, G.; De Giuli, V.; Mary, D.; Pollesello, P.; Minisini, R.; et al. Levosimendan inhibits peroxidation in hepatocytes by modulating apoptosis/autophagy interplay. *PLoS ONE* **2015**, *10*, e0124742. [CrossRef] [PubMed]
25. López Farré, A.; Casado, S. Heart failure, redox alterations, and endothelial dysfunction. *Hypertension* **2001**, *38*, 1400–1405. [CrossRef] [PubMed]
26. Keith, M.; Geranmayegan, A.; Sole, M.J.; Kurian, R.; Robinson, A.; Omran, A.S.; Jeejeebhoy, K.N. Increased oxidative stress in patients with congestive heart failure. *J. Am. Coll. Cardiol.* **1998**, *31*, 1352–1356. [CrossRef]
27. Polidori, M.C.; Savino, K.; Alunni, G.; Freddio, M.; Senin, U.; Sies, H.; Stahl, W.; Mecocci, P. Plasma lipophilic antioxidants and malondialdehyde in congestive heart failure patients: Relationship to disease severity. *Free Radic. Biol. Med.* **2002**, *32*, 148–152. [CrossRef]
28. Avgeropoulou, C.; Andreadou, I.; Markantonis-Kyroudis, S.; Demopoulou, M.; Missovoulos, P.; Androulakis, A.; Kallikazaros, I. The Ca^{2+}-sensitizer levosimendan improves oxidative damage, BNP and pro-inflammatory cytokine levels in patients with advanced decompensated heart failure in comparison to dobutamine. *Eur. J. Heart Fail.* **2005**, *7*, 882–887. [CrossRef]
29. Delle Karth, G.; Buberl, A.; Geppert, A.; Neunteufl, T.; Huelsmann, M.; Kopp, C.; Nikfardjam, M.; Berger, R.; Heinz, G. Hemodynamic effects of a continuous infusion of levosimendan in critically ill patients with cardiogenic shock requiring catecholamines. *Acta Anaesthesiol. Scand.* **2003**, *47*, 1251–1256. [CrossRef]
30. Wilkman, E.; Kaukonen, K.M.; Pettilä, V.; Kuitunen, A.; Varpula, M. Association between inotrope treatment and 90-day mortality in patients with septic shock. *Acta Anaesthesiol. Scand.* **2013**, *57*, 431–442. [CrossRef]
31. Lang, R.M.; Badano, L.P.; Mor-Avi, V.; Afilalo, J.; Armstrong, A.; Ernande, L.; Flachskampf, F.A.; Foster, E.; Goldstein, S.A.; Kuznetsova, T. Guidelines and standrards. Recommendations for Cardiac Chamber Quantification by Echocardiography in Adults: An Update from the American Society of Echocardiography and the European Association of Cardiovascular Imaging. *J. Am. Soc. Echocardiogr.* **2015**, *28*, 1–39. [CrossRef] [PubMed]
32. Rudski, L.G.; Lai, W.W.; Afilalo, J.; Hua, L.; Handschumacher, M.D.; Chandrasekaran, K.; Solomon, S.D.; Louie, E.K.; Schiller, N.B. Guidelines and standards. Guidelines for the Echocardiographic Assessment of the Right Heart in Adults: A Report from the American Society of Echocardiography Endorsed by the European Association of Echocardiography, a registered branch of the European Society of Cardiology, and the Canadian Society of Echocardiography. *J. Am. Soc. Echocardiogr.* **2010**, *23*, 685–713.
33. Nagueh, S.F.; Smiseth, O.A.; Appleton, C.P.; Byrd, B.F.; Dokainish, H.; Edvardsen, T.; Flachskampf, F.A.; Gillebert, T.C.; Klein, A.L.; Lancellotti, P.; et al. Lancellotti PASE/EACVI Guidelines and standards. Recommendations for the Evaluation of Left Ventricular Diastolic Function by Echocardiography: An Update from the American Society of Echocardiography and the European Association of Cardiovascular Imaging. *J. Am. Soc. Echocardiogr.* **2016**, *29*, 277–314. [CrossRef]
34. Cholley, B.; Caruba, T.; Grosjean, S.; Amour, J.; Ouattara, A.; Villacorta, J.; Miguet, B.; Guinet, P.; Lévy, F.; Squara, P.; et al. Effect of Levosimendan on Low Cardiac Output Syndrome in Patients with Low Ejection Fraction Undergoing Coronary Artery Bypass Grafting with Cardiopulmonary Bypass: The LICORN Randomized Clinical Trial. *JAMA* **2017**, *318*, 548–556. [CrossRef] [PubMed]
35. Sangalli, F.; Avalli, L.; Laratta, M.; Formica, F.; Maggioni, E.; Caruso, R.; Cristina Costa, M.; Guazzi, M.; Fumagalli, R. Effects of Levosimendan on Endothelial Function and Hemodynamics During Weaning from Veno-Arterial Extracorporeal Life Support. *J. Cardiothorac. Vasc. Anesth.* **2016**, *30*, 1449–1453. [CrossRef] [PubMed]
36. De Cillà, S.; Vezzola, D.; Farruggio, S.; Vujosevic, S.; Clemente, N.; Raina, G.; Mary, D.; Casini, G.; Rossetti, L.; Avagliano, L.; et al. The subthreshold micropulse laser treatment of the retina restores the oxidant/antioxidant balance and counteracts programmed forms of cell death in the mice eyes. *Acta Ophthalmol.* **2017**, *42*, 1725–1738. [CrossRef]
37. Farruggio, S.; Raina, G.; Cocomazzi, G.; Librasi, C.; Mary, D.; Gentilli, S.; Grossini, E. Genistein improves viability, proliferation and mitochondrial function of cardiomyoblasts cultured in physiologic and peroxidative conditions. *Int. J. Mol. Med.* **2019**, *44*, 2298–2310. [CrossRef]

38. Surico, D.; Bordino, V.; Cantaluppi, V.; Mary, D.; Gentilli, S.; Oldani, A.; Farruggio, S.; Melluzza, C.; Raina, G.; Grossini, E. Preeclampsia and intrauterine growth restriction: Role of human umbilical cord mesenchymal stem cells-trophoblast cross-talk. *PLoS ONE* **2019**, *14*, e0218437. [CrossRef]
39. Leong, L.N. Targeting oxidative stress in HF. *Heart Metab.* **2009**, *42*, 21–24.
40. Mochizuki, M.; Yano, M.; Oda, T.; Tateishi, H.; Kobayashi, S.; Yamamoto, T.; Ikeda, Y.; Ohkusa, T.; Ikemoto, N.; Matsuzaki, M. Scavenging free radicals by low-dose carvedilol prevents redox-dependent Ca^{2+} leak via stabilization of ryanodine receptor in heart failure. *J. Am. Coll Cardiol.* **2007**, *49*, 1722–1732. [CrossRef]
41. Oe, H.; Nakamura, K.; Kihara, H.; Shimada, K.; Fukuda, S.; Takagi, T.; Miyoshi, T.; Hirata, K.; Yoshikawa, J.; Ito, H. FESC, for Effect of a DPP-4 inhibitor on left ventricular diastolic dysfunction in patients with type 2 diabetes and diabetic cardiomyopathy (3D) study investigators. Comparison of effects of sitagliptin and voglibose on left ventricular diastolic dysfunction in patients with type 2 diabetes: Results of the 3D trial. *Cardiovasc Diabetol.* **2015**, *14*, 83. [CrossRef] [PubMed]
42. Jeong, E.M.; Dudley, S.C. Diastolic dysfunction. *Circ. J.* **2015**, *79*, 470–477. [CrossRef] [PubMed]
43. Kuznetsov, A.V.; Javadov, S.; Margreiter, R.; Grimm, M.; Hagenbuchner, J.; Ausserlechner, M.J. The Role of Mitochondria in the Mechanisms of Cardiac Ischemia-Reperfusion Injury. *Antioxidants* **2019**, *8*, 454. [CrossRef] [PubMed]
44. Liang, W.; Chen, J.; Mo, L.; Ke, X.; Zhang, W.; Zheng, D.; Pan, W.; Wu, S.; Feng, J.; Song, M.; et al. ATP-sensitive K^+ channels contribute to the protective effects of exogenous hydrogen sulfide against high glucose-induced injury in H9c2 cardiac cells. *Int. J. Mol. Med.* **2016**, *37*, 763–772. [CrossRef]
45. Zhang, D.M.; Chai, Y.; Erickson, J.R.; Brown, J.H.; Bers, D.M.; Lin, Y.F. Intracellular signalling mechanism responsible for modulation of sarcolemmal ATP-sensitive potassium channels by nitric oxide in ventricular cardiomyocytes. *J. Physiol.* **2014**, *592*, 971–990. [CrossRef]
46. Holmuhamedov, E.L.; Jovanović, S.; Dzeja, P.P.; Jovanović, A.; Terzic, A. Mitochondrial ATP-sensitive K+ channels modulate cardiac mitochondrial function. *Am. J. Physiol.* **1998**, *275*, 1567–1576. [CrossRef]
47. Bouchez, S.; Fedele, F.; Giannakoulas, G.; Gustafsson, F.; Harjola, V.P.; Karason, K.; Kivikko, M.; Von Lewinski, D.; Oliva, F.; Papp, Z.; et al. Levosimendan in Acute and Advanced Heart Failure: An Expert Perspective on Posology and Therapeutic Application. *Cardiovasc. Drugs Ther.* **2018**, *32*, 617–624. [CrossRef]
48. Goldenthal, M.J. Mitochondrial involvement in myocyte death and heart failure. *Heart Fail. Rev.* **2016**, *21*, 137–155. [CrossRef]
49. Uberti, F.; Caimmi, P.P.; Molinari, C.; Mary, D.; Vacca, G.; Grossini, E. Levosimendan modulates programmed forms of cell death through K(ATP) channels and nitric oxide. *J. Cardiovasc. Pharmacol.* **2011**, *57*, 246–258. [CrossRef]
50. Hemodynamic Evaluation of Levosimendan in Patients with PH-HFpEF (HELP). Available online: https://clinicaltrials.gov/ct2/show/NCT03541603 (accessed on 4 December 2019).
51. Al-Chalabi, A.; Heunks, L.M.A.; Papp, Z.; Pollesello, P. Potential of the Cardiovascular Drug Levosimendan in the Management of Amyotrophic Lateral Sclerosis: An Overview of a Working Hypothesis. *J. Cardiovasc. Pharmacol.* **2019**, *74*, 389–399. [CrossRef]

11

Increased Lymphangiogenesis and Lymphangiogenic Growth Factor Expression in Perivascular Adipose Tissue of Patients with Coronary Artery Disease

Ioannis Drosos [1], Maria Pavlaki [2], Maria Del Pilar Ortega Carrillo [1], Adriani Kourkouli [2], Katja Buschmann [3], Fotios Konstantinou [4], Rajinikanth Gogiraju [1], Magdalena L. Bochenek [1,5], Georgios Chalikias [2], Christos Tortopidis [2], Christian F. Vahl [3], Dimitrios Mikroulis [4], Dimitrios Tziakas [2], Thomas Münzel [1], Stavros Konstantinides [2,5] and Katrin Schäfer [1,*]

1. Center for Cardiology, Cardiology 1, University Medical Center of the Johannes Gutenberg University Mainz, 55130 Mainz, Germany
2. Department of Cardiology, Democritus University of Thrace, 68100 Alexandroupolis, Greece
3. Department of Cardiothoracic and Vascular Surgery, University Medical Center of the Johannes Gutenberg University Mainz, 55130 Mainz, Germany
4. Department of Cardiothoracic Surgery, Democritus University of Thrace, 68100 Alexandroupolis, Greece
5. Center for Thrombosis and Hemostasis, University Medical Center of the Johannes Gutenberg University Mainz, 55130 Mainz, Germany

* Correspondence: katrin.schaefer@unimedizin-mainz.de

Abstract: Experimental and human autopsy studies have associated adventitial lymphangiogenesis with atherosclerosis. An analysis of perivascular lymphangiogenesis in patients with coronary artery disease is lacking. Here, we examined lymphangiogenesis and its potential regulators in perivascular adipose tissue (PVAT) surrounding the heart (C-PVAT) and compared it with PVAT of the internal mammary artery (IMA-PVAT). Forty-six patients undergoing coronary artery bypass graft surgery were included. Perioperatively collected C-PVAT and IMA-PVAT were analyzed using histology, immunohistochemistry, real time PCR, and PVAT-conditioned medium using cytokine arrays. C-PVAT exhibited increased PECAM-1 (platelet endothelial cell adhesion molecule 1)-positive vessel density. The number of lymphatic vessels expressing lymphatic vessel endothelial hyaluronan receptor-1 or podoplanin was also elevated in C-PVAT and associated with higher inflammatory cell numbers, increased intercellular adhesion molecule 1 (ICAM1) expression, and fibrosis. Significantly higher expression of regulators of lymphangiogenesis such as vascular endothelial growth factor (VEGF)-C, VEGF-D, and VEGF receptor-3 was observed in C-PVAT compared to IMA-PVAT. Cytokine arrays identified angiopoietin-2 as more highly expressed in C-PVAT vs. IMA-PVAT. Findings were confirmed histologically and at the mRNA level. Stimulation of human lymphatic endothelial cells with recombinant angiopoietin-2 in combination with VEGF-C enhanced sprout formation. Our study shows that PVAT surrounding atherosclerotic arteries exhibits more extensive lymphangiogenesis, inflammation, and fibrosis compared to PVAT surrounding a non-diseased vessel, possibly due to local angiopoietin-2, VEGF-C, and VEGF-D overexpression.

Keywords: coronary artery disease; human; inflammation; lymphangiogenesis; perivascular adipose tissue

1. Introduction

Accumulating clinical and experimental data suggest an active contribution of the adventitia to remodeling processes in the vascular wall, including neointima formation and atherosclerosis.

For example, preclinical studies in hypercholesterolemic animal models have shown that adventitial angiogenesis promotes atherosclerotic plaque progression, whereas inhibition of plaque neovascularization reduced lesion growth [1–3]. The expansion of thin-walled, leaky vasa vasorum and microvessels within atherosclerotic lesions has been pathophysiologically linked to plaque instability by increasing inflammatory cell infiltration and intraplaque hemorrhage [4–6], among others.

In addition to arteries and veins, lymphatic vessels exist and develop in parallel with blood vessels in most organs. Although the extent and complexity of the lymphatic vasculature has been known for more than a century [7], its role in the pathogenesis of cardiovascular disease processes has received little attention. Lymph vessels control the drainage of interstitial fluids and macromolecules (proteins, lipids) leaking from capillaries back to the venous circulation and are thus critical for the maintenance of tissue homeostasis [8]. In addition, they have an important function in immune surveillance and may accelerate the resolution of inflammation by removing inflammatory mediators or trafficking immune cells to draining lymph nodes. Lymph vessel dysfunction results in lymphedema, but also may play a role during inflammation, cancer, obesity, or hypertension (reviewed in [9]).

Regarding atherosclerosis, which is characterized by chronic inflammation and cholesterol accumulation in the arterial wall, the possibility of a direct contribution of adventitial lymphangiogenesis has only been recently addressed. Studies in animal models after experimentally induced lymphostasis or genetic modulation of lymphatic vessel formation suggested a protective role of the lymphatic vasculature during atherosclerosis [10,11]. Moreover, cardiac lymphangiogenesis has been shown to take part in the clearance of immune cells and resolution of inflammation after myocardial infarction [12,13]. A causal role of lymph vessel dysfunction in the pathophysiology of atherosclerosis is further supported by findings in mice that excessive cholesterol accumulation is associated with structural and functional alterations of lymphatic vessels [14], and that lymphatic dysfunction develops before atherosclerotic lesion formation [15]. As far as human atherosclerosis is concerned, the available knowledge is limited to autopsy studies of large arteries from organ donors and the clinical observation that (adventitial) lymphangiogenesis correlates with atherosclerosis severity [11,16–18]. Similar findings were obtained in 21 endarterectomy samples from patients with internal carotid artery stenosis showing a more developed lymphatic network in the adventitia of atherosclerotic lesions compared to healthy arteries [19]. Whether these observations reflect lymphatic dysfunction or the reactive enlargement of perivascular lymphatic networks to local cues or systemic differences between patients at risk and control individuals remains unknown.

Given the anatomical proximity of perivascular adipose tissue (PVAT) with the adventitia and its known paracrine activities on the underlying vessel, studied by our group [20] and others (reviewed in [21]), we hypothesized that differences may exist in the extent of the lymphatic vasculature and the expression of lymphangiogenic growth factors between PVAT surrounding the aortic root and coronaries of patients with coronary artery disease (CAD) and PVAT of the internal mammary artery (IMA), an artery protected from the development of atherosclerosis [22].

2. Materials and Methods

2.1. Study Patients

Forty-six patients (76% male; mean age, 68.6 ± 9.8 years; mean body mass index, 29.1 ± 5.4 kg/m^2) undergoing elective coronary artery bypass graft surgery in two university medical centers were included in the study. All patients had been diagnosed with multivessel CAD via coronary angiography. The left (and in some cases also the right) IMA was used as an aortocoronary bypass in all patients. The study complied with the declaration of Helsinki and was approved by the Ethics Committee of the University General Hospital of Alexandroupolis, Greece, and the University Medical Center of the Johannes Gutenberg University Mainz, Germany, respectively. All patients signed a written informed consent prior to inclusion in the study. Due to the limited amount of tissue from each patient, not all analyses could be performed in all patients, and samples had to be split into groups.

2.2. Tissue Specimen Collection

'Cardiac' perivascular adipose tissue (C-PVAT), located adjacent to the aortic root and around the coronary arteries, and PVAT surrounding the IMA (IMA-PVAT) was collected perioperatively and immediately transferred to the laboratory in ice-cold sterile saline solution (Braun). IMA-PVAT was collected immediately after preparation of the arterial bypass graft and before establishing the extracorporeal circulation. C-PVAT was collected during extracorporeal circulation, immediately after removing the aortic cross-clamp, from the same position in all patients, regardless of the localization of atherosclerotic lesions within the coronary tree. PVAT specimens were briefly rinsed with sterile saline and visible connective tissue or blood vessels removed. PVAT samples were then either directly processed under sterile conditions for the preparation of conditioned medium (CM) or stored at −80 °C pending protein or RNA isolation. Specimens intended for RNA isolation were transferred to TRI Reagent®Solution (ThermoFisher Scientific; Dreieich, Germany) before storage at −80 °C. PVAT samples intended for histology/immunohistochemistry were fixed in 10% zinc formalin (Sigma-Aldrich; Darmstadt, Germany), embedded in paraffin wax (Leica; Wetzlar, Germany) and cut into 5-μm-thick sections.

2.3. Generation of Perivascular Adipose Tissue Conditioned Medium

For the generation of PVAT-derived CM, C-PVAT and IMA-PVAT specimens were cut into pieces under sterile conditions and then transferred into Dulbecco's Modified Eagle's medium (ThermoFisher Scientific) supplemented with 1% penicillin/streptomycin and 0.5% fetal bovine serum (both Biosera). A standard culture medium volume/tissue mass proportion of 2 μL per mg of tissue was employed. Culture medium and PVAT were then incubated in a cell culture incubator (New Brunswick, Eppendorf; Wesseling-Berzdorf, Germany; 37 °C, 5% CO_2) for 24 h. Control medium was prepared in parallel by incubating medium without PVAT tissue. After removal of PVAT pieces, CM was centrifuged at 20,000 *g* for 10 min and the supernatant kept at −80°C pending analysis.

2.4. Membrane-Based Protein Array

C-PVAT- and IMA-PVAT-derived CM (1 mL) from five patients with CAD was examined for secreted proteins using a customized RayBio®membrane-based antibody array against 29 target proteins (RayBiotech, Hölzel Diagnostika Handels GmbH; Köln, Germany), following the instructions of the manual. Chemiluminescence detection was performed using a ChemiDoc™ MP imaging system (Bio-Rad; Rüdigheim, Germany). Semi-quantitative analysis was performed by densitrometry using ImageJ software (version 1.52, NIH) and Gilles Carpentier's Protein Array Analyser for ImageJ macro (rsb.info.nih.gov/ij/macros/toolsets/ProteinArrayAnalyzer.txt). Negative control dots were used for background subtraction and positive control dots to normalize values and to allow comparison among array membranes. Quantitative data were expressed as fold change vs. IMA-PVAT.

2.5. Reverse Transcription Quantitative Real-time PCR

PVAT was homogenized in TRI Reagent®solution using a rotating homogenizer (ART Prozess and Labortechnik GmbH; Müllheim, Germany). For RNA isolation from human dermal lymphatic endothelial cells (HDLECs), cells were directly harvested from the culture plate using TRI Reagent®solution and a cell scraper. RNA isolation was performed using a standard protocol. For PVAT samples, an additional purification step was performed using NucleoSpin®RNA columns (Macherey-Nagel; Düren, Germany). The amount of RNA was quantified on a NanoDrop™ 2000 spectrophotometer (ThermoFisher Scientific). Reverse transcription was performed using M-MLV reverse transcriptase (Promega; Mannheim, Germany) or iScript™ cDNA Synthesis Kit (Bio-Rad). For quantitative real-time PCR (qPCR), SsoAdvanced™ Universal SYBR®Green Supermix (Bio-Rad) and a CFX Connect™ Real-Time PCR Detection System (Bio-Rad) were used. Two technical replicates were prepared for each sample. For PVAT gene expression analysis, LRP10 was used as endogenous reference gene [20]. For HDLECs, preliminary analysis of common reference genes indicated 18S as the most stably expressed gene. The sequences of all primers that were used are shown in Table S1. Data were normalized to the respective reference gene and are expressed as $2^{(-DCq)}$ values for C-PVAT and IMA-PVAT or as $2^{(-DDCq)}$ (fold change vs. control-treated samples) for HDLECs.

2.6. *Spheroid Lymphangiogenesis Assay*

HDLECs were cultured in Endothelial Cell Growth Medium MV2 (PromoCell; Heidelberg, Germany) and analyzed up to passage 5. Spheroids of HDLECs were prepared on day one following a standard protocol. In short, cultured HDLECs were detached using 0.05% trypsin-EDTA (ThermoFisher Scientific) and resuspended at a density of 400 cells per 100 μL Endothelial Cell Growth Medium MV2 containing 20% methylcellulose in Medium 199 (both Sigma-Aldrich). Subsequently, 100 μL of the cell suspension were transferred to the wells of a round-bottom 96-well suspension culture plate and incubated for 24 h at 5% CO_2, 37 °C in order for HDLEC spheroids to form. On day two, spheroids were collected from the 96-well plate. After centrifugation at 390 *g* for three minutes, the supernatant was discarded and spheroids resuspended at a 1:1 mixture of 50% rat tail collagen I (Corning; Wiesbaden, Germany), 0.05% acetic acid (in Medium 199) and 5% fetal bovine serum in methylcellulose/Medium 199 solution. The suspension was transferred to the wells of a 24-well plate and incubated for 30 min before adding Endothelial Cell Growth Medium MV2. Spheroids were stimulated with recombinant human angiopoietin-2 (ANGPT2; 100 ng/mL) and/or recombinant human vascular endothelial growth factor (VEGF)-C (100 ng/mL; both from R&D Systems) for 24 h. Images of five randomly selected spheroids per well were captured using an inverted microscope (Motic AE31; Wetzlar, Germany). The number of sprouts was manually counted and the cumulative sprout length measured using ImageJ software.

2.7. *Histology and Immunohistochemistry*

Masson's trichrome stain was used for the histological examination of PVAT specimens. For the immunohistochemical staining of the paraffin-embedded tissue sections, a standardized protocol was used. Briefly, paraffin sections were deparaffinized and epitopes were retrieved by heating in 10 mM Tris buffer containing 1 mM EDTA or in 0.1 M citrate buffer (pH 6.0), depending on the target epitope. Unspecific binding sites were blocked using 10% normal goat serum (Abcam; Cambridge, UK). Vessel endothelium was stained using an anti-PECAM-1 antibody (mouse monoclonal; Dako; Santa Clara, CA, USA). Anti-podoplanin (PDPN; rabbit polyclonal; Novus Biologicals) and anti-lymphatic vessel endothelial hyaluronan receptor 1 (LYVE-1; rabbit polyclonal; Novus Biologicals) antibodies were used to selectively stain lymphatic endothelium. Tissue macrophages were visualized using anti-CD68 antibodies (mouse monoclonal; Dako), ANGPT2-expressing cells using anti-ANGPT2 antibody (rabbit polyclonal; Novus Biologicals; Wiesbaden, Germany). After incubating with biotinylated secondary goat anti-mouse or anti-rabbit antibodies (ThermoFisher Scientific), sections were incubated with avidin–biotin complex (Vector Laboratories; Burlingame, CA, USA). Diaminobenzidine or aminoethylcarbazole (Vector Laboratories) substrate was used for visualization, followed by brief counterstaining using Gill's hematoxyline (Sigma-Aldrich). Negative controls were prepared for all immunohistochemical stainings by omitting the primary antibody (representative images shown in Figure S1).

2.8. Image Acquisition and Analysis

Histology and immunohistochemistry sections were examined and representative images were captured using an Olympus BX51 microscope (Hamburg, Germany). The number of total vessels and lymphatic collector vessels was quantified by manually counting PECAM-1- and PDPN-immunopositive vessel-like structures per 200× microscope field, respectively. The number of lymphatic capillaries was quantified by manually counting LYVE-1-immunopositive structures per 200× microscope field. The number of tissue macrophages was determined by manually counting CD68-immunopositive cells per 400× microscope field. Results were expressed as number of immunopositive vessel-like structures or cells per mm^2. Sections stained with Masson's trichrome stain were used for the assessment of fibrosis, which was performed by quantifying the blue-stained collagen area relative to total tissue area at 100× magnification. For all quantitative image analyses, three optical fields were randomly selected and measurements averaged.

2.9. Statistical Analysis

Data are presented as mean ± standard deviation (SD), if normally distributed, or as median (25% and 75% interquartile range (IQR)), if not. Normal distribution was examined with the D'Agostino–Pearson omnibus normality test. Paired comparison analyses between PVAT samples from one patient were performed using Student's paired *t*-test if values were normally distributed, or the Wilcoxon matched-pairs signed rank test if not. Multiple comparisons were performed using one-way ANOVA with Turkey's multiple comparisons test. Differences were considered statistically significant if $p < 0.05$. All statistical analyses were performed using GraphPad PRISM version 8.0.

3. Results

3.1. C-PVAT Contains More Lymphatic Vessels than IMA-PVAT

We had previously shown that C-PVAT from patients with CAD is characterized by more pronounced angiogenesis and higher numbers of blood vessels compared to IMA-PVAT [20]. Immunohistochemical detection of PECAM-1 in paired PVAT tissue specimens from 10 patients with CAD confirmed those previous findings by showing a significantly higher density of PECAM-1-immunopositive vessels in C-PVAT compared to IMA-PVAT (25.4 ± 2.75 vs. 12.9 ± 1.79 per mm^2, $p = 0.004$; Figure 1A,D; for findings in negative controls please see Figure S1A). To distinguish lymphatic vessels, we used markers expressed on lymphatic endothelium, namely LYVE-1 and PDPN. LYVE-1 has been shown to be mainly expressed in lymphatic capillaries, PDPN in lymphatic collector vessels [23]. These analyses revealed that both the number of LYVE-1 (24.7 (0.61–32.3) vs. 2.97 (0–6.58) per mm^2, $p = 0.027$; Figure 1B,E; Figure S1B) and PDPN (5.45 ± 1.54 vs. 0.74 ± 0.34 per mm^2, $p = 0.023$; Figure 1C,F; Figure S1C) -immunopositive vessels was significantly increased in C-PVAT compared to IMA-PVAT. Of note, neither the anti-LYVE-1 nor the anti-PDPN antibody showed any immunoreactivity for endothelium lining blood vessels. Interestingly, the mean diameter of PDPN-positive vessels was significantly increased in C-PVAT compared to IMA-PVAT ($p = 0.008$), in line with lymphatic dysfunction [14,15].

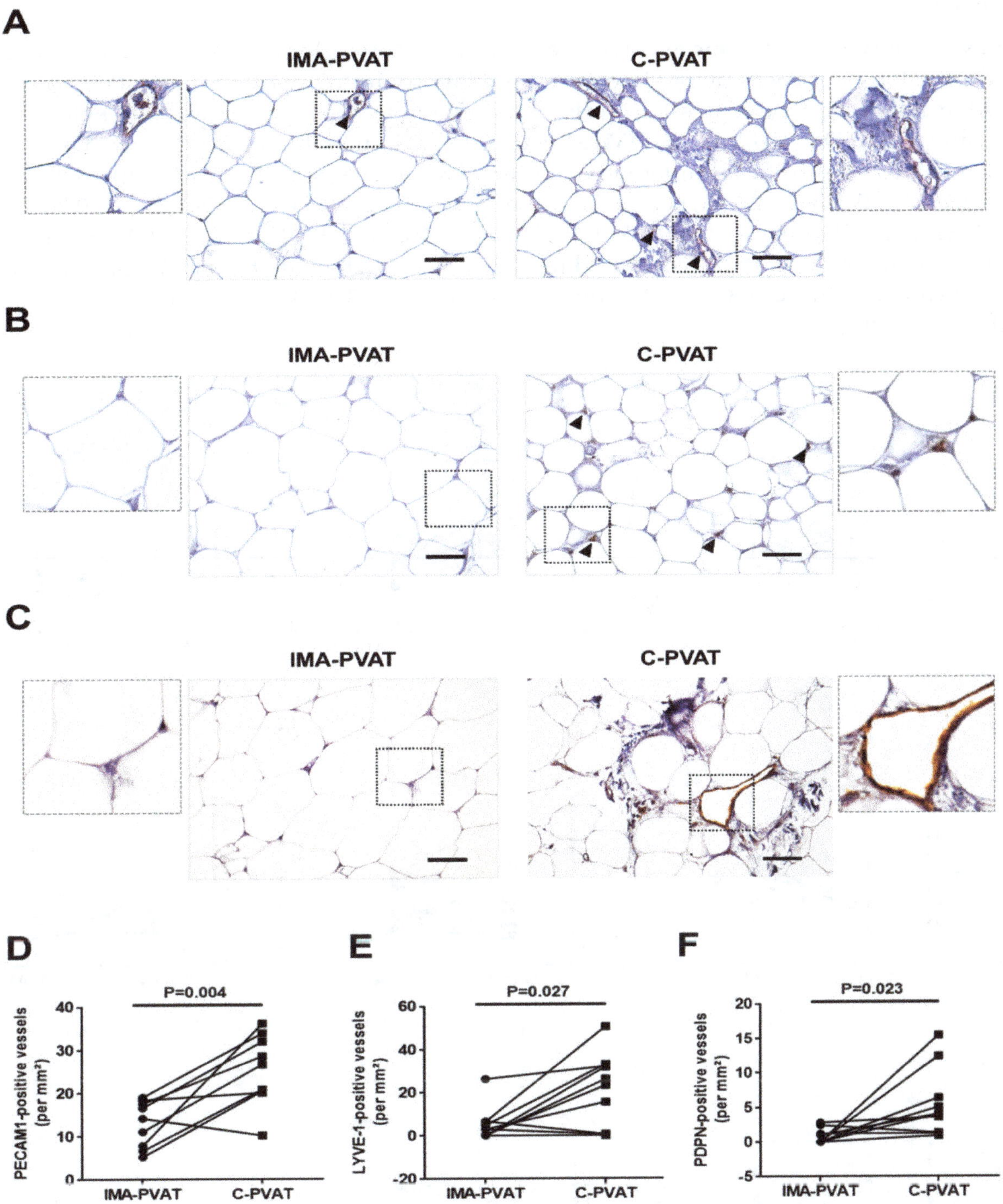

Figure 1. Angiogenesis and lymphangiogenesis in perivascular adipose tissue (PVAT). (**A–C**) Immunohistochemical detection of platelet endothelial cell adhesion molecule 1 (PECAM-1) (**A**), anti-lymphatic vessel endothelial hyaluronan receptor 1 (LYVE-1) (**B**), and anti-podoplanin (PDPN) (**C**) in internal mammary artery (IMA)-PVAT and cardiac (C)-PVAT. Inserts show higher magnification. Size bars represent 100 µm. (**D–F**) Quantification of the number of PECAM-1 (**D**), LYVE-1 (**E**), and PDPN (**F**) immunopositive vessels per mm^2 in $n = 10$ patients with coronary artery disease (CAD). Paired IMA-PVAT (●) and C-PVAT (■) values in individual patients are connected with a line. Statistical analysis was performed using Student's paired t-test (**D**,**F**) or Wilcoxon matched-pairs signed rank test (**E**).

3.2. Lymphangiogenic Growth Factors and Their Receptors Are Expressed at Higher Levels in C-PVAT Compared to IMA-PVAT

To examine whether the more extensive lymphatic network in C-PVAT is accompanied by a higher expression of growth factors known to mediate (lymph-) angiogenesis, qPCR analysis was employed to determine gene expression levels of vascular endothelial growth factor (VEGF)-A, VEGF-B, VEGF-C, and VEGF-D in C-PVAT and IMA-PVAT (paired tissue samples from 16–18 patients). These analyses revealed no significant differences in the mRNA levels of *VEGF-A* (0.85 (0.68–1.21) vs. 0.72 (0.41–1.02), $p = 0.421$; Figure 2A), whereas the expression of *VEGF-C* (0.83 (0.55–1.25) vs. 0.36 (0.22–0.72), $p = 0.022$; Figure 2C) and *VEGF-D* (0.58 (0.42–0.87) vs. 0.25 (0.21–0.31), $p = 0.007$; Figure 2D) was significantly increased in C-PVAT compared to IMA-PVAT. On the other hand, *VEGF-B* mRNA levels were significantly reduced in C-PVAT compared to IMA-PVAT (5.38 (3.92–7.53) vs. 2.99 (2.72–4.13), $p = 0.002$; Figure 2B).

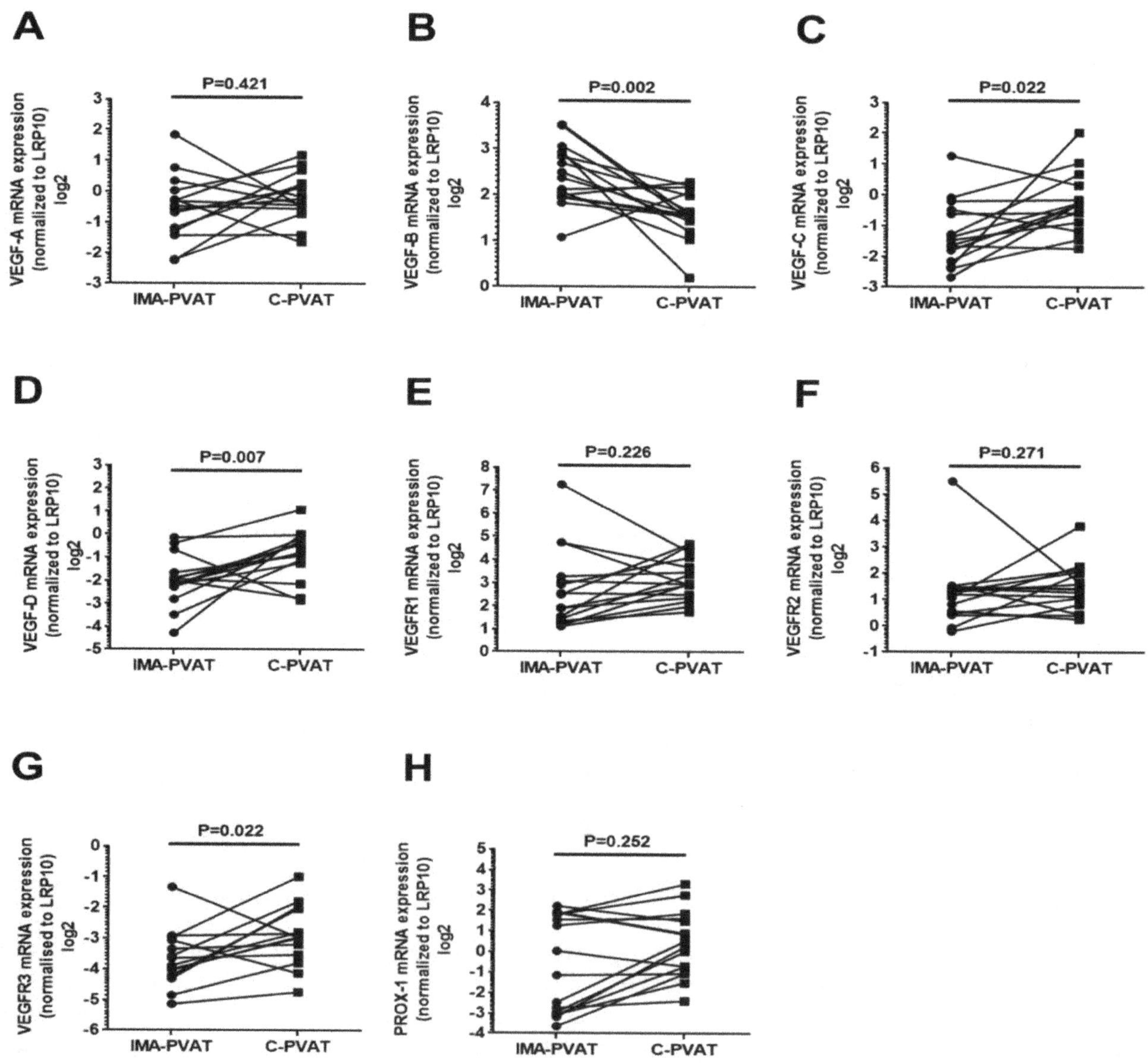

Figure 2. Analysis of growth factors involved in angiogenesis and lymphangiogenesis. Quantification of mRNA expression of vascular endothelial growth factor (*VEGF*)*-A* (**A**), *VEGF-B* (**B**), *VEGF-C* (**C**), *VEGF-D* (**D**), VEGF receptor (*VEGFR*)*-1* (**E**), *VEGFR2* (**F**), *VEGFR3* (**G**), and prospero homeobox-1 (*PROX-1*) (**H**) in IMA-PVAT and C-PVAT of $n = 15–16$ patients with CAD. Paired IMA-PVAT (●) and C-PVAT (■) values in individual patients are connected with a line. Statistical analysis was performed using Wilcoxon matched-pairs signed rank test.

We then also examined the mRNA expression of the receptors for VEGF, namely VEGF receptor (VEGFR)-1, VEGFR2, and VEGFR3. In agreement with our findings of a significantly higher VEGF-C and VEGF-D expression in C-PVAT, mRNA levels of *VEGFR3* were significantly increased in C-PVAT compared to IMA-PVAT (0.13 (0.09–0.25) vs. 0.07 (0.05–0.12), $p = 0.022$; Figure 2G), whereas no differences in the mRNA expression of *VEGFR1* (7.78 (5.29–16.2) vs. 4.70 (2.59–9.37), $p = 0.226$; Figure 2E) and *VEGFR2* (2.68 (1.85–4.15) vs. 2.38 (1.41–2.79), $p = 0.271$; Figure 2F) were observed between both PVAT depots. These results suggested a higher state of VEGF-C/VEGF-D-mediated VEGFR3 signaling which may be responsible for the observed differences in the lymphatic endothelial cell density between C-PVAT and IMA-PVAT.

Analysis of the transcription factor prospero-related homeobox (PROX)-1, a master regulator of embryonic lymphatic development [24,25], revealed similar *PROX-1* mRNA levels in C-PVAT and IMA-PVAT (1.31 (0.51–3.01) vs. 0.74 (0.12–3.50), $p = 0.252$; Figure 2H) suggesting that the observed differences in the number of lymphatic vessels was not the result of a different embryonically defined lymphangiogenic potential in both adipose tissue depots.

3.3. *Increased Inflammation and Fibrosis in PVAT Surrounding Atherosclerotic Arteries*

Previous studies have shown that inflammation triggers lymphangiogenesis and identified macrophages as main cellular source of VEGF-C and VEGF-D [26,27]. Higher numbers of CD68-immunopositive macrophages were observed in human C-PVAT compared to IMA-PVAT of patients with CAD (207 ± 35.8 vs. 52.9 ± 7.32 per mm^2, $p = 0.001$; Figure 3A,C; Figure S1D). Because of the complex interplay between lymphangiogenesis, inflammation and fibrosis, we next examined both PVAT depots after staining with Masson's trichrome stain. These analyses revealed a significantly higher degree of fibrosis in C-PVAT compared to IMA-PVAT (0.83 (0.02–4.63) vs. 0.02 (0.01–0.11) % per microscope field, $p = 0.027$; Figure 3B,D). Of note, real time PCR analysis did not reveal differences of transforming growth factor-beta (*TGFβ*) mRNA levels between both adipose tissue depots ($p = 0.151$).

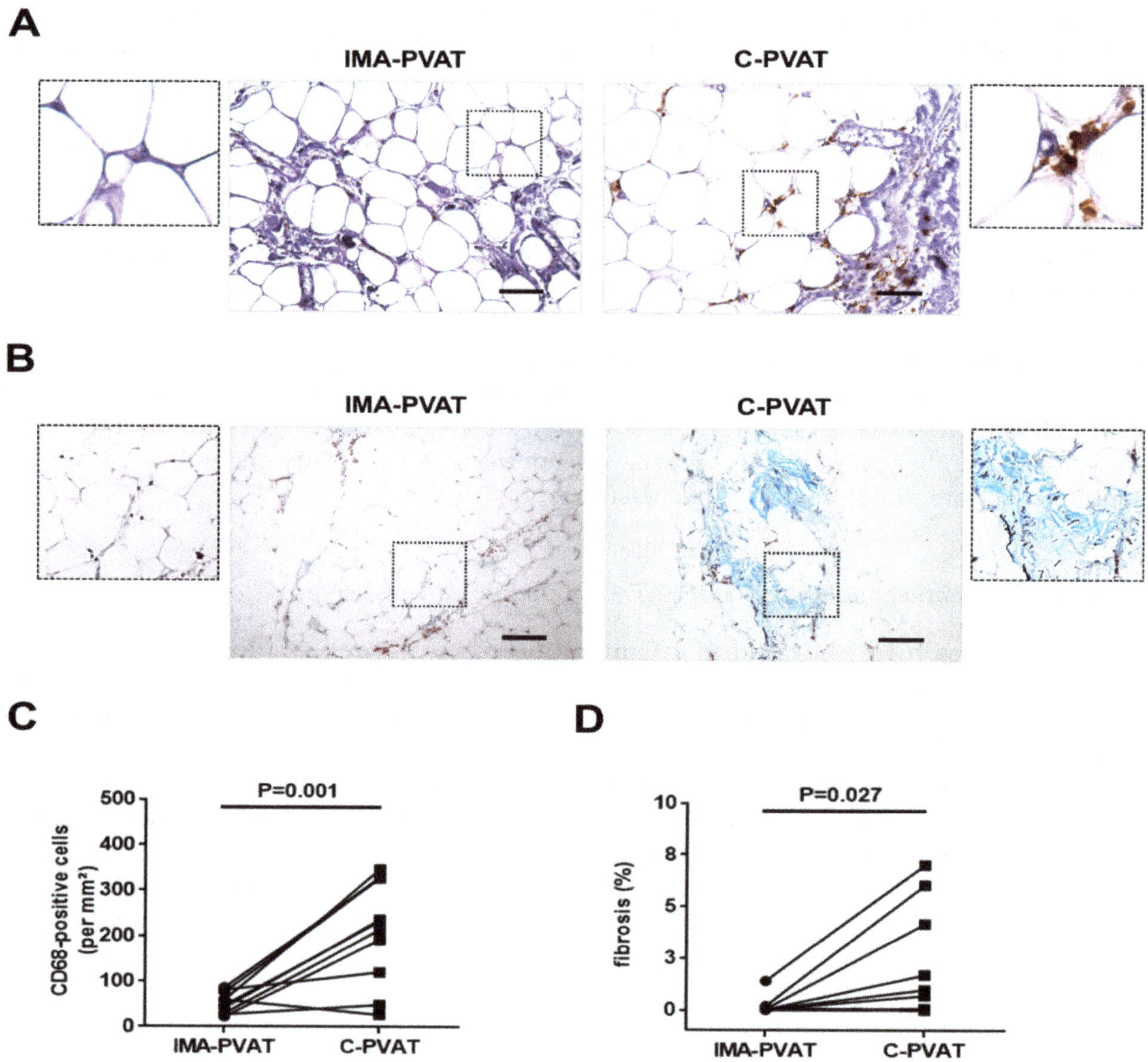

Figure 3. Fibrosis and inflammation in PVAT. (**A**) Immunohistochemical detection of CD68 in IMA-PVAT and C-PVAT. Size bars represent 50 µm. (**B**) Masson trichrome stain in IMA-PVAT and C-PVAT. Size bars represent 200 µm. (**C**) Quantification of the number of CD68-immunopositive cells per mm^2. (**D**) Quantification of the percentage of fibrotic area in $n = 10$ patients with coronary artery disease (CAD). Paired IMA-PVAT (●) and C-PVAT (■) values in individual patients are connected with a line. Statistical analysis was performed using Student's paired *t*-test (**C**) or Wilcoxon matched-pairs signed rank test (**D**).

3.4. Protein Array Analysis Reveals Significantly Higher Angiopoietin-2 and Intercellular Adhesion Molecule-1 Levels in C-PVAT Compared to IMA-PVAT

PVAT has been shown to express and secrete a number of cytokines and other factors, which may act locally or in a paracrine manner on the neighboring vessel wall (reviewed in [28]). For this reason and given our findings, we next aimed at investigating a broader spectrum of PVAT-secreted factors, with particular focus on potential candidates involved in (lymph)angiogenesis, inflammation and fibrosis. A semiquantitative paired expression analysis of 29 target proteins was performed in conditioned medium (CM) derived from C-PVAT and IMA-PVAT of five patients with CAD using a membrane-based antibody array (representative results are shown in Figure 4A, the position of all target proteins on the membranes is given in Figure S2). Among those, inflammatory factors (interleukin-6, interleukin-8, monocyte chemoattractant protein-1), matrix metalloproteinases (MMP1, MMP9) and their inhibitors (tissue inhibitor of metalloproteinases TIMP1, TIMP2), adipokines (adiponectin, leptin) and growth factors (angiopoietin-1 and -2, basic fibroblast growth factor) were detected in CM from both adipose tissue depots (heat map in Figure 4B, quantitative analyses for all 29 target proteins in Figure S3A–D).

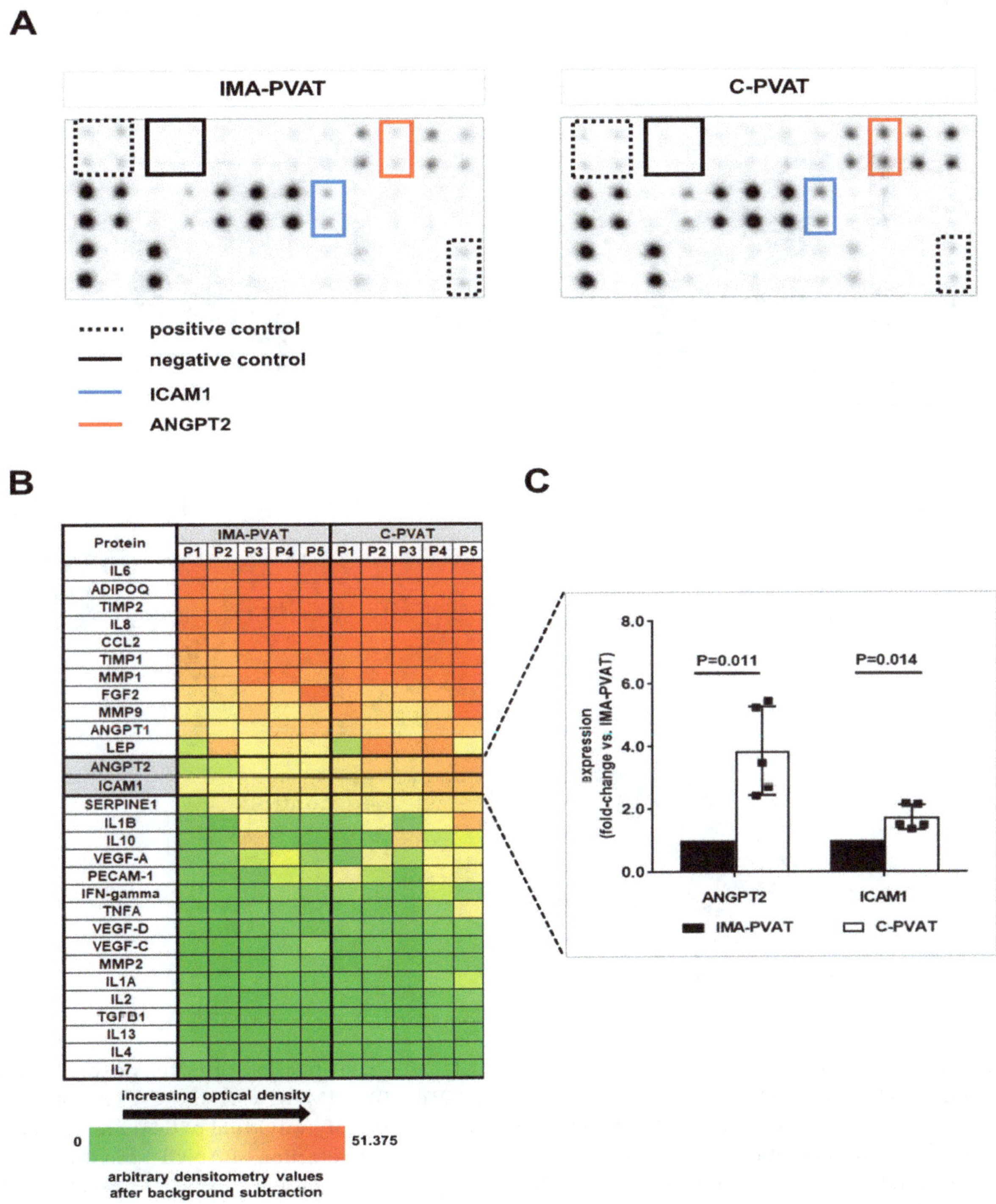

Figure 4. Protein array analysis of factors potentially involved in perivascular lymphangiogenesis. (**A**) Representative chemiluminescence detection images of a protein membrane array in IMA-PVAT- and C-PVAT-derived conditioned medium from one patient with CAD. A commercially available membrane-based antibody protein array was used. Each vertical pair of dots represents one protein.

Boxes of the same color on both membranes mark the respective dot pairs for each protein. Positive and negative control dots are also marked. (**B**) Heat map representation of the expression of 29 proteins quantified using membrane-based protein array analysis in IMA-PVAT- and C-PVAT-derived conditioned medium of $n = 5$ patients with CAD. Each column represents one patient (P1, P2, etc.). (**C**) Quantitative analysis shown for proteins exhibiting a statistically significant difference in expression between IMA-PVAT and C-PVAT. Bars represent fold change of mean protein expression compared to IMA-PVAT. Error bars represent standard deviation. Statistical analysis was performed using Student's paired t-test.

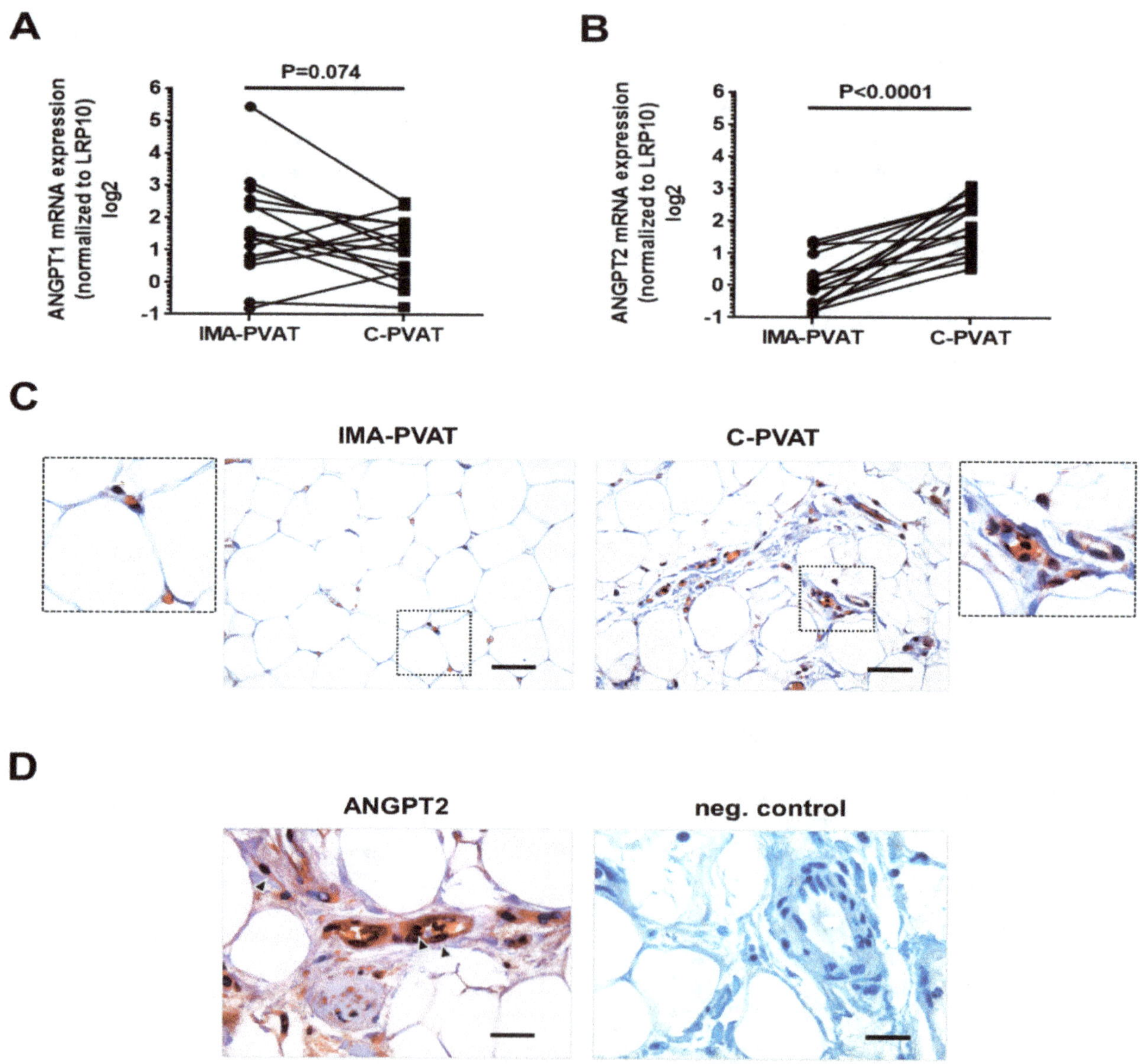

Figure 5. Expression of angiopoietin-1 and -2 in PVAT. (**A**) Quantification of mRNA expression of angiopoietin-1 (ANGPT1) (**A**) and angiopoietin-2, ANGPT2 (**B**) in IMA-PVAT and C-PVAT of $n = 16$ patients with CAD. Paired IMA-PVAT (●) and C-PVAT (■) values of individual patient are connected with a line. (**C**) Representative image after immunohistochemical detection of ANGPT2 in IMA-PVAT and C-PVAT. Size bars represent 50 μm. (**D**) Higher magnification showing ANGPT2-positive cells (arrows). Negative control after omitting the primary antibody is also shown. Size bars represent 20 μm. Statistical analysis was performed using Wilcoxon matched-pairs signed rank test.

Among the most abundant factors, ANGPT2 ($p = 0.011$) and ICAM1 ($p = 0.014$) protein levels were found to significantly differ, with higher levels in C-PVAT compared to IMA-PVAT (Figure 4B). ANGPT2 overexpression in C-PVAT could be confirmed on the transcriptional level by qPCR analysis in 16 patients with CAD, showing significantly higher *ANGPT2* mRNA levels in C-PVAT compared to IMA-PVAT (1.31 (0.51–3.01) vs. 0.74 (0.12–3.50), $p < 0.0001$; Figure 5B). On the other hand, *ANGPT1* mRNA levels did not significantly differ between C-PVAT and IMA-PVAT (2.18 (1.28–5.73) vs. 2.70 (1.63–5.73), $p = 0.074$; Figure 5A). Immunohistochemical staining of ANGPT2 identified endothelium, but also infiltrating immune cells and fibroblasts as possible cellular source of ANGPT2 in PVAT specimens (Figure 5D), both of which were more abundant in C-PVAT (Figure 5C). These findings suggested that the increased expression of ANGPT2 in C-PVAT compared to IMA-PVAT represents the composite result of increased vascularization, inflammation, and fibrosis. Protein levels of ICAM1 were significantly elevated in C-PVAT compared to IMA-PVAT (Figure 4B), in line with the presence of inflamed lymphatic endothelium [29]. Moreover, VEGF-D levels were also significantly increased in C-PVAT compared to IMA-PVAT, in accordance with the difference at mRNA level, whereas no statistically significant increase was detected for VEGF-C (Figure S3A). The expression of MMP9 was also found to be increased in C-PVAT compared to IMA-PVAT, the difference approaching but not reaching statistical significance ($p = 0.057$).

3.5. Recombinant ANGPT2 Stimulates Sprouting Angiogenesis of Human Lymphatic Endothelial Cells

To further study the importance of the above observations for perivascular adipose tissue lymphangiogenesis, the effect of recombinant human ANGPT2 was examined employing the three-dimensional spheroid angiogenesis assay in human lymphatic endothelial cells (HDLECs). Of note, total CM from C-PVAT and IMA-PVAT did not differ in its ability to promote HDLECs angiogenesis in the matrigel™ (Figure S4A–C) or the spheroid assay (Figure S4D–F); however, due to the fact that PVAT-derived conditioned medium contains a mixture of numerous factors, the effects of one specific factor on cultivated cells in vitro may have been obscured.

Flow cytometry analysis confirmed that HDLECs express (lymphatic) endothelial cell markers, including VEGFR3, the receptor for VEGF-C, and TIE2 (TEK receptor tyrosine kinase), the receptor for ANGPT2 (Figure S5). Stimulation of HDLEC spheroids with ANGPT2 (100 ng/mL) for 24 h did not alter the number of sprouts (Figure 6A,B) or the cumulative sprout length (Figure 6A,C) compared to control-treated spheroids. Stimulation of HDLECs spheroids with ANGPT2 together with VEGF-C (100 ng/mL each), both overexpressed (ANGPT2 on the mRNA and the protein level, VEGF-C on the mRNA level) in C-PVAT, significantly increased both the number of sprouts ($p = 0.005$ vs. control, $p = 0.021$ vs. VEGF-C; Figure 6B) and the cumulative sprout length ($p = 0.004$ vs. control and ANGPT2, $p = 0.006$ vs. VEGF-C; Figure 6C). These findings are in agreement with the more extended lymphatic network in C-PVAT compared to IMA-PVAT observed in this study and previous findings on the role of ANGPT2 and VEGF-C as important regulators of functional lymphatic vessel formation [30–32].

Previous studies have shown that inflammatory cytokines, in particular TNFα, is capable of inducing ANPGT2, but also ICAM1 expression suggesting a role of ANGPT2 in inflammatory lymphangiogenesis [33]. Because TNFα levels did not differ in CM from either of the PVAT depots (Figure S3C), we examined the possible role of perivascular hypoxia in the observed overexpression of ANGPT2 and ICAM1. Chemical hypoxia was induced on cultured HDLECs by stimulation with 1 mM cobalt chloride ($CoCl_2$) for 4 h (eight independent experiments). The mRNA expression of ICAM1 was found to be significantly increased in $CoCl_2$-treated compared to control-treated HDLECs (5.4 fold increase vs. control; $p < 0.0001$; Figure 6D). VEGF-D mRNA levels were also significantly increased (8.7 fold increase vs. control; $p = 0.001$; Figure 6E), whereas no significant differences were found in the mRNA expression of ANGPT2, VEGF-C, TIE2 and VEGFR3.

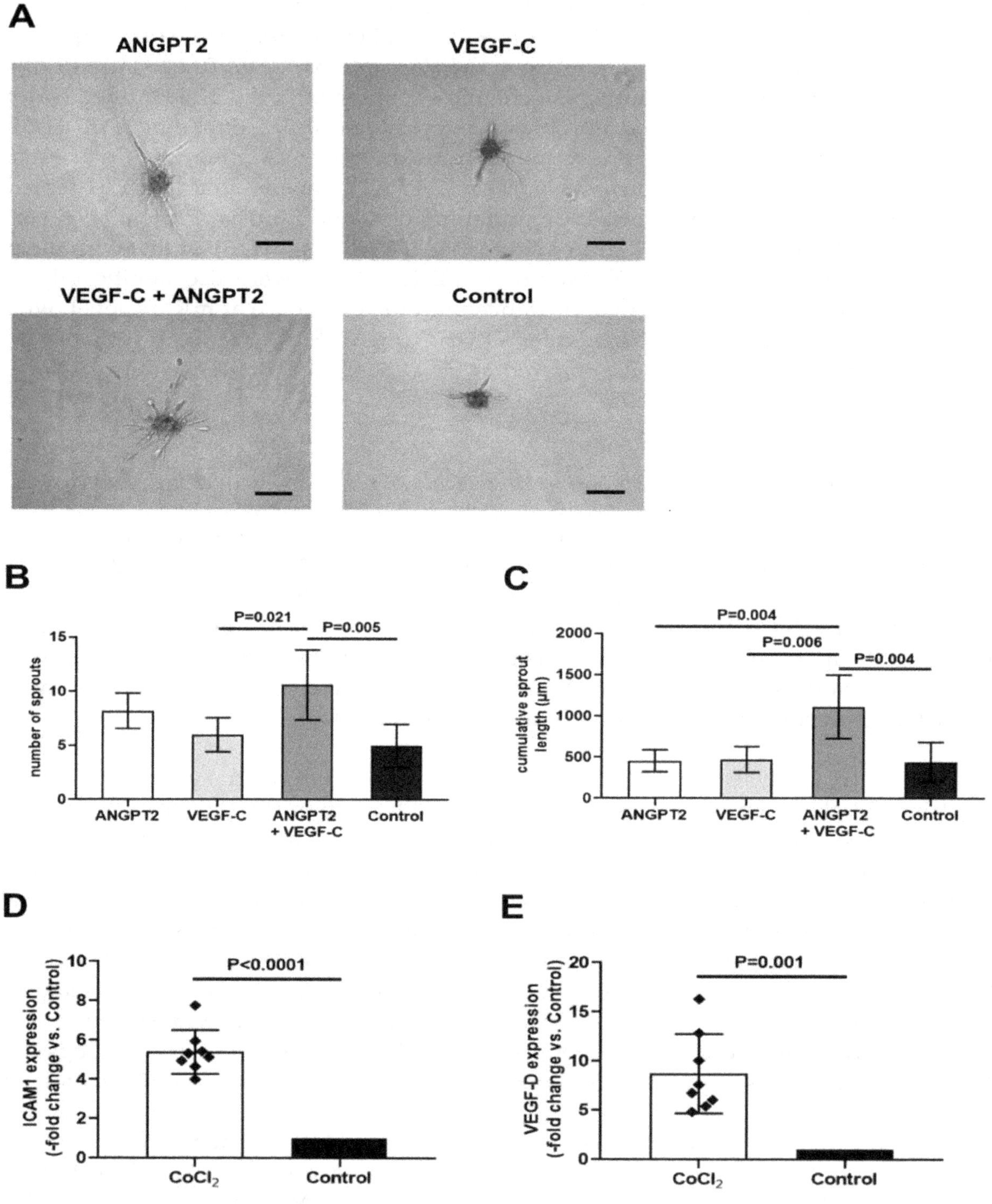

Figure 6. Effects of ANGPT2 and VEGF-C on human sprouting lymphangiogenesis. Representative images of human dermal lymphatic endothelial cell (HDLEC) spheroids (**A**) as well as the results after quantitative analysis of the number of sprouts (per spheroid) (**B**) and the cumulative sprout length (µm) in $n = 5$ spheroids (**C**) after stimulation with recombinant human ANGPT2; (100 ng/mL) and/or VEGF-C (100 ng/mL) or control (CTL). Size bars represent 200 µm. (**D–E**) Quantification of mRNA expression of ICAM1 (**D**) and VEGF-D (**E**) in HDLECs, after induction of chemical hypoxia using 1 mM of $CoCl_2$ for 4 h in $n = 8$ independent experiments. Bars represent fold change of mean mRNA expression compared to Control. Error bars represent standard deviation. Statistical analysis was performed using one-way ANOVA with Turkey's multiple comparisons test (**B,C**) and Student's paired t-test (**D,E**).

4. Discussion

The main findings of our study are that (1) PVAT surrounding the aortic root and the coronary arteries of patients with CAD exhibits a denser lymphatic vessel network compared to PVAT surrounding the IMA, an 'atherosclerosis-resistant' artery; (2) The expression of lymphangiogenic growth factors (VEGF-C and VEGF-D) and their primary receptor (VEGFR3) is significantly increased in C-PVAT compared to IMA-PVAT, both at the mRNA (VEGF-C and VEGF-D) and the protein level (VEGF-D); (3) Increased lymphangiogenesis was accompanied with increased expression of ICAM1, infiltration with macrophages and more extensive fibrosis; and (4) Elevated levels of ANGPT2 in C-PVAT could be identified as one potential factor contributing to the observed increase in perivascular lymphangiogenesis. To the best of our knowledge, the present study is the first to compare lymphangiogenesis and its regulators in the perivascular fat surrounding an atherosclerotic and a non-diseased vessel in patients with coronary artery disease. Regarding the use of the IMA as 'control' artery it should be noted that, although the reason for the observed resistance of this artery to atherosclerosis is unclear [34], PVAT surrounding the IMA has been reported to exert vasodilatatory effects on the underlying vessel [35], which supports the hypothesis that IMA-PVAT may in part be responsible for the protection of this artery against atherosclerosis. Previous findings of marked gene expression heterogeneity between PVAT surrounding the coronary artery and the IMA in patients with CAD also support the contribution of differences in perivascular fat composition to the susceptibility to atherosclerosis [36,37]. On the other hand, C-PVAT from healthy individuals cannot be surgically obtained and is therefore not available as 'control' PVAT depot in patients with CAD undergoing bypass surgery.

The possible role of the adventitia and perivascular adipose tissue in the pathophysiology of atherosclerosis has only recently received attention. Several studies, including from our own group, identified factors expressed and released in the perivascular fat as important local mediators of vascular repair processes and atherosclerotic lesion formation (reviewed in [28]). Some of the factors overexpressed in PVAT possess angiogenic activities, such as leptin [38] or CCL2 [39], and adventitial neoangiogenesis may contribute to atherosclerotic plaque progression and instability [1–6]. In contrast to perivascular networks created by blood endothelial cells, studies on the possible role of adventitial lymphangiogenesis in atherosclerosis are limited. For example, dissection of the plaque draining lymph node in apolipoprotein E-knockout mice aggravated atherosclerotic burden [11], whereas restoration of lymphatic drainage in hypercholesterolemic mice improved reverse cholesterol transport. On the other hand, and to the best of our knowledge, animal studies have so far not addressed the importance of coronary perivascular lymphangiogenesis during atherosclerosis. On the other hand, post-mortem analyses in humans and a clinical study found a more extended lymphatic vasculature in the adventitia of atherosclerotic vessels [11,16–19]. Although contradictory at first, both observations may reflect different stages of a chronic disease process in which perivascular lymph vessels reactively develop to accelerate the removal of lipids and the exit of inflammatory cells, but become exhausted and dysfunctional at later stages due to chronic overactivation [8,15]. Although our study cannot provide a definite answer to the important question of whether the observed increased lymphangiogenesis in C-PVAT is the consequence of the existing atherosclerosis in human coronary arteries or one of its causes, the increased expression of ICAM1, infiltration with macrophages, and fibrosis observed in C-PVAT appear to be in accordance with the concept of reactive, i.e. inflammation- or fibrosis-induced, adventitial lymphangiogenesis.

Overall, the findings of this and previous studies emphasize that the connections among (peri)vascular inflammation, fibrosis and (lymph)angiogenesis are rather complex and that the pathophysiological pathways underlying our observations are probably not unidirectional. Available data rather propose a circular mechanism with multiple shortcuts among various biological processes (schematically depicted in Figure 7), in which advanced atherosclerosis with arterial wall inflammation and fibrosis promote perivascular angiogenesis and lymphangiogenesis.

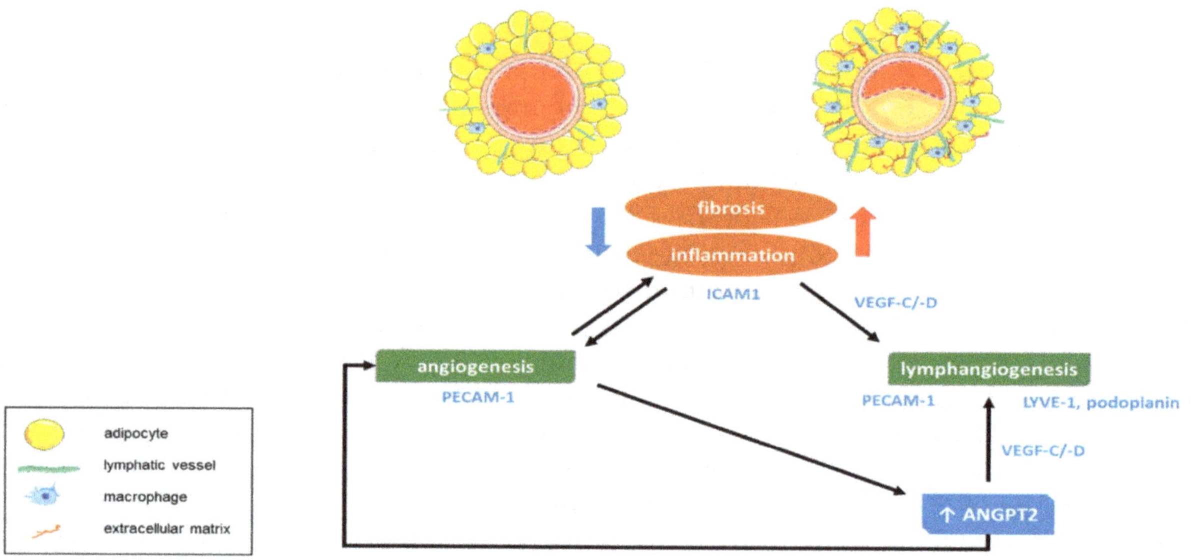

Figure 7. Schematic drawing depicting the main findings of this study.

Regarding the signals mediating perivascular lymphangiogenesis, the increase in lymphatic vessels in C-PVAT compared to IMA-PVAT was accompanied with elevated mRNA levels of two major regulators of lymphangiogenesis, namely VEGF-C and VEGF-D, as well as their receptor VEGFR3. Increased numbers of intimal cells expressing VEGF-C were also reported in patients with atherosclerosis of the iliac arteries and found to correlate with atherosclerotic lesion severity and the number of LYVE1-positive lymphatic vessels, whereas similar associations were not observed for VEGF-D [18]. Macrophages are an important source of VEGF-C and VEGF-D, as shown in tumors [26,27,40], and both growth factors may also act as chemoattractant by upregulating the expression of VEGFR3 on M1 polarized macrophages, as shown in visceral adipose tissue of mice [41]. TGFβ [42,43] and proinflammatory cytokines, such as interleukin (IL) 1β and TNFα [44], have been shown to further enhance the expression of VEGF-C and to promote lymphangiogenesis, although we did not detect differences in their expression levels between both adipose tissue depots.

The importance of VEGF-C–VEGFR3 in the regulation of lymphangiogenesis is well established [31,45,46]. However, under some circumstances VEGF-C may also bind to VEGFR2, expressed on lymphatic and blood endothelial cells [47,48]. VEGF-C was shown to promote angiogenesis in the developing embryo [49] or following ischemia [50]. Others found that VEGF-C overexpression selectively induced lymphangiogenesis without altering accompanying angiogenesis [45,51]. The net result of VEGF-C signaling in terms of (lymph)angiogenesis may depend on the local abundance of VEGFR2 and VEGFR3 receptors, as findings in mice expressing a VEGFR3-specific mutant of VEGF-C exhibited growth of lymphatic, but not of blood vessels [52]. VEGF-D also binds both VEGFR2 and VEGFR3 with high affinity [53] and has angiogenic as well as lymphangiogenic activities [54,55]. On the other hand, the expression of VEGF-A, an essential hemangiogenic factor, did not significantly differ between C-PVAT and IMA-PVAT, whereas VEGF-B, a specific ligand for VEGFR1 with limited angiogenic potential, was markedly reduced in our study. Although VEGF-B is dispensable for blood vessel growth, it was found to have pro-survival effects on endothelial cells, vascular smooth muscle cells and pericytes [56]. Interestingly, VEGF-B is highly expressed in brown adipose tissue [57] and was shown to control endothelial fatty acid uptake [58]. The significantly reduced expression observed in C-PVAT may reflect the loss of protective (brown) adipose tissue properties compared to IMA-PVAT, as suggested by findings in rodents [59].

ANGPT2 holds a significant role in postnatal angiogenic remodeling, but also the proper development of lymphatic vessels [30,60]. Here, we show that the expression of ANGPT2 is increased in C-PVAT compared to IMA-PVAT in patients with CAD, and findings could be confirmed at the protein level in the secretome of C-PVAT and IMA-PVAT. Others have shown that ANGPT2 overexpression leads to lymphatic hyperplasia [30], suggesting that increased ANGPT2 levels may have contributed to the enhanced lymphangiogenic vessel density observed in this PVAT depot. In agreement with the described synergistic effect of VEGF and ANGPT2 in promoting lymphangiogenesis [60,61], we could show that stimulation of HDLEC spheroids using a combination of ANGPT2 and VEGF-C results in lymphangiogenic sprouting, whereas stimulation with ANPGT2 or VEGF-C alone had weak or no effects at all. Although ANGPT2 is mainly expressed in endothelial cells [62], immunohistochemical analysis revealed ANGPT2 protein expression also in infiltrating immune cells and myofibroblasts, in line with their role as important source of lymphangiogenic growth factors. Binding of ANGPT2 to TIE2 receptors may activate NFκB (nuclear factor 'kappa-light-chain-enhancer' of activated B-cells) signaling and the expression of adhesion receptors on endothelial cells, including ICAM1 [63]. NFkB may also upregulate the expression of VEGFR3 on lymphatic endothelial cells and increase their sensitivity to VEGF-C and -D [64], and analyses in mice or human endothelial cells lacking ANGPT2 showed that it may increase the responsiveness of vascular endothelial cells to inflammatory stimuli [65].

In addition to inflammatory signals, hypoxia may be a relevant factor underlying the observed elevated lymphangiogenic growth factor levels in C-PVAT. Hypoxic cells, such as those present in tumors or atherosclerotic plaques, may release angiogenic growth factors, and we have previously shown that hypoxia levels are higher in C-PVAT compared to IMA-PVAT and that this difference may underlie the increased expression of leptin, an adipokine with proangiogenic properties, in the C-PVAT of CAD patients [20]. Hypoxia is also a major stimulus inducing the expression of VEGF. In the present study, inhibition of hypoxia-inducible factor 1-alpha (HIF1α) degradation by $CoCl_2$ did not alter the expression of ANGPT2 and VEGF-C or their receptors, but significantly increased the expression of VEGF-D and ICAM-1. A previous study showed that the VEGF-C promotor does not contain hypoxia-responsive elements, and that hypoxia may induces VEGF-C via HIF1α-independent mechanisms [66]. Interestingly, lymphatic vessels respond to the same angiogenic cues as endothelial cells lining blood vessels, although they exhibit unidirectional flow and do not transport erythrocytes and thus will not improve oxygen supply to hypoxic tissues. The parallel increase of blood and lymph vessel formation could represent a mechanism to remove excess interstitial fluid and cells extravasated from immature and leaky angiogenic blood vessels during hypoxia.

Our study has some limitations. Due to the small amount of tissue available from each patient, the total study collective had to be split into groups for different types of assays, which may have influenced our observations. It should also be noted that 'only' PVAT but not specimens from the underlying vascular wall were available for analysis, and that we could not directly associate our findings in PVAT with the severity of the atherosclerotic lesion in the underlying artery. Also, perioperative C-PVAT sampling was performed in a standardized manner (near the aortic root), regardless of the localization of atherosclerotic lesions within the coronary tree. All individuals included in the present study were diagnosed with advanced coronary atherosclerosis with indication for a bypass graft surgery, and our study could therefore not examine earlier stages of this chronic vascular wall disease evolving over many years. Also, C-PVAT from healthy individuals is not available for analysis and thus the distribution of lymphatic vessels in C-PVAT under 'normal' conditions is unknown. On the other hand, using the IMA as an internal 'healthy' control artery may have helped to provide additional insights into the pathophysiological role of local processes, in particular perivascular lymphangiogenesis during atherosclerosis, whereas the possible impact of systemic effects on the composition and expression patterns should have been minimized by the direct comparison of these two PVAT depots from the same patient. However, it cannot be excluded that differences in the local microenvironment between the two PVAT depots may have contributed to the observed differences.

In conclusion, our findings show an increased lymphangiogenic activity in PVAT surrounding atherosclerotic coronary arteries compared to PVAT surrounding the IMA, an artery free of atherosclerosis, in patients with CAD. Increased ANGPT2 expression and activated VEGF-C/VEGF-D-mediated VEGFR3 signaling, in combination with a local proinflammatory and hypoxic environment, may pathophysiologically underlie these observations.

Author Contributions: Conceptualization of the study, I.D., S.K., and K.S.; validation, I.D., M.P., and K.S.; formal analysis, I.D., G.C., and K.S.; investigation, I.D., M.P., M.O.C., A.K., R.G., M.L.B., G.C., and C.T.; resources, K.B., F.K., C.F.V., D.M., D.T., and T.M.; data curation, I.D., M.P., M.O.C., and A.K.; writing—original draft preparation, I.D. and K.S.; writing—review and editing, I.D., M.P., K.B., S.K., and K.S.; visualization, I.D.; supervision, S.K. and K.S.; project administration, K.S.; funding acquisition, I.D., S.K., and K.S.

Acknowledgments: The authors acknowledge the expert technical assistance of Marina Janocha, Anna Kern, and Michaela Moisch.

References

1. Moulton, K.S.; Vakili, K.; Zurakowski, D.; Soliman, M.; Butterfield, C.; Sylvin, E.; Lo, K.M.; Gillies, S.; Javaherian, K.; Folkman, J. Inhibition of plaque neovascularization reduces macrophage accumulation and progression of advanced atherosclerosis. *Proc. Natl. Acad. Sci. USA* **2003**, *100*, 4736–4741. [CrossRef] [PubMed]
2. Tanaka, K.; Nagata, D.; Hirata, Y.; Tabata, Y.; Nagai, R.; Sata, M. Augmented angiogenesis in adventitia promotes growth of atherosclerotic plaque in apolipoprotein E-deficient mice. *Atherosclerosis* **2011**, *215*, 366–373. [CrossRef] [PubMed]
3. Xu, X.; Mao, W.; Chai, Y.; Dai, J.; Chen, Q.; Wang, L.; Zhuang, Q.; Pan, Y.; Chen, M.; Ni, G.; et al. Angiogenesis Inhibitor, Endostar, Prevents Vasa Vasorum Neovascularization in a Swine Atherosclerosis Model. *J. Atheroscler. Thromb.* **2015**, *22*, 1100–1112. [CrossRef] [PubMed]
4. Dunmore, B.J.; McCarthy, M.J.; Naylor, A.R.; Brindle, N.P. Carotid plaque instability and ischemic symptoms are linked to immaturity of microvessels within plaques. *J. Vasc. Surg.* **2007**, *45*, 155–159. [CrossRef] [PubMed]
5. Sluimer, J.C.; Kolodgie, F.D.; Bijnens, A.P.; Maxfield, K.; Pacheco, E.; Kutys, B.; Duimel, H.; Frederik, P.M.; van Hinsbergh, V.W.; Virmani, R.; et al. Thin-walled microvessels in human coronary atherosclerotic plaques show incomplete endothelial junctions relevance of compromised structural integrity for intraplaque microvascular leakage. *J. Am. Coll. Cardiol.* **2009**, *53*, 1517–1527. [CrossRef] [PubMed]
6. Michel, J.B.; Virmani, R.; Arbustini, E.; Pasterkamp, G. Intraplaque haemorrhages as the trigger of plaque vulnerability. *Eur. Heart J.* **2011**, *32*, 1977–1985. [CrossRef]
7. Hoggan, G.; Hoggan, F.E. The Lymphatics of the Walls of the Larger Blood-Vessels and Lymphatics. *J. Anat. Physiol.* **1882**, *17*, 1–23. [PubMed]
8. Lim, H.Y.; Thiam, C.H.; Yeo, K.P.; Bisoendial, R.; Hii, C.S.; McGrath, K.C.; Tan, K.W.; Heather, A.; Alexander, J.S.; Angeli, V. Lymphatic vessels are essential for the removal of cholesterol from peripheral tissues by SR-BI-mediated transport of HDL. *Cell Metab.* **2013**, *17*, 671–684. [CrossRef]
9. Coso, S.; Bovay, E.; Petrova, T.V. Pressing the right buttons: Signaling in lymphangiogenesis. *Blood* **2014**, *123*, 2614–2624. [CrossRef]
10. Martel, C.; Li, W.; Fulp, B.; Platt, A.M.; Gautier, E.L.; Westerterp, M.; Bittman, R.; Tall, A.R.; Chen, S.H.; Thomas, M.J.; et al. Lymphatic vasculature mediates macrophage reverse cholesterol transport in mice. *J. Clin. Invest.* **2013**, *123*, 1571–1579. [CrossRef]
11. Rademakers, T.; van der Vorst, E.P.; Daissormont, I.T.; Otten, J.J.; Theodorou, K.; Theelen, T.L.; Gijbels, M.; Anisimov, A.; Nurmi, H.; Lindeman, J.H.; et al. Adventitial lymphatic capillary expansion impacts on plaque T cell accumulation in atherosclerosis. *Sci. Rep.* **2017**, *7*. [CrossRef] [PubMed]
12. Santulli, G. The lymphatic border patrol outwits inflammatory cells in myocardial infarction. *Sci. Transl. Med.* **2018**, *10*. [CrossRef] [PubMed]
13. Vieira, J.M.; Norman, S.; Villa Del Campo, C.; Cahill, T.J.; Barnette, D.N.; Gunadasa-Rohling, M.; Johnson, L.A.; Greaves, D.R.; Carr, C.A.; Jackson, D.G.; et al. The cardiac lymphatic system stimulates resolution of inflammation following myocardial infarction. *J. Clin. Invest.* **2018**, *128*, 3402–3412. [CrossRef] [PubMed]
14. Lim, H.Y.; Rutkowski, J.M.; Helft, J.; Reddy, S.T.; Swartz, M.A.; Randolph, G.J.; Angeli, V. Hypercholesterolemic mice exhibit lymphatic vessel dysfunction and degeneration. *Am. J. Pathol.* **2009**, *175*, 1328–1337. [CrossRef] [PubMed]
15. Milasan, A.; Dallaire, F.; Mayer, G.; Martel, C. Effects of LDL Receptor Modulation on Lymphatic Function. *Sci. Rep.* **2016**, *6*. [CrossRef] [PubMed]

16. Kholova, I.; Dragneva, G.; Cermakova, P.; Laidinen, S.; Kaskenpaa, N.; Hazes, T.; Cermakova, E.; Steiner, I.; Yla-Herttuala, S. Lymphatic vasculature is increased in heart valves, ischaemic and inflamed hearts and in cholesterol-rich and calcified atherosclerotic lesions. *Eur. J. Clin. Invest.* **2011**, *41*, 487–497. [CrossRef] [PubMed]
17. Drozdz, K.; Janczak, D.; Dziegiel, P.; Podhorska, M.; Piotrowska, A.; Patrzalek, D.; Andrzejak, R.; Szuba, A. Adventitial lymphatics and atherosclerosis. *Lymphology* **2012**, *45*, 26–33.
18. Grzegorek, I.; Drozdz, K.; Chmielewska, M.; Gomulkiewicz, A.; Jablonska, K.; Piotrowska, A.; Karczewski, M.; Janczak, D.; Podhorska-Okolow, M.; Dziegiel, P.; et al. Arterial wall lymphangiogenesis is increased in the human iliac atherosclerotic arteries: Involvement of CCR7 receptor. *Lymphat. Res. Biol.* **2014**, *12*, 222–231. [CrossRef]
19. Drozdz, K.; Janczak, D.; Dziegiel, P.; Podhorska, M.; Patrzalek, D.; Ziolkowski, P.; Andrzejak, R.; Szuba, A. Adventitial lymphatics of internal carotid artery in healthy and atherosclerotic vessels. *Folia. Histochem. Cytobiol.* **2008**, *46*, 433–436. [CrossRef]
20. Drosos, I.; Chalikias, G.; Pavlaki, M.; Kareli, D.; Epitropou, G.; Bougioukas, G.; Mikroulis, D.; Konstantinou, F.; Giatromanolaki, A.; Ritis, K.; et al. Differences between perivascular adipose tissue surrounding the heart and the internal mammary artery: Possible role for the leptin-inflammation-fibrosis-hypoxia axis. *Clin. Res. Cardiol.* **2016**, *105*, 887–900. [CrossRef]
21. Tanaka, K.; Sata, M. Roles of Perivascular Adipose Tissue in the Pathogenesis of Atherosclerosis. *Front. Physiol.* **2018**, *9*. [CrossRef] [PubMed]
22. Sims, F.H. A comparison of coronary and internal mammary arteries and implications of the results in the etiology of arteriosclerosis. *Am. Heart J.* **1983**, *105*, 560–566. [CrossRef]
23. Kilarski, W.W. Physiological Perspective on Therapies of Lymphatic Vessels. *Adv. Wound Care* **2018**, *7*, 189–208. [CrossRef] [PubMed]
24. Hong, Y.K.; Harvey, N.; Noh, Y.H.; Schacht, V.; Hirakawa, S.; Detmar, M.; Oliver, G. Prox1 is a master control gene in the program specifying lymphatic endothelial cell fate. *Dev. Dyn.* **2002**, *225*, 351–357. [CrossRef] [PubMed]
25. Wigle, J.T.; Harvey, N.; Detmar, M.; Lagutina, I.; Grosveld, G.; Gunn, M.D.; Jackson, D.G.; Oliver, G. An essential role for Prox1 in the induction of the lymphatic endothelial cell phenotype. *EMBO J.* **2002**, *21*, 1505–1513. [CrossRef] [PubMed]
26. Schoppmann, S.F.; Birner, P.; Stockl, J.; Kalt, R.; Ullrich, R.; Caucig, C.; Kriehuber, E.; Nagy, K.; Alitalo, K.; Kerjaschki, D. Tumor-associated macrophages express lymphatic endothelial growth factors and are related to peritumoral lymphangiogenesis. *Am. J. Pathol.* **2002**, *161*, 947–956. [CrossRef]
27. Gousopoulos, E.; Proulx, S.T.; Bachmann, S.B.; Dieterich, L.C.; Scholl, J.; Karaman, S.; Bianchi, R.; Detmar, M. An Important Role of VEGF-C in Promoting Lymphedema Development. *J. Invest. Dermatol.* **2017**, *137*, 1995–2004. [CrossRef]
28. Schäfer, K.; Drosos, I.; Konstantinides, S. Perivascular adipose tissue: Epiphenomenon or local risk factor? *Int. J. Obes. (Lond.)* **2017**, *41*, 1311–1323. [CrossRef]
29. Podgrabinska, S.; Kamalu, O.; Mayer, L.; Shimaoka, M.; Snoeck, H.; Randolph, G.J.; Skobe, M. Inflamed lymphatic endothelium suppresses dendritic cell maturation and function via Mac-1/ICAM-1-dependent mechanism. *J. Immunol.* **2009**, *183*, 1767–1779. [CrossRef]
30. Zheng, W.; Nurmi, H.; Appak, S.; Sabine, A.; Bovay, E.; Korhonen, E.A.; Orsenigo, F.; Lohela, M.; D'Amico, G.; Holopainen, T.; et al. Angiopoietin 2 regulates the transformation and integrity of lymphatic endothelial cell junctions. *Genes Dev.* **2014**, *28*, 1592–1603. [CrossRef]
31. Kuchler, A.M.; Gjini, E.; Peterson-Maduro, J.; Cancilla, B.; Wolburg, H.; Schulte-Merker, S. Development of the zebrafish lymphatic system requires VEGFC signaling. *Curr. Biol.* **2006**, *16*, 1244–1248. [CrossRef] [PubMed]
32. Sweat, R.S.; Sloas, D.C.; Murfee, W.L. VEGF-C induces lymphangiogenesis and angiogenesis in the rat mesentery culture model. *Microcirculation* **2014**, *21*, 532–540. [CrossRef] [PubMed]
33. Yan, Z.X.; Jiang, Z.H.; Liu, N.F. Angiopoietin-2 promotes inflammatory lymphangiogenesis and its effect can be blocked by the specific inhibitor L1-10. *Am. J. Physiol. Heart Circ. Physiol.* **2012**, *302*, H215–H223. [CrossRef] [PubMed]

34. Otsuka, F.; Yahagi, K.; Sakakura, K.; Virmani, R. Why is the mammary artery so special and what protects it from atherosclerosis? *Ann. Cardiothorac. Surg.* **2013**, *2*, 519–526. [CrossRef]
35. Malinowski, M.; Deja, M.A.; Janusiewicz, P.; Golba, K.S.; Roleder, T.; Wos, S. Mechanisms of vasodilatatory effect of perivascular tissue of human internal thoracic artery. *J. Physiol. Pharmacol.* **2013**, *64*, 309–316. [PubMed]
36. Lu, D.; Wang, W.; Xia, L.; Xia, P.; Yan, Y. Gene expression profiling reveals heterogeneity of perivascular adipose tissues surrounding coronary and internal thoracic arteries. *Acta. Biochim. Biophys. Sin. (Shanghai)* **2017**, *49*, 1075–1082. [CrossRef]
37. Numaguchi, R.; Furuhashi, M.; Matsumoto, M.; Sato, H.; Yanase, Y.; Kuroda, Y.; Harada, R.; Ito, T.; Higashiura, Y.; Koyama, M.; et al. Differential Phenotypes in Perivascular Adipose Tissue Surrounding the Internal Thoracic Artery and Diseased Coronary Artery. *J. Am. Heart Assoc.* **2019**, *8*. [CrossRef]
38. Schroeter, M.R.; Stein, S.; Heida, N.M.; Leifheit-Nestler, M.; Cheng, I.F.; Gogiraju, R.; Christiansen, H.; Maier, L.S.; Shah, A.M.; Hasenfuss, G.; et al. Leptin promotes the mobilization of vascular progenitor cells and neovascularization by NOX2-mediated activation of MMP9. *Cardiovasc. Res.* **2012**, *93*, 170–180. [CrossRef]
39. Salcedo, R.; Ponce, M.L.; Young, H.A.; Wasserman, K.; Ward, J.M.; Kleinman, H.K.; Oppenheim, J.J.; Murphy, W.J. Human endothelial cells express CCR2 and respond to MCP-1: Direct role of MCP-1 in angiogenesis and tumor progression. *Blood* **2000**, *96*, 34–40.
40. Nakano, T.; Nakashima, Y.; Yonemitsu, Y.; Sumiyoshi, S.; Chen, Y.X.; Akishima, Y.; Ishii, T.; Iida, M.; Sueishi, K. Angiogenesis and lymphangiogenesis and expression of lymphangiogenic factors in the atherosclerotic intima of human coronary arteries. *Hum. Pathol.* **2005**, *36*, 330–340. [CrossRef]
41. Karaman, S.; Hollmen, M.; Robciuc, M.R.; Alitalo, A.; Nurmi, H.; Morf, B.; Buschle, D.; Alkan, H.F.; Ochsenbein, A.M.; Alitalo, K.; et al. Blockade of VEGF-C and VEGF-D modulates adipose tissue inflammation and improves metabolic parameters under high-fat diet. *Mol. Metab.* **2015**, *4*, 93–105. [CrossRef] [PubMed]
42. Kinashi, H.; Falke, L.L.; Nguyen, T.Q.; Bovenschen, N.; Aten, J.; Leask, A.; Ito, Y.; Goldschmeding, R. Connective tissue growth factor regulates fibrosis-associated renal lymphangiogenesis. *Kidney Int.* **2017**, *92*, 850–863. [CrossRef] [PubMed]
43. Kinashi, H.; Ito, Y.; Sun, T.; Katsuno, T.; Takei, Y. Roles of the TGF-beta(-)VEGF-C Pathway in Fibrosis-Related Lymphangiogenesis. *Int. J. Mol. Sci.* **2018**, *19*, 2487. [CrossRef]
44. Ristimaki, A.; Narko, K.; Enholm, B.; Joukov, V.; Alitalo, K. Proinflammatory cytokines regulate expression of the lymphatic endothelial mitogen vascular endothelial growth factor-C. *J. Biol. Chem.* **1998**, *273*, 8413–8418. [CrossRef] [PubMed]
45. Jeltsch, M.; Kaipainen, A.; Joukov, V.; Meng, X.; Lakso, M.; Rauvala, H.; Swartz, M.; Fukumura, D.; Jain, R.K.; Alitalo, K. Hyperplasia of lymphatic vessels in VEGF-C transgenic mice. *Science* **1997**, *276*, 1423–1425. [CrossRef] [PubMed]
46. Karkkainen, M.J.; Haiko, P.; Sainio, K.; Partanen, J.; Taipale, J.; Petrova, T.V.; Jeltsch, M.; Jackson, D.G.; Talikka, M.; Rauvala, H.; et al. Vascular endothelial growth factor C is required for sprouting of the first lymphatic vessels from embryonic veins. *Nat. Immunol.* **2004**, *5*, 74–80. [CrossRef]
47. Joukov, V.; Pajusola, K.; Kaipainen, A.; Chilov, D.; Lahtinen, I.; Kukk, E.; Saksela, O.; Kalkkinen, N.; Alitalo, K. A novel vascular endothelial growth factor, VEGF-C, is a ligand for the Flt4 (VEGFR-3) and KDR (VEGFR-2) receptor tyrosine kinases. *EMBO J.* **1996**, *15*, 1751. [CrossRef]
48. Kriehuber, E.; Breiteneder-Geleff, S.; Groeger, M.; Soleiman, A.; Schoppmann, S.F.; Stingl, G.; Kerjaschki, D.; Maurer, D. Isolation and characterization of dermal lymphatic and blood endothelial cells reveal stable and functionally specialized cell lineages. *J. Exp. Med.* **2001**, *194*, 797–808. [CrossRef]
49. Cao, Y.; Linden, P.; Farnebo, J.; Cao, R.; Eriksson, A.; Kumar, V.; Qi, J.H.; Claesson-Welsh, L.; Alitalo, K. Vascular endothelial growth factor C induces angiogenesis in vivo. *Proc. Natl. Acad. Sci. USA* **1998**, *95*, 14389–14394. [CrossRef]
50. Witzenbichler, B.; Asahara, T.; Murohara, T.; Silver, M.; Spyridopoulos, I.; Magner, M.; Principe, N.; Kearney, M.; Hu, J.S.; Isner, J.M. Vascular endothelial growth factor-C (VEGF-C/VEGF-2) promotes angiogenesis in the setting of tissue ischemia. *Am. J. Pathol.* **1998**, *153*, 381–394. [CrossRef]

51. Enholm, B.; Karpanen, T.; Jeltsch, M.; Kubo, H.; Stenback, F.; Prevo, R.; Jackson, D.G.; Yla-Herttuala, S.; Alitalo, K. Adenoviral expression of vascular endothelial growth factor-C induces lymphangiogenesis in the skin. *Circ. Res.* **2001**, *88*, 623–629. [CrossRef] [PubMed]
52. Veikkola, T.; Jussila, L.; Makinen, T.; Karpanen, T.; Jeltsch, M.; Petrova, T.V.; Kubo, H.; Thurston, G.; McDonald, D.M.; Achen, M.G.; et al. Signalling via vascular endothelial growth factor receptor-3 is sufficient for lymphangiogenesis in transgenic mice. *EMBO J.* **2001**, *20*, 1223–1231. [CrossRef] [PubMed]
53. Achen, M.G.; Jeltsch, M.; Kukk, E.; Makinen, T.; Vitali, A.; Wilks, A.F.; Alitalo, K.; Stacker, S.A. Vascular endothelial growth factor D (VEGF-D) is a ligand for the tyrosine kinases VEGF receptor 2 (Flk1) and VEGF receptor 3 (Flt4). *Proc. Natl. Acad. Sci. USA* **1998**, *95*, 548–553. [CrossRef] [PubMed]
54. Marconcini, L.; Marchio, S.; Morbidelli, L.; Cartocci, E.; Albini, A.; Ziche, M.; Bussolino, F.; Oliviero, S. c-fos-induced growth factor/vascular endothelial growth factor D induces angiogenesis in vivo and in vitro. *Proc. Natl. Acad. Sci. USA* **1999**, *96*, 9671–9676. [CrossRef] [PubMed]
55. Byzova, T.V.; Goldman, C.K.; Jankau, J.; Chen, J.; Cabrera, G.; Achen, M.G.; Stacker, S.A.; Carnevale, K.A.; Siemionow, M.; Deitcher, S.R.; et al. Adenovirus encoding vascular endothelial growth factor-D induces tissue-specific vascular patterns in vivo. *Blood* **2002**, *99*, 4434–4442. [CrossRef] [PubMed]
56. Zhang, F.; Tang, Z.; Hou, X.; Lennartsson, J.; Li, Y.; Koch, A.W.; Scotney, P.; Lee, C.; Arjunan, P.; Dong, L.; et al. VEGF-B is dispensable for blood vessel growth but critical for their survival, and VEGF-B targeting inhibits pathological angiogenesis. *Proc. Natl. Acad. Sci. USA* **2009**, *106*, 6152–6157. [CrossRef] [PubMed]
57. Asano, A.; Irie, Y.; Saito, M. Isoform-specific regulation of vascular endothelial growth factor (VEGF) family mRNA expression in cultured mouse brown adipocytes. *Mol. Cell Endocrinol.* **2001**, *174*, 71–76. [CrossRef]
58. Hagberg, C.E.; Falkevall, A.; Wang, X.; Larsson, E.; Huusko, J.; Nilsson, I.; van Meeteren, L.A.; Samen, E.; Lu, L.; Vanwildemeersch, M.; et al. Vascular endothelial growth factor B controls endothelial fatty acid uptake. *Nature* **2010**, *464*, 917–921. [CrossRef]
59. Berbee, J.F.; Boon, M.R.; Khedoe, P.P.; Bartelt, A.; Schlein, C.; Worthmann, A.; Kooijman, S.; Hoeke, G.; Mol, I.M.; John, C.; et al. Brown fat activation reduces hypercholesterolaemia and protects from atherosclerosis development. *Nat. Commun.* **2015**, *6*. [CrossRef]
60. Gale, N.W.; Thurston, G.; Hackett, S.F.; Renard, R.; Wang, Q.; McClain, J.; Martin, C.; Witte, C.; Witte, M.H.; Jackson, D.; et al. Angiopoietin-2 is required for postnatal angiogenesis and lymphatic patterning, and only the latter role is rescued by Angiopoietin-1. *Dev. Cell* **2002**, *3*, 411–423. [CrossRef]
61. Holash, J.; Maisonpierre, P.C.; Compton, D.; Boland, P.; Alexander, C.R.; Zagzag, D.; Yancopoulos, G.D.; Wiegand, S.J. Vessel cooption, regression, and growth in tumors mediated by angiopoietins and VEGF. *Science* **1999**, *284*, 1994–1998. [CrossRef] [PubMed]
62. Scholz, A.; Plate, K.H.; Reiss, Y. Angiopoietin-2: A multifaceted cytokine that functions in both angiogenesis and inflammation. *Ann. N. Y. Acad. Sci.* **2015**, *1347*, 45–51. [CrossRef] [PubMed]
63. Rathnakumar, K.; Savant, S.; Giri, H.; Ghosh, A.; Fisslthaler, B.; Fleming, I.; Ram, U.; Bera, A.K.; Augustin, H.G.; Dixit, M. Angiopoietin-2 mediates thrombin-induced monocyte adhesion and endothelial permeability. *J. Thromb. Haemost.* **2016**, *14*, 1655–1667. [CrossRef] [PubMed]
64. Flister, M.J.; Wilber, A.; Hall, K.L.; Iwata, C.; Miyazono, K.; Nisato, R.E.; Pepper, M.S.; Zawieja, D.C.; Ran, S. Inflammation induces lymphangiogenesis through up-regulation of VEGFR-3 mediated by NF-kappaB and Prox1. *Blood* **2010**, *115*, 418–429. [CrossRef] [PubMed]
65. Fiedler, U.; Reiss, Y.; Scharpfenecker, M.; Grunow, V.; Koidl, S.; Thurston, G.; Gale, N.W.; Witzenrath, M.; Rosseau, S.; Suttorp, N.; et al. Angiopoietin-2 sensitizes endothelial cells to TNF-alpha and has a crucial role in the induction of inflammation. *Nat. Med.* **2006**, *12*, 235–239. [CrossRef] [PubMed]
66. Morfoisse, F.; Kuchnio, A.; Frainay, C.; Gomez-Brouchet, A.; Delisle, M.B.; Marzi, S.; Helfer, A.C.; Hantelys, F.; Pujol, F.; Guillermet-Guibert, J.; et al. Hypoxia induces VEGF-C expression in metastatic tumor cells via a HIF-1alpha-independent translation-mediated mechanism. *Cell Rep.* **2014**, *6*, 155–167. [CrossRef] [PubMed]

12

The Impact of the Circadian Genes *CLOCK* and *ARNTL* on Myocardial Infarction

Ivana Škrlec [1,*], Jakov Milić [2] and Robert Steiner [2,3]

1 Histology, Genetics, Cellular, and Molecular Biology Laboratory, Department of Biology and Chemistry, Faculty of Dental Medicine and Health, Josip Juraj Strossmayer University of Osijek, Crkvena 21, HR-31000 Osijek, Croatia
2 Faculty of Medicine, Josip Juraj Strossmayer University of Osijek, Josipa Huttlera 4, HR-31000 Osijek, Croatia; milic.jakov@gmail.com (J.M.); steiner_robert5@hotmail.com (R.S.)
3 Clinical Department of Cardiovascular Diseases and Intensive Care, Clinic for Internal Medicine, University Hospital Osijek, Josipa Huttlera 4, HR-31000 Osijek, Croatia
* Correspondence: iskrlec@fdmz.hr

Abstract: The circadian rhythm regulates various physiological mechanisms, and its disruption can promote many disorders. Disturbance of endogenous circadian rhythms enhances the chance of myocardial infarction (MI), showing that circadian clock genes could have a crucial function in the onset of the disease. This case-control study was performed on 1057 participants. It was hypothesized that the polymorphisms of one nucleotide (SNP) in three circadian clock genes (*CLOCK*, *ARNTL*, and *PER2*) could be associated with MI. Statistically significant differences, estimated by the Chi-square test, were found in the distribution of alleles and genotypes between MI and no-MI groups of the *CLOCK* (rs6811520 and rs13124436) and *ARNTL* (rs3789327 and rs12363415) genes. According to the results of the present study, the polymorphisms in the *CLOCK* and *ARNTL* genes could be related to MI.

Keywords: cardiovascular diseases; circadian rhythm; clock genes; myocardial infarction; polymorphisms

1. Introduction

Today, there is a global epidemic of cardiovascular diseases (CVDs). The World Health Organization (WHO) data for 2017 shows that CVDs caused 19.9 million deaths globally, and around 80% of CVDs deaths were because of stroke and myocardial infarction (MI) [1]. In recent decades, mortality from CVDs has decreased in developed countries, but CVDs remains one of the principal causes of death worldwide [2]. However, CVDs continue to be the third major cause of death in Croatia, with 45% of total mortality in 2016 [3,4]. Various pathophysiological processes stimulate and lead to the onset of MI. MI is an inflammatory disease. Thrombotic obstruction of the coronary arteries occurs at the position of initiated atherosclerotic plaque. It promotes total coronary circulation arrest, which leads to the death of cardiomyocytes and MI [5]. The etiology of MI is mainly unknown, in spite of the many studies conducted.

The circadian rhythm regulates many physiological mechanisms, and its disruption can result in many physiopathological disorders [6]. The circadian clock is integrated within approximately 24 h [7]. It regulates physiological processes at several levels, from gene transcription to sophisticated performance [8]. Cardiovascular incidents happen in a circadian fashion, with a significant incidence in the morning after rising [9]. Many cardiovascular events show morning circadian preferences, such as myocardial infarction [10], dissection of aortic aneurysms [11], and stroke [12]. Additionally, the incidence of MI is higher during the winter months, especially in the elderly [13]. The circadian rhythm adjusts the feedback of endothelial cells to damage the circulatory system [14]. Some physiological factors that oscillate with the circadian rhythms might trigger the onset of MI [15]. Those physiological factors are glucose homeostasis, blood pressure [16], myocardial contractions, vascular endothelial function, fibrinolytic activity, and metabolism [17,18].

In the peripheral clocks of cardiovascular cells or tissue, the central clock synchronizes and controls the everyday transcription of clock-controlled genes (CCGs) [19]. The primary circadian clock is placed in the SCN (suprachiasmatic nucleus) in the hypothalamus and is controlled by many circadian rhythm genes. Light drives the central clock. Decreased daylight exposure and overexposure to light at night impairs the circadian organization of sleep. Sleep disorders can lead to increased energy input, decreased energy expenditure, and insulin resistance [20]. Short sleep is associated with hypertension, diabetes mellitus, obesity, and mortality. Daylight saving time also causes a modest increase in MI occurrence [21]. Peripheral clocks are found in the cardiomyocyte, blood vessels, and vascular endothelial cells [22]. The circadian clock within cardiomyocytes regulates cardiac metabolic gene expression. It has the function of synchronizing cardiomyocyte metabolic activity with the availability of nutrients [22,23]. Polymorphisms in clock genes are associated with obesity, sleep disturbances, psychological and metabolic complications, plus cardiovascular disorders, such as stroke, vascular death, and myocardial infarction [6]. Desynchronization of the circadian rhythm can cause metabolic disorders and various other issues. Some of those are dyslipidemia, glucose intolerance, hypertension, type 2 diabetes mellitus (T2DM), and CVDs [24,25]. Whole-genome studies have detected numerous genes variants related to the elevated risk of myocardial infarction [26]. Genes included in the metabolic processes of lipid metabolism and the progress of T2DM have been the most investigated genes so far in relation to an enhanced risk of myocardial infarction [7].

Through the transcription and translation feedback loops, circadian rhythm genes control the cyclic transcription of mRNA and protein synthesis. There are some essential proteins in the SCN. The activators are CLOCK (Circadian Locomotor Output Cycles Kaput) and ARNTL (Aryl Hydrocarbon Receptor Nuclear Translocator-Like), while the inhibitors of transcription are PER (Period) and CRY (Cryptochrome) proteins. The day-to-night shift is generated by circadian oscillations that are maintained at the transcriptional and posttranscriptional levels in a single cell by the feedback loop of the circadian clock genes. ARNTL/CLOCK protein heterodimers trigger the expression of PER, CRY, and other clock-controlled genes. CRY/PER protein heterodimers serve as a negative feedback loop and repress the action of ARNTL and CLOCK [8,27]. The entire procedure of activating and suppressing gene transcription in a loop persists for approximately 24 h. Transcription factors stimulate the transcription of clock genes and other clock-controlled genes, initiating numerous physiological processes [7,28].

This research is a continuation of the preliminary study from 2018 [29]. The present study was aimed at searching for a potential correlation between the SNPs of the *CLOCK*, *ARNTL*, and *PER2* genes in patients with myocardial infarction. It was carried out as a case-referent study, comparing participants with myocardial infarction versus the participants without myocardial infarction.

2. Experimental Section

2.1. Participants

The data presented here were collected as part of previously reported studies on circadian rhythm variations in patients with myocardial infarction [25,29,30]. The sample included 431 patients (243 males, 188 females) of Croatian origin with non-fatal acute myocardial infarction at the Clinical Department of Cardiovascular Diseases and Intensive Care at the University Hospital Osijek, from August 2012 to December 2018. Inclusion criteria for type 1 and 2 MI patients, according to Thygesen et al., were elevated cardiac troponin T above the 99th percentile and one of the following factors: symptoms of myocardial ischemia, electrocardiogram (ECG) changes, pathological Q waves, evidence of loss of viable myocardium, and coronary thrombus [31,32]. Patients were eliminated from the analysis if they did not satisfy these requirements. Patients were excluded if they had undergone percutaneous coronary intervention or a coronary artery bypass, because those are not clinical characteristics of acute MI. Patients with type 4 and 5 MI were excluded, and also patients with type 1 and 2 MI who underwent PCI (percutaneous coronary intervention). A total of 125 patients were eliminated from the study: 35 due to percutaneous coronary intervention, 42 due to coronary artery bypass, 37 refused to participate, and 11 withdrew from the study (Figure 1).

Participants (total of 626) whose medical records did not present a history of cardiovascular disease were included in the control no-MI group. Their general physician selected them in the outpatient clinic after a checkup. Patients with cardiovascular disease or MI were eliminated. Due to the complex inheritance of cardiovascular risk factors identified in monozygotic twins, the relatives of the patient were eliminated from the no-MI group [33].

Systematic data on their medical history were obtained from all participants. Data on age, smoking, hypertension, and diabetes mellitus were included in the questionnaire. The patient's medical record confirms all of the above information.

This study was authorized by the Ethics Committees of the University Hospital Osijek (No. 25-1:3160-3/2012) and the Faculty of Medicine Osijek (No. 2158-61-07-12-2). It was performed following the Declaration of Helsinki and its amendments. All participants signed informed consent.

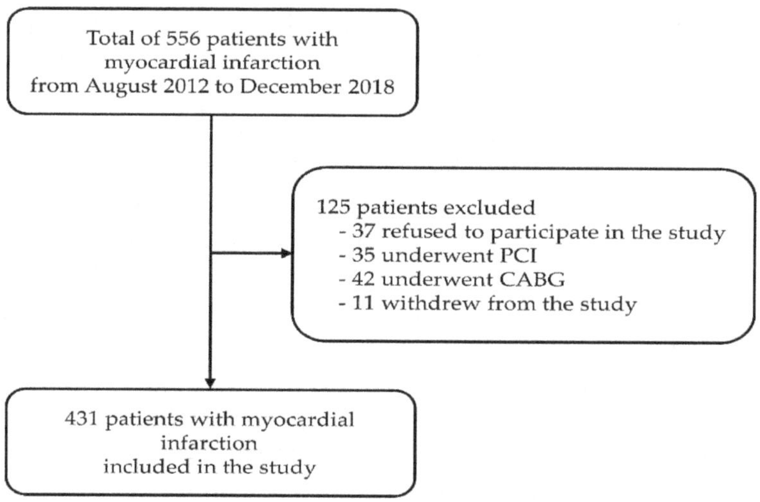

Figure 1. Patient selection flow chart. CABG—coronary artery bypass grafting, PCI—percutaneous coronary intervention.

2.2. SNP Selection and Genotyping

SNPs in three circadian rhythm genes, CLOCK, ARNTL, and PER2, were genotyped in this study. SNPs were selected on the basis of the familiar genetic linkage, consistent with HapMap Phase 3 (http://www.hapmap.org). The collection of the most specific polymorphisms for *CLOCK* (rs11932595, rs6811520, and rs13124436), *ARNTL* (rs3789327, rs4757144, and rs12363415), and *PER2* (rs35333999 and rs934945) genes were acquired using the Tagger algorithm accessible within the Haploview software (Haploview, version 4.2) [34]. Additionally, selected circadian rhythm gene SNPs had been associated with cardiovascular risk factors in previous studies [14,16,18].

The extraction of genomic DNA was made from lymphocytes using conventional methods (QIAamp DNA Blood Mini Kit, Qiagen, Hilden, Germany). Genotyping was performed using TaqMan SNP genotyping assays by the real-time PCR method, performed using a 7500 Real-Time PCR System (Applied Biosystems, Foster City, CA, USA). Details of the selected TaqMan probes are shown in Table 1. Allele discrimination analyses were carried out using SDS 7500 Software Version 2.3 (Applied Biosystems, Foster City, CA, USA).

Table 1. Selected TaqMan probe details.

Gene	SNP	SNP ID	Location	SNP Type
ARNTL	rs3789327	C_2160503_20	Chromosome 11	intronic region
ARNTL	rs4757144	C_1870683_20	Chromosome 11	intronic region
ARNTL	rs12363415	C_31248677_10	Chromosome 11	intronic region
CLOCK	rs11932595	C_296556_10	Chromosome 4	intronic region
CLOCK	rs6811520	C_31137409_30	Chromosome 4	intronic region
CLOCK	rs13124436	C_11821304_10	Chromosome 4	intronic region
PER2	rs35333999	C_25992030_10	Chromosome 2	Coding (Iso/Val)
PER2	rs934945	C_8740718_20	Chromosome 2	Coding (Glu/Gly)

2.3. Statistical Analysis

All analyses were performed using SPSS software (version 22.0, SPSS Inc., Chicago, IL, USA) for Windows). Quantitative demographic and clinical variables are presented as mean and standard deviation, while categorical variables are presented as frequency and percentages. Chi-square tests (χ^2) on contingency tables were applied to analyze allele and genotype frequencies in both groups. By comparing the distribution of genotypes with those expected by the Hardy–Weinberg equilibrium, a further level of quality control of genotyping was accomplished applying the Chi-square goodness-of-fit test. Analyses were performed using SNPStats [35] and the SHEsis web tools [36]. The relationship between genotypes and cardiovascular risk factors were studied applying the Mann–Whitney U test. Logistic regression, for the likelihood of a patient having a manifestation of myocardial infarction, was applied to evaluate the outcome of *CLOCK* (rs11932595, rs6811520, rs13124436), *ARNTL* (rs3789327, rs4757144, rs12363415), and *PER2* (rs35333999 and rs934945) genotypes. Age, hypertension history, diastolic and systolic blood pressure, and BMI were applied as covariates. The Kruskal–Wallis test was applied to establish the association within genotypes and risk factors. When the p-value was equal to or less than 0.05, the associations were marked significant. Appling the Benjamini–Hochberg (false detection rate—FDR value) correction method, significant value corrections were made due to the many SNPs studied. Q-values less than 0.05 were deemed significant. Pairwise linkage disequilibrium (LD) and haplotypes were calculated applying the SHEsis web tool [37] and Haploview (version 4.2) because the participants in the present study were not related.

3. Results

Table 2 shows the prevalence of cardiovascular risk factors in the 1057 study participants. In the present study, the mean age of all participants was 64 ± 10 years, and 53.4% were males. Table 3 presents allele frequencies, while Table 4 shows the genotype distribution of the *CLOCK*, *ARNTL*, and *PER2* SNPs. In the patients' group, the *ARNTL* gene SNPs rs3789327 and rs12363415, and rs6811520 and rs13124436 of the *CLOCK* gene deviated from the Hardy–Weinberg equilibrium.

Table 2. Prevalence of cardiovascular risk factors of myocardial infarction (MI) and no-MI participants.

	MI	no-MI	p-Value *
Number	431	626	
Male sex (%)	243 (56.4%)	321 (51.3%)	0.102
Age (years)	66 ±11	62 ± 10	**<0.001**
History of hypertension (%)	351 (73.1%)	408 (65.2%)	**0.007**
Smokers (%)	119 (27.6%)	193 (30.8%)	**<0.001**
History of type 2 diabetes mellitus (%)	275 (63.8%)	426 (68.1%)	0.151
Diastolic blood pressure (mm Hg)	79.12 ± 11.39	83.46 ± 11.13	**<0.001**
Systolic blood pressure (mm Hg)	140.04 ± 22.20	142.3 ± 21.42	0.085
BMI (kg/m^2)	29.78 ± 4.46	29.37 ± 4.59	0.198

BMI, body mass index. *Mann–Whitney U test p-value.

Table 3. Allele frequencies of the *ARNTL, CLOCK,* and *PER2* polymorphisms (N = 1057).

Gene	SNP	Minor Allele	MAF MI	MAF no-MI	*p*-Value	*q*-Value
ARNTL	rs3789327 *	G	0.425	0.518	**2.27×10^{-5}**	**6.05×10^{-5}**
	rs4757144	G	0.420	0.442	0.324	0.432
	rs12363415 *	A	0.413	0.338	**4.37×10^{-4}**	**8.74×10^{-4}**
CLOCK	rs11932595	G	0.428	0.437	0.685	0.782
	rs6811520 *	C	0.444	0.620	**7.11×10^{-15}**	**5.68×10^{-14}**
	rs13124436 *	A	0.200	0.301	**1.72×10^{-7}**	**6.88×10^{-7}**
PER2	rs35333999	T	0.038	0.055	0.077	0.123
	rs934945	T	0.172	0.174	0.885	0.885

MAF, minor allele frequency; *q*-value, corrected significant *p*-value by the Benjamini–Hochberg method. * Deviation from the Hardy–Weinberg equilibrium in the MI group.

Table 4. Genotype distribution and frequencies of the *ARNTL, CLOCK,* and *PER2* polymorphisms.

Gene	SNP	Genotype	Genotype Frequency, N (%)				
			MI	no-MI	*p*-value	χ^2	*q*-Value
ARNTL	rs3789327 *	AA	161 (37.4%)	164 (26.3%)	**2.7×10^{-4}**	16.46	**7.2×10^{-4}**
		AG	174 (40.4%)	237 (43.8%)			
		GG	96 (22.3%)	187 (30%)			
	rs4757144	AA	153 (35.5%)	199 (31.8%)	0.456	1.57	0.608
		AG	194 (45%)	300 (48%)			
		GG	84 (19.5%)	126 (20.2%)			
	rs12363415 *	AA	142 (32.9%)	151 (24.1%)	**0.007**	9.95	**0.014**
		AG	72 (16.7%)	121 (19.3%)			
		GG	217 (50.3%)	354 (56.5%)			
CLOCK	rs11932595	AA	142 (33%)	191 (30.6%)	0.589	1.06	0.673
		AG	208 (48.4%)	322 (51.5%)			
		GG	80 (18.6%)	112 (17.9%)			
	rs6811520 *	CC	123 (28.5%)	255 (40.8%)	**3.44×10^{-15}**	69.33	**2.75×10^{-14}**
		CT	137 (31.8%)	265 (42.4%)			
		TT	171 (39.7%)	105 (16.8%)			
	rs13124436 *	AA	39 (9%)	123 (19.6%)	**1.26×10^{-5}**	22.61	**5.04×10^{-5}**
		AG	94 (21.8%)	131 (20.9%)			
		GG	298 (69.1%)	372 (59.4%)			
PER2	rs35333999	CC	399 (92.8%)	560 (89.6%)	0.208	3.14	0.333
		CT	29 (6.7%)	61 (9.8%)			
		TT	2 (0.5%)	4 (0.6%)			
	rs934945	CC	296 (68.7%)	427 (68.2%)	0.986	0.03	0.986
		CT	122 (28.3%)	180 (28.8%)			
		TT	13 (3%)	19 (3%)			

χ^2, Chi-square; *q*-value, corrected significant *p* value by the Benjamini–Hochberg method. * Deviation from the Hardy–Weinberg equilibrium in the MI group.

Logistic regression was adjusted to evaluate the independent impact of the chosen polymorphism after modification for cardiovascular risk factors. All tested SNPs showed a significant interaction between age, diastolic blood pressure, and the risk of myocardial infarction ($p < 0.001$) (Table 5). Under the dominant genotype model, a considerable difference was for the rs3789327 and rs12363415 SNPs in the *ARNTL* gene (AA + AG versus GG, $p = 0.003$, OR = 1.52 with 95% CI = 1.12–1.95, and AA + AG versus GG, $p < 0.001$, OR = 3.14 with 95% CI = 2.13–4.62, respectively). Under the recessive genotype model notable difference was for the rs6811520 and rs13124436 SNPs in the *CLOCK* gene (CC versus CT + TT, $p < 0.001$, OR = 0.35 with 95% CI = 0.26–0.47, and GG versus AG + AA, $p = 0.006$, OR = 1.76 with 95% CI = 1.17–2.65, respectively). The significant difference was detected under the dominant genotype model for the *PER2* gene polymorphism rs35333999 (TT + CT versus CC, $p = 0.005$, OR = 1.93 with 95% CI = 1.19-3.11).

Table 5. Odds ratios for myocardial infarction adjusted for cardiovascular risk factors included in the logistic regression model.

Risk Factor	OR (95% CI)	*p*-Value
Age	0.96 (0.95–0.97)	**<0.001**
History of hypertension	1.23 (0.91–1.68)	0.182
Diastolic blood pressure	1.36 (1.02–1.05)	**<0.001**
Systolic blood pressure	1.01 (0.99–1.01)	0.217
BMI	0.98 (0.95–1.07)	0.114

OR, odds ratio; CI, confidence interval.

The association between circadian rhythm gene polymorphisms and cardiovascular risk factors in patients with MI is shown in Table 6.

Table 6. The association between cardiovascular risk factors and circadian rhythm gene polymorphisms in patients with MI.

Gene	Sex	Age	History of Hypertension	Smoking	History of T2DM	Diastolic Blood Pressure	Systolic Blood Pressure	BMI
ARNTL								
rs3789327	**0.045**	0.953	0.247	0.133	**0.006**	0.309	0.113	0.561
rs4757144	0.844	0.818	0.319	0.273	0.537	0.129	0.121	0.777
rs12363415	0.071	0.872	**<0.001**	0.168	**<0.001**	**0.005**	**<0.001**	**<0.001**
CLOCK								
rs11932595	0.177	0.487	0.263	0.319	0.118	0.266	**0.029**	0.229
rs6811520	**<0.001**	0.641	**<0.001**	0.950	**<0.001**	0.820	**<0.001**	0.200
rs13124436	**0.003**	0.665	**<0.001**	0.309	**<0.001**	0.402	**<0.001**	0.028
PER2								
rs35333999	0.956	**0.002**	0.720	0.422	0.102	0.521	0.934	0.772
rs934945	0.156	0.104	0.085	**0.048**	0.518	0.734	0.589	0.302

Kruskal–Wallis test *p*-values. T2DM, type 2 diabetes mellitus; BMI, body mass index.

The completed haplotypes were analyzed in the three circadian rhythm genes. The frequencies of the predicted haplotypes of the tested circadian rhythm gene genetic variants in MI and no-MI participants are presented in Table S1.

There was no linkage disequilibrium (LD) between SNPs in the *ARNTL* gene. The LD between rs3789327 and rs4757144 was D′ = 0.039, $R^2 = 0.001$, between rs3789327 and rs12363415 D′ = 0.216, $R^2 = 0.025$, and between rs4757144 and rs12363415 D′ = 0.109, $R^2 = 0.005$. The LD for the *CLOCK* gene polymorphisms was as follows: the LD between rs1192595 and rs6811520 was D′ = 0.414, $R^2 = 0.108$, between rs1192595 and rs13124436 D′ = 0.062, $R^2 = 0.001$, and between rs6811520 and rs13124436 D′ = 0.596, $R^2 = 0.103$. The LD calculated for polymorphisms in the *PER2* gene (rs35333999 and rs934945) was D′ = 0.986, $R^2 = 0.010$ (Figure S1).

4. Discussion

In the present study, given the findings of the investigated SNPs of the *CLOCK*, *ARNTL*, and *PER2* genes, it was noted that polymorphisms in those clock genes might be an extra risk factor for myocardial infarction. An association between MI and polymorphisms of the *CLOCK* (rs6811520 and rs13124436) and *ARNTL* (rs37389327 and rs12363415) genes were found in a sample of 1057 participants in this case-referent study. *ARNTL*, rs3789327, was connected with T2DM in MI patients, while rs13124436 and rs6811520 of the *CLOCK* gene were connected with hypertension, T2DM, and systolic blood pressure in MI patients. In the present study, patients with MI had substantially reduced diastolic blood pressure as opposed to the no-MI group.

The circadian rhythm is a network that enables a person to manage environmental variations and adjust to them. Accordingly, the circadian rhythm controls a range of physiological and metabolic activities, and any obstruction of that rhythm may impact a person's health. The role of circadian rhythm in MI has been investigated in several studies. Cardiomyocyte circadian gene expression regulates the myocardial contractile purpose, metabolism, and gene expression [38]. The fundamental idea is that acute cardiovascular events do not happen randomly throughout the day but are accelerated partially by circadian controlled factors [39]. An increasing amount of experimental and clinical evidence shows an essential connection between cardiac dysfunction and intrinsic circadian biology. Virtually all tissues of the body have a circadian clock that regulates the timing of many critical biological reactions in response to a diversity of environmental signals. The molecular machinery for the regulation of circadian rhythms is very conserved and found in virtually every cell type [40].

Human research has recognized polymorphisms and transcription motifs of circadian rhythm genes, such as *CRY2, CLOCK, ARNTL, PER2,* or *NPAS2,* which are linked with hypertension, metabolic syndrome, or T2DM [30,41]. Circadian rhythm genes play a significant part in homeostatic equilibrium. They adjust the fibrinolytic system, and the *CRY* and *CLOCK* genes are precisely engaged in this action and, accordingly, raise the CVD risk. The purpose of the circadian clock in cardiovascular activity has been strongly emphasized in many studies. However, this research showed an association of MI with some circadian clock polymorphisms. This is relevant because approximately 43% of all protein-coding genes have circadian transcription in an organ-specific way [40].

Circadian rhythm genes play a crucial role in many physiological activities. The *ARNTL* gene is an integral part of lipid metabolism due to its influences on the transcription of genes included in lipogenesis in adipocytes in a circadian fashion, as shown in animal models [24]. In humans, *CLOCK* gene SNPs are connected to body weight, metabolic syndrome risk, and insomnia [24,42], while *PER2* and *PER3* gene SNPs are linked to sleep disturbances [43]. Different polymorphisms of circadian clock genes are connected with various cardiovascular disease risk factors [44]. Thus, metabolic syndrome, T2DM, and stroke are associated with *CLOCK* gene variants [29,45,46], while myocardial infarction is associated with *CRY2* and *PER2* gene variations [29]. Metabolic syndrome in humans is associated with the transcription of *CRY1* and *PER2* in adipose tissue [41,47]. Patients with diabetes have more severe atherosclerotic changes in their blood vessels [48] and have a two to three times higher risk of developing cardiovascular disease than healthy subjects [46]. Lifestyle and metabolic disorders are directly related, as indicated by biological and epidemiological studies [49], although the biochemical and genetic connection of the circadian clock with metabolic disorders has not been investigated in detail. Therefore, the significance of the circadian rhythm in the preservation of "energetic" equilibrium and metabolism is obvious.

Tsai et al. showed the significance of the circadian clock in cardiomyocytes in mice with mutated clock genes. They pointed out that the circadian rhythm is a primary controller of cardiac triglyceride metabolism [50], whereas *ARNTL* gene deletion in adipocyte causes obesity [51]. Polymorphisms of the *BMAL1* gene, which is the mouse equivalent of the human *ARNTL* gene, are connected with hypertension and T2DM [52,53], just as in this study where we found an association of rs3789327 and rs12363415 with T2DM in MI patients. All these data confirm the responsibility of *ARNTL* polymorphisms in the metabolic disorders in humans. The *ARNTL* gene SNPs are associated with hypertension, diabetes mellitus, and metabolic syndrome. All these conditions increase the risk of MI [54]. *BMAL1* was shown to be responsible for the daily variations in blood pressure [40], and here, we found an association of rs12363415 with diastolic and systolic blood pressure. Physiological rhythms of heart rate and blood pressure are lost in *Bmal1* knockout mice [55], and such mice developed dilated cardiomyopathy [56]. *BMAL1* knockout mice had depressed cardiovascular circadian rhythms and developed age-dependent dilated cardiomyopathy. The knockout of *BMAL1* or deletion of all three isoforms of *Cry* in mice contributed to arterial stiffness and the impairment of extracellular matrix composition [40].

Genetic variations in the *CLOCK* gene are connected with T2DM and cardiovascular disorders in humans [29,30,41,53,57]. Here, an association of rs6811520 and rs13124436 with T2DM was found in MI patients. Studies using *CLOCK* mutant mice show the crucial function of the *CLOCK* in myocardial contractility, basal metabolism, and daily pulse rate control [41]. Mutation of the *Clock* gene in mouse cardiomyocytes only disrupts circadian rhythm in cardiomyocytes. This *Clock* mutation leads to physiological changes in cardiomyocytes. Some of these are heart rate, cardiac metabolism, response to external signals, contractility, and cardiac growth and regeneration [38]. CLOCK is a transcription factor and one of the primary regulators of the transcription of the circadian clock gene. It is also the regulator of expression of the various transcription factors required for control of the diverse physiological and behavioral processes that occur in a circadian fashion [58]. In this study, rs11932595 SNP of the *CLOCK* gene was connected with systolic blood pressure in MI patients. CLOCK, thrombomodulin, and plasminogen activator-1 inhibitor are required for the endothelial homeostasis. The circadian rhythm regulates genes in vascular endothelial cells [41], and disorder of clock could cause atherosclerosis and MI. Specific *CLOCK* gene polymorphisms are linked to excess weight [59,60], metabolic syndrome, and CVD [61]. A mutation in *CLOCK* leads to the development of age-dependent cardiomyopathy in male mice [40].

PER2 polymorphisms could be connected with myocardial infarction [29]. In this study, the *PER2* genetic variant rs35333999 is connected with age in MI patients. PER2 in the heart plays a crucial part in myocardial ischemia and fatty acid metabolism [62]. In contrast, mutations in the *PER2* gene are connected with a shortened circadian period during constant darkness [63]. In the mouse heart, PER2 has a protective function during myocardial ischemia [62,64]. It is included in the control of fatty acid metabolism with raised utilization of oxygen. In the hearts of mice with clock gene mutations, lipolysis is considerably reduced, which can accelerate the development of metabolic disorders, such as atherosclerosis, which could result in MI [50]. *PER2* knockout mice had more extensive infarct sizes, and the *PER2* in the heart exhibits an essential function during inflammation in myocardial ischemia and reperfusion [64]. The reduction of glycogen storage leads to enlarged infarct areas in mice with *PER2* mutation as a result of lowered glycolysis during myocardial ischemia. Suarez-Barrientos et al. observed that the infarct area was more extensive early in the morning [61], which is similar to the conclusion of Eckle et al. that PER2 stabilization dependent on light had a cardioprotective function in ischemia [65]. The deletion of the *Per2* gene in mice reduces the severity of MI because it limits inflammatory processes, reduces apoptosis, and promotes cardiomyocyte hypertrophy. Therefore, *Per2* gene disruption has a protective function in MI [66]. Activation of PER2 at the time of ischemia controls the beta-oxidation of fatty acids and inflammatory processes. Inflammation and metabolism are related, and inflammation might be an outcome of a disturbed metabolism [61]. Patients with raised inflammatory markers and metabolic syndrome have a higher chance of developing CVD. Disturbance of the circadian rhythm is involved in the development of a CVD, and hypertension is an essential element [30,53]. Furthermore, a mutation in the *PER2* gene was connected with aortic endothelial dysfunction, it reduces the production of nitric oxide, and other vasodilatory prostaglandins [40]. Per1 was also found to control the expression of many genes linked to sodium transport in the kidneys [40].

Genetic factors may explain, at least in part, some susceptibility to MI in individuals exposed to chronic or even short-term disorders. Thus, shift work is associated with a small but significant increase in the risk of developing CVD, which means that sleep disorders make an essential contribution to the risk of developing CVD [67]. Shift work and physical inactivity are associated with CVD risk factors such as increased triglyceride levels, which can lead to increased risk for MI [68]. A family history of CVD is another risk factor for developing CVD, especially premature CVD, and sudden cardiac death. In addition to genetic factors, a lifestyle passed on from generation to generation has a significant impact on the development of CVD. The increased genetic predisposition for MI, along with inherited life patterns of physical inactivity, may explain to some extent the increase in the incidence of MI [69]. Studies have shown an association between daylight saving time and the incidence of myocardial infarction. A particularly significant increase in the incidence of MI was observed in the first week after the spring shift [21]. The shift to daylight saving time causes circadian rhythm disturbance and sleep disruption, thereby increasing the risk of MI. Therefore, the abolition of daylight saving time is considered to be good for human health and might reduce the risk of CVD [70].

Cardiovascular disease and metabolic disorders are associated with circadian rhythm disturbances in humans [71]. It is crucial to know the ethnic structure of the investigated population since the frequency of circadian rhythm gene polymorphisms differs significantly between different populations [72]. This study investigated the relationship between myocardial infarction patients and various circadian clock genes polymorphisms. The present study examined the prevalence of genetic variants and several genotype models within two groups, patients with myocardial infarction and no-MI participants. Specific genetic variants of circadian rhythm genes might affect the ability of individuals to adapt their circadian rhythm to changing environmental conditions. The results of the present study are compatible with new presumptions, where circadian rhythm aberrations play an essential part in the onset of MI.

A possible explanation for the lack of correlation of all the studied polymorphisms of the circadian rhythm genes with MI is that individual SNPs have a minor input in the onset of MI. Only when certain combinations of specific SNPs are considered together, a significant association might be obtained. It is significant because the circadian rhythm genes are closely connected in a complex clock mechanism. As MI is a complex trait, the humble contributions of numerous genes affect the phenotypic presentation.

Limitations of the Study

The sample size is a limitation of this research. A more significant association between phenotype and genotype might be obtained with more patients involved. The number of participants was limited and might produce a false-positive result. The inadequate statistical capability to distinguish positive relationships is a result of the small frequency of some genotypes, as well as the excessive ORs and an extensive range of 95% CI. There is a chance of developing some of the CVDs in the no-MI group. A limitation of the study might be the age discrepancy between the MI patients and the no-MI group. However, a significant association only exists for age and one SNP in the *PER2* gene, rs35333999, in MI patients. Moreover, it is plausible that the *CLOCK*, *ARNTL*, and *PER2* gene SNPs studied are not usefully associated with MI. In the present case, useful polymorphisms or a collection of usefully relevant SNPs that could be better related to MI should be identified. This strategy of approaching the MI problem produces the chance to proceed with the investigation in multicenter studies with more participants. An advantage of the sample in this research is that it was nearly homogeneous in demographic variables such as sex, ethnicity, and cultural background.

5. Conclusions

The physiological activities of the individual are coordinated daily by the circadian rhythm. The circadian rhythm plays a significant part in numerous features of normal cardiovascular homeostasis and disease pathogenesis and pathophysiology. Circadian clock gene SNPs might be valuable in assessing the risk, prediction, or evaluating the feedback to therapy of CVD patients. Data are presented here indicating that the *ARNTL* and *CLOCK* gene polymorphisms could be associated with MI and therefore suggest the involvement of the circadian clock in the development of MI. These findings might increase knowledge of the physiopathological processes implicated in MI, and need replication in different individuals with MI. Additional confirmation and systematic study of the circadian rhythm in MI are achievable. In this age of personalized medicine, understanding of the genetic background of the circadian rhythm of a person could be essential for therapy and should be incorporated into diagnostic procedures.

Author Contributions: I.Š. and J.M. performed experiments, analyzed data, and managed the specimens. I.Š. and R.S. were responsible for the design, collection, and quality control of the human specimen. R.S. supervised the study. I.Š. wrote the manuscript. All authors have read and agreed to the published version of the manuscript.

Acknowledgments: The authors acknowledge the contribution of the medical staff who helped with this study.

References

1. World Health Organization. *Noncommunicable Diseases Progress Monitor, 2017*; WHO: Geneva, Switzerland, 2017.
2. Kralj, V.; Brkić Biloš, I. Cardiovascular diseases – mortality and morbidity trends in Croatia, Europe and worldwide. *Cardiol. Croat.* **2016**, *11*, 504. [CrossRef]
3. World Health Organization. *Noncommunicable Diseases Country Profiles 2018*; WHO: Geneva, Switzerland, 2018.
4. Stevanovic, R.; Capak, K.; Brkic, K. *Croatian Health Statistics Yearbook 2016*; Croatian Institute of Public Health: Zagreb, Croatia, 2017.
5. Thygesen, K.; Alpert, J.S.; White, H.D. Universal definition of myocardial infarction. *Eur. Heart J.* **2007**, *28*, 2525–2538. [CrossRef]
6. Škrlec, I. Circadian rhythm and myocardial infarction. *Med. Flum.* **2019**, *55*, 32–42. [CrossRef]
7. Škrlec, I.; Marić, S.; Včev, A. Myocardial infarction and circadian rhythm. In *Visions Cardiomyocyte-Fundamental Concepts of Heart and Life Disease*; Tsipis, A., Ed.; IntechOpen: London, UK, 2019; pp. 60–75. [CrossRef]
8. Partch, C.L.; Green, C.B.; Takahashi, J.S. Molecular architecture of the mammalian circadian clock. *Trends Cell Biol.* **2014**, *24*, 90–99. [CrossRef]
9. Touitou, Y.; Bogdan, A. Circadian and seasonal variations of physiological and biochemical determinants of acute myocardial infarction. *Biol. Rhythm Res.* **2007**, *38*, 169–179. [CrossRef]
10. Muller, J.E.; Stone, P.H.; Turi, Z.G.; Rutherford, J.D.; Czeisler, C.A.; Parker, C.; Poole, W.K.; Passamani, E.; Roberts, R.; Robertson, T.; et al. Circadian variation in the frequency of onset of acute myocardial infarction. *N. Engl. J. Med.* **1985**, *313*, 1315–1322. [CrossRef]
11. Mehta, R.H.; Manfredini, R.; Hassan, F.; Sechtem, U.; Bossone, E.; Oh, J.K.; Cooper, J.V.; Smith, D.E.; Portaluppi, F.; Penn, M.; et al. Chronobiological patterns of acute aortic dissection. *Circulation* **2002**, *106*, 1110–1115. [CrossRef]
12. Elliott, W.J. Circadian variation in the timing of stroke onset: A meta-analysis. *Stroke* **1998**, *29*, 992–996. [CrossRef]
13. Manfredini, R.; Boari, B.; Smolensky, M.H.; Salmi, R.; Gallerani, M.; Guerzoni, F.; Guerra, V.; Malagoni, A.M.; Manfredini, F. Seasonal variation in onset of myocardial infarction—A 7-year single-center study in Italy. *Chronobiol. Int.* **2005**, *22*, 1121–1135. [CrossRef]
14. Garaulet, M.; Madrid, J.A. Chronobiology, genetics and metabolic syndrome. *Curr. Opin. Lipidol.* **2009**, *20*, 127–134. [CrossRef]
15. Virag, J.A.I.; Lust, R.M. Circadian influences on myocardial infarction. *Front. Physiol.* **2014**, *5*, 422. [CrossRef]
16. Leu, H.B.; Chung, C.M.; Lin, S.J.; Chiang, K.M.; Yang, H.C.; Ho, H.Y.; Ting, C.T.; Lin, T.H.; Sheu, S.H.; Tsai, W.C.; et al. Association of circadian genes with diurnal blood pressure changes and non-dipper essential hypertension: A genetic association with young-onset hypertension. *Hypertens. Res.* **2015**, *38*, 155–162. [CrossRef]
17. Kelly, M.A.; Rees, S.D.; Hydrie, M.Z.I.; Shera, A.S.; Bellary, S.; O'Hare, J.P.; Kumar, S.; Taheri, S.; Basit, A.; Barnett, A.H.; et al. Circadian gene variants and susceptibility to type 2 diabetes: A pilot study. *PLoS ONE* **2012**, *7*, e32670. [CrossRef]
18. Englund, A.; Kovanen, L.; Saarikoski, S.T.; Haukka, J.; Reunanen, A.; Aromaa, A.; Lönnqvist, J.; Partonen, T. NPAS2 and PER2 are linked to risk factors of the metabolic syndrome. *J. Circadian Rhythm.* **2009**, *7*, 5. [CrossRef]
19. Suzuki, S.; Ishii, H.; Ichimiya, S.; Kanashiro, M.; Watanabe, J.; Uchida, Y.; Yoshikawa, D.; Maeda, K.; Matsubara, T.; Murohara, T. Impact of the circadian rhythm on microvascular function in patients with ST-elevation myocardial infarction. *Int. J. Cardiol.* **2013**, *168*, 4948–4949. [CrossRef]

20. Poggiogalle, E.; Jamshed, H.; Peterson, C.M. Circadian regulation of glucose, lipid, and energy metabolism in humans. *Metabolism* **2018**, *84*, 11–27. [CrossRef]
21. Manfredini, R.; Fabbian, F.; Cappadona, R.; Modesti, P.A. Daylight saving time, circadian rhythms, and cardiovascular health. *Intern. Emerg. Med.* **2018**, *13*, 641–646. [CrossRef]
22. Martino, T.A.; Young, M.E. Influence of the cardiomyocyte circadian clock on cardiac physiology and pathophysiology. *J. Biol. Rhythm.* **2015**, *30*, 183–205. [CrossRef]
23. Durgan, D.J.; Young, M.E. The cardiomyocyte circadian clock: Emerging roles in health and disease. *Circ. Res.* **2010**, *106*, 647–658. [CrossRef]
24. Gómez-Abellán, P.; Madrid, J.A.; Ordovás, J.M.; Garaulet, M. Chronobiological aspects of obesity and metabolic syndrome. *Endocrinol. Nutr.* **2012**, *59*, 50–61. [CrossRef]
25. Škrlec, I.; Milić, J.; Heffer, M.; Steiner, R.; Peterlin, B.; Wagner, J. Association of Circadian Rhythm with Myocardial Infarction. *Acta Clin. Croat.* **2018**, *57*, 480–485. [CrossRef] [PubMed]
26. Erdmann, J.; Linsel-Nitschke, P.; Schunkert, H. Genetic causes of myocardial infarction: New insights from genome-wide association studies. *Dtsch. Arztebl. Int.* **2010**, *107*, 694–699. [CrossRef] [PubMed]
27. Takeda, N.; Maemura, K. Circadian clock and the onset of cardiovascular events. *Hypertens. Res.* **2016**, *39*, 383–390. [CrossRef] [PubMed]
28. Kelleher, F.C.; Rao, A.; Maguire, A. Circadian molecular clocks and cancer. *Cancer Lett.* **2014**, *342*, 9–18. [CrossRef] [PubMed]
29. Škrlec, I.; Milić, J.; Heffer, M.; Peterlin, B.; Wagner, J. Genetic variations in circadian rhythm genes and susceptibility for myocardial infarction. *Genet. Mol. Biol.* **2018**, *41*, 403–409. [CrossRef]
30. Škrlec, I.; Milić, J.; Heffer, M.; Wagner, J.; Peterlin, B. Circadian clock genes and circadian phenotypes in patients with myocardial infarction. *Adv. Med. Sci.* **2019**, *64*, 224–229. [CrossRef]
31. Thygesen, K.; Alpert, J.S.; Jaffe, A.S.; Simoons, M.L.; Chaitman, B.R.; White, H.D. Third universal definition of myocardial infarction. *Nat. Rev. Cardiol.* **2012**, *9*, 620–633. [CrossRef]
32. Thygesen, K.; Alpert, J.S.; Jaffe, A.S.; Chaitman, B.R.; Bax, J.J.; Morrow, D.A.; White, H.D.; Mickley, H.; Crea, F.; Van de Werf, F.; et al. Fourth universal definition of myocardial infarction (2018). *Eur. Heart J.* **2019**, *40*, 237–269. [CrossRef]
33. Elder, S.J.; Lichtenstein, A.H.; Pittas, A.G.; Roberts, S.B.; Fuss, P.J.; Greenberg, A.S.; McCrory, MA.; Bouchard, T.J., Jr.; Saltzman, E.; Neale, M.C. Genetic and environmental influences on factors associated with cardiovascular disease and the metabolic syndrome. *J. Lipid Res.* **2009**, *50*, 1917–1926. [CrossRef]
34. de Bakker, P.I.W.; Yelensky, R.; Pe'er, I.; Gabriel, S.B.; Daly, M.J.; Altshuler, D. Efficiency and power in genetic association studies. *Nat. Genet.* **2005**, *37*, 1217–1223. [CrossRef]
35. Solé, X.; Guinó, E.; Valls, J.; Iniesta, R.; Moreno, V. SNPStats: A web tool for the analysis of association studies. *Bioinformatics* **2006**, *22*, 1928–1929. [CrossRef] [PubMed]
36. Shi, Y.Y.; He, L. SHEsis, a powerful software platform for analyses of linkage disequilibrium, haplotype construction, and genetic association at polymorphism loci. *Cell Res.* **2005**, *15*, 97–98. [CrossRef]
37. Li, Z.; Zhang, Z.; He, Z.; Tang, W.; Li, T.; Zeng, Z.; He, L.; Shi, Y.Y. A partition-ligation-combination-subdivision EM algorithm for haplotype inference with multiallelic markers: Update of the SHEsis (http://analysis.bio-x.cn). *Cell Res.* **2009**, *19*, 519–523. [CrossRef] [PubMed]
38. Bray, M.S.; Shaw, C.A.; Moore, M.W.S.; Garcia, R.A.P.; Zanquetta, M.M.; Durgan, D.J.; Jeong, W.J.; Tsai, Ju.; Bugger, H.; Zhang, D.; et al. Disruption of the circadian clock within the cardiomyocyte influences myocardial contractile function, metabolism, and gene expression. *Am. J. Physiol. Heart Circ. Physiol.* **2008**, *294*, H1036–H1047. [CrossRef] [PubMed]
39. Khaper, N.; Bailey, C.D.C.; Ghugre, N.R.; Reitz, C.; Awosanmi, Z.; Waines, R.; Martino, T.A. Implications of disturbances in circadian rhythms for cardiovascular health: A new frontier in free radical biology. *Free Radic. Biol. Med.* **2017**, *119*, 85–92. [CrossRef] [PubMed]
40. Rabinovich-Nikitin, I.; Lieberman, B.; Martino, T.A.; Kirshenbaum, L.A. Circadian-Regulated Cell Death in Cardiovascular Diseases. *Circulation* **2019**, *139*, 965–980. [CrossRef] [PubMed]
41. Scott, E.M. Circadian clocks, obesity and cardiometabolic function. *Diabetes Obes. Metab.* **2015**, *17*, 84–89. [CrossRef]
42. Huang, W.; Ramsey, K.M.; Marcheva, B.; Bass, J. Circadian rhythms, sleep, and metabolism. *J. Clin. Investig.* **2011**, *121*, 2133–2141. [CrossRef]

43. Pedrazzoli, M.; Secolin, R.; Esteves, L.O.B.; Pereira, D.S.; Koike, B.D.V.; Louzada, F.M.; Lopes-Cendes, I.; Tufik, S. Interactions of polymorphisms in different clock genes associated with circadian phenotypes in humans. *Genet. Mol. Biol.* **2010**, *33*, 627–632. [CrossRef]
44. Dashti, H.S.; Smith, C.E.; Lee, Y.C.; Parnell, L.D.; Lai, C.Q.; Arnett, D.K.; Ordovás, JM.; Garaulet, M. CRY1 circadian gene variant interacts with carbohydrate intake for insulin resistance in two independent populations: Mediterranean and North American. *Chronobiol. Int.* **2014**, *31*, 660–667. [CrossRef]
45. Prasai, M.J.; George, J.T.; Scott, E.M. Molecular clocks, type 2 diabetes and cardiovascular disease. *Diabetes Vasc. Dis. Res.* **2008**, *5*, 89–95. [CrossRef]
46. Martín-Timón, I.; Sevillano-Collantes, C.; Segura-Galindo, A.; Del Cañizo-Gómez, F.J. Type 2 diabetes and cardiovascular disease: Have all risk factors the same strength? *World J. Diabetes* **2014**, *5*, 444–470. [CrossRef]
47. Gómez-Abellán, P.; Hernández-Morante, J.J.; Luján, J.A.; Madrid, J.A.; Garaulet, M. Clock genes are implicated in the human metabolic syndrome. *Int. J. Obes.* **2008**, *32*, 121–128. [CrossRef]
48. Paneni, F.; Beckman, J.A.; Creager, M.A.; Cosentino, F. Diabetes and vascular disease: Pathophysiology, clinical consequences, and medical therapy: Part I. *Eur. Heart J.* **2013**, *34*, 2436–2443. [CrossRef]
49. Dibner, C.; Schibler, U. Circadian timing of metabolism in animal models and humans. *J. Intern. Med.* **2015**, *277*, 513–527. [CrossRef]
50. Tsai, J.Y.; Kienesberger, P.C.; Pulinilkunnil, T.; Sailors, M.H.; Durgan, D.J.; Villegas-Montoya, C.; Jahoor, A.; Gonzalez, R.; Garvey, M.E.; Boland, B.; et al. Direct Regulation of Myocardial Triglyceride Metabolism by the Cardiomyocyte Circadian Clock. *J. Biol. Chem.* **2010**, *285*, 2918–2929. [CrossRef]
51. Paschos, G.K.; Ibrahim, S.; Song, W.L.; Kunieda, T.; Grant, G.; Reyes, T.M.; Bradfield, C.A.; Vaughan, C.H.; Eiden, M.; Masoodi, M.; et al. Obesity in mice with adipocyte-specific deletion of clock component Arntl. *Nat. Med.* **2012**, *18*, 1768–1777. [CrossRef]
52. Woon, P.Y.; Kaisaki, P.J.; Bragança, J.; Bihoreau, M.; Levy, J.C.; Farrall, M.; Gauguier, D. Aryl hydrocarbon receptor nuclear translocator-like (BMAL1) is associated with susceptibility to hypertension and type 2 diabetes. *Proc. Natl. Acad. Sci. USA* **2007**, *104*, 14412–14417. [CrossRef]
53. Škrlec, I.; Milić, J.; Cilenšek, I.; Petrovič, D.; Wagner, J.; Peterlin, B. Circadian clock genes and myocardial infarction in patients with type 2 diabetes mellitus. *Gene* **2019**, *701*, 98–103. [CrossRef]
54. Crnko, S.; Du Pré, B.C.; Sluijter, J.P.G.; Van Laake, L.W. Circadian rhythms and the molecular clock in cardiovascular biology and disease. *Nat. Rev. Cardiol.* **2019**, *16*, 437–447. [CrossRef]
55. Curtis, A.M.; Cheng, Y.; Kapoor, S.; Reilly, D.; Price, T.S.; Fitzgerald, G.A. Circadian variation of blood pressure and the vascular response to asynchronous stress. *Proc. Natl. Acad. Sci. USA* **2007**, *104*, 3450–3455. [CrossRef]
56. Lefta, M.; Campbell, K.S.; Feng, H.Z.; Jin, J.P.; Esser, K.A. Development of dilated cardiomyopathy in Bmal1-deficient mice. *Am. J. Physiol.-Heart Circ. Physiol.* **2012**, *303*, H475–H485. [CrossRef]
57. Corella, D.; Asensio, E.M.; Coltell, O.; Sorlí, J.V.; Estruch, R.; Martínez-González, M.Á.; Salas-Salvadó, J.; Castañer, O.; Arós, F.; Lapetra, J.; et al. CLOCK gene variation is associated with incidence of type-2 diabetes and cardiovascular diseases in type-2 diabetic subjects: Dietary modulation in the PREDIMED randomized trial. *Cardiovasc. Diabetol.* **2016**, *15*, 4. [CrossRef]
58. Riestra, P.; Gebreab, S.Y.; Xu, R.; Khan, R.J.; Gaye, A.; Correa, A.; Min, N.; Sims, M.; Davis, S.K. Circadian CLOCK gene polymorphisms in relation to sleep patterns and obesity in African Americans: Findings from the Jackson heart study. *BMC Genet.* **2017**, *18*, 58. [CrossRef]
59. Bandín, C.; Martinez-Nicolas, A.; Ordovás, J.M.; Ros Lucas, J.A.; Castell, P.; Silvente, T.; Madrid, J.A.; Garaulet, M. Differences in circadian rhythmicity in CLOCK 3111T/C genetic variants in moderate obese women as assessed by thermometry, actimetry and body position. *Int. J. Obes.* **2013**, *37*, 1044–1050. [CrossRef]
60. Garcia-Rios, A.; Gomez-Delgado, F.J.; Garaulet, M.; Alcala-Diaz, J.F.; Delgado-Lista, F.J.; Marin, C.; Rangel-Zuniga, O.A.; Rodriguez-Cantalejo, F.; Gomez-Luna, P.; Ordovas, J.M.; et al. Beneficial effect of CLOCK gene polymorphism rs1801260 in combination with low-fat diet on insulin metabolism in the patients with metabolic syndrome. *Chronobiol. Int.* **2014**, *31*, 401–408. [CrossRef]
61. Suarez-Barrientos, A.; Lopez-Romero, P.; Vivas, D.; Castro-Ferreira, F.; Nunez-Gil, I.; Franco, E.; Ruiz-Mateos, B.; Garcia-Rubira, J.C.; Fernandez-Ortiz, A.; Macaya, C.; et al. Circadian variations of infarct size in acute myocardial infarction. *Heart* **2011**, *97*, 970–976. [CrossRef]

62. Bonney, S.; Kominsky, D.; Brodsky, K.; Eltzschig, H.; Walker, L.; Eckle, T. Cardiac Per2 functions as novel link between fatty acid metabolism and myocardial inflammation during ischemia and reperfusion injury of the heart. *PLoS ONE* **2013**, *8*, e71493. [CrossRef]
63. Vukolic, A.; Antic, V.; Van Vliet, B.N.; Yang, Z.; Albrecht, U.; Montani, J. Role of mutation of the circadian clock gene Per2 in cardiovascular circadian rhythms. *Am. J. Physiol.-Regul. Integr. Comp. Physiol.* **2010**, *298*, 627–634. [CrossRef]
64. Bonney, S.; Hughes, K.; Harter, P.N.; Mittelbronn, M.; Walker, L.; Eckle, T. Cardiac period 2 in myocardial ischemia: Clinical implications of a light dependent protein. *Int. J. Biochem. Cell Biol.* **2013**, *45*, 667–671. [CrossRef]
65. Eckle, T.; Hartmann, K.; Bonney, S.; Reithel, S.; Mittelbronn, M.; Walker, L.A.; Lowes, B.D.; Han, J.; Borchers, C.H.; Buttrick, PM.; et al. Adora2b-elicited Per2 stabilization promotes a HIF-dependent metabolic switch crucial for myocardial adaptation to ischemia. *Nat. Med.* **2012**, *18*, 774–782. [CrossRef]
66. Virag, J.A.I.; Dries, J.L.; Easton, P.R.; Friesland, A.M.; Deantonio, J.H.; Chintalgattu, V.; DeAntonio, J.H.; Chintalgattu, V.; Cozzi, E.; Lehmann, B.D.; et al. Attenuation of myocardial injury in mice with functional deletion of the circadian rhythm gene mPer2. *Am. J. Physiol. Heart Cric. Physiol.* **2010**, *198*, H1088–H1095. [CrossRef]
67. Vetter, C.; Devore, E.E.; Wegrzyn, L.R.; Massa, J.; Speizer, F.E.; Kawachi, I.; Rosner, B.; Stampfer, M.J.; Schernhammer, E.S. Association between rotating night shiftwork and risk of coronary heart disease among women. *JAMA* **2016**, *315*, 1726–1734. [CrossRef]
68. Hermansson, J.; Bøggild, H.; Hallqvist, J.; Karlsson, B.; Knutsson, A.; Nilsson, T.; Reuterwall, C.; Gillander Gådin, K. Interaction between shift work and established coronary risk factors. *Int. J. Occup. Environ. Med.* **2019**, *10*, 57–65. [CrossRef]
69. Hermansson, J.; Hallqvist, J.; Karlsson, B.; Knutsson, A.; Gillander Gådin, K. Shift work, parental cardiovascular disease and myocardial infarction in males. *Occup. Med.* **2018**, *68*, 120–125. [CrossRef]
70. Manfredini, R.; Fabbian, F.; Cappadona, R.; De Giorgi, A.; Bravi, F.; Carradori, T.; Flacco, M.E.; Manzoli, L. Daylight Saving Time and Acute Myocardial Infarction: A Meta-Analysis. *J. Clin. Med.* **2019**, *8*, 404. [CrossRef]
71. Kurose, T.; Yabe, D.; Inagaki, N. Circadian rhythms and diabetes. *J. Diabetes Investig.* **2011**, *2*, 176–177. [CrossRef]
72. Allebrandt, K.V.; Roenneberg, T. The search for circadian clock components in humans: New perspectives for association studies. *Braz. J. Med. Biol. Res.* **2008**, *41*, 716–721. [CrossRef]

13

Short-Term Therapies for Treatment of Acute and Advanced Heart Failure—Why so Few Drugs Available in Clinical Use, Why Even Fewer in the Pipeline?

Piero Pollesello [1,*], Tuvia Ben Gal [2], Dominique Bettex [3], Vladimir Cerny [4], Josep Comin-Colet [5], Alexandr A. Eremenko [6], Dimitrios Farmakis [7], Francesco Fedele [8], Cândida Fonseca [9], Veli-Pekka Harjola [10], Antoine Herpain [11], Matthias Heringlake [12], Leo Heunks [13], Trygve Husebye [14], Visnja Ivancan [15], Kristjan Karason [16], Sundeep Kaul [17], Jacek Kubica [18], Alexandre Mebazaa [19], Henning Mølgaard [20], John Parissis [21], Alexander Parkhomenko [22], Pentti Põder [23], Gerhard Pölzl [24], Bojan Vrtovec [25], Mehmet B. Yilmaz [26] and Zoltan Papp [27,28]

1. Critical Care, Orion Pharma, 02101 Espoo, Finland
2. Heart Failure Unit, Rabin Medical Center, Tel Aviv University, Petah Tikva 4941492d, Israel; bengalt@clalit.org.il
3. Institute of Anaesthesiology, University Hospital of Zurich, University of Zurich, 8091 Zurich, Switzerland; dominique.bettex@usz.ch
4. Department of Anesthesiology, Perioperative Medicine and Intensive Care, Masaryk Hospital, J.E. Purkinje University, 400 96 Usti nad Labem, Czech Republic; vladimir.cerny@fnhk.cz
5. Heart Diseases Institute, Hospital Universitari de Bellvitge, 08015 Barcelona, Spain; josepcomin@gmail.com
6. Department of Cardiac Intensive Care, Petrovskii National Research Centre of Surgery, Sechenov University, 119146 Moscow, Russia; aeremenko54@mail.ru
7. Department of Cardiology, Medical School, University of Cyprus, 1678 Nicosia, Cyprus; dimitrios_farmakis@yahoo.com
8. Department of Cardiovascular, Respiratory, Nephrology, Anesthesiology and Geriatric Sciences, 'La Sapienza' University of Rome, 00185 Rome, Italy; Francesco.Fedele@uniroma1.it
9. Heart Failure Clinic of S. Francisco Xavier Hospital, CHLO, 1449-005 Lisbon, Portugal; mcandidafonseca@gmail.com
10. Emergency Medicine, Department of Emergency Medicine and Services, Helsinki University Hospital, University of Helsinki, 00014 Helsinki, Finland; Veli-Pekka.Harjola@hus.fi
11. Department of Intensive Care, Experimental Laboratory of Intensive Care, Erasme Hospital, Université Libre de Bruxelles, 1050 Bruxelles, Belgium; Antoine.Herpain@erasme.ulb.ac.be
12. Department of Anesthesiology and Intensive Care Medicine, University of Lübeck, 23562 Lübeck, Germany; Matthias.Heringlake@uksh.de
13. Department of Intensive Care Medicine, Amsterdam UMC, Location VUmc 081 HV, The Netherlands; l.heunks@vumc.nl
14. Department of Cardiology, Oslo University Hospital Ullevaal, 0372 Oslo, Norway; tr-huse@online.no
15. Department of Anesthesiology, Reanimatology and Intensive Care, University Hospital Centre, 10000 Zagreb, Croatia; vivancan@kbc-zagreb.hr
16. Transplant Institute, Sahlgrenska University Hospital, 413 45 Gothenburg, Sweden; kristjan.karason@medfak.gu.se
17. Intensive Care Unit, National Health Service, Leeds LS2 9JT, UK; sunnykaul@aol.com
18. Department of Cardiology and Internal Medicine, Nicolaus Copernicus University, 87-100 Torun, Poland; jkubica@cm.umk.pl
19. Department of Anaesthesiology and Critical Care Medicine, AP-HP, Saint Louis and Lariboisière University Hospitals, Université de Paris and INSERM UMR-S 942-MASCOT, 75010 Paris, France; alexandre.mebazaa@aphp.fr
20. Department of Cardiology, Århus University Hospital, 8200 Århus, Denmark; hennmoel@rm.dk
21. Emergency Department, Attikon University Hospital, National and Kapodistrian University of Athens, 157 72 Athens, Greece; jparissis@yahoo.com

[22] Emergency Cardiology Department, National Scientific Center M.D. Strazhesko Institute of Cardiology, 02000 Kiev, Ukraine; aparkhomenko@yahoo.com
[23] Department of Cardiology, North Estonia Medical Center, 13419 Tallinn, Estonia; Pentti.Poder@regionaalhaigla.ee
[24] Department of Internal Medicine III, Cardiology and Angiology, Medical University of Innsbruck, 6020 Innsbruck, Austria; gerhard.poelzl@tirol-kliniken.at
[25] Advanced Heart Failure and Transplantation Center, Department of Cardiology, Ljubljana University Medical Center, SI-1000 Ljubljana, Slovenia; bojan.vrtovec@gmail.com
[26] Department of Cardiology, Dokuz Eylul University Faculty of Medicine, 35340 Izmir, Turkey; cardioceptor@gmail.com
[27] Division of Clinical Physiology, Department of Cardiology, Faculty of Medicine, University of Debrecen, H-4032 Debrecen, Hungary; pappz@med.unideb.hu
[28] HAS-UD Vascular Biology and Myocardial Pathophysiology Research Group, Hungarian Academy of Sciences, 4001 Debrecen, Hungary
* Correspondence: piero.pollesello@orionpharma.com

Abstract: Both acute and advanced heart failure are an increasing threat in term of survival, quality of life and socio-economical burdens. Paradoxically, the use of successful treatments for chronic heart failure can prolong life but—per definition—causes the rise in age of patients experiencing acute decompensations, since nothing at the moment helps avoiding an acute or final stage in the elderly population. To complicate the picture, acute heart failure syndromes are a collection of symptoms, signs and markers, with different aetiologies and different courses, also due to overlapping morbidities and to the plethora of chronic medications. The palette of cardio- and vasoactive drugs used in the hospitalization phase to stabilize the patient's hemodynamic is scarce and even scarcer is the evidence for the agents commonly used in the practice (e.g., catecholamines). The pipeline in this field is poor and the clinical development chronically unsuccessful. Recent set backs in expected clinical trials for new agents in acute heart failure (AHF) (omecamtiv, serelaxine, ularitide) left a field desolately empty, where only few drugs have been approved for clinical use, for example, levosimendan and nesiritide. In this consensus opinion paper, experts from 26 European countries (Austria, Belgium, Croatia, Cyprus, Czech Republic, Denmark, Estonia, Finland, France, Germany, Greece, Hungary, Israel, Italy, The Netherlands, Norway, Poland, Portugal, Russia, Slovenia, Spain, Sweden, Switzerland, Turkey, U.K. and Ukraine) analyse the situation in details also by help of artificial intelligence applied to bibliographic searches, try to distil some lesson-learned to avoid that future projects would make the same mistakes as in the past and recommend how to lead a successful development project in this field in dire need of new agents.

Keywords: acute heart failure; advanced heart failure; short-term hemodynamic therapy; regulatory clinical trials; clinical development; levosimendan

---

1. Introduction

Despite the availability of successful treatments for chronic heart failure (CHF), acute heart failure (AHF) and advanced heart failure (AdHF) still impose considerable and rising health burdens in their impact on life expectancy and quality of life of an increasingly elderly population and the associated social and economic burdens.

AHF and AdHF syndromes are a collection of symptoms, signs and markers with different aetiologies, different clinical courses and different cardiac reserve. The innately complex nature of these conditions is further exacerbated by the fact that they are preponderantly encountered in an elderly population with overlapping morbidities and a plethora of chronic medications including drugs for serious co-morbidities.

In an acute episode, when a patient decompensates despite optimal p.o. medications, intravenous cardio- and vasoactive drugs are used to stabilize the situation. However, the repertoire of such drugs is relatively narrow—diuretics, vasodilators and inotropes—and evidence for sustained benefit of these agents is often strikingly thin—demonstration of mortality and morbidity gains in the long term remain elusive. Disappointingly, the number of successful innovations in recent years has been small.

Recent experiences with an array of innovative cardio- and vasoactive drugs in acute heart failure were recently summarized in a review by Machaj et al. [1] (see Table 1 for studies on AHF).

Table 1. Recent large-scale regulatory Phase III trials testing novel therapies for acute heart failure. Data extracted from Machaj et al. [1].

Agent Name	Omecamtiv Mecarbil	Ularitide	Serelaxin	
Trial name	ATOMIC-AHF	TRUE-AHF	RELAX-AHF	RELAX-AHF-2
Registry number	NCT01300013	NCT01661634	NCT00520806	NCT01870778
Sample size	614 AHF patients	2.157 AHF patients	1.161 pts hospitalized for AHF	6.600 AHF patients
Outcomes	• failed to meet the primary endpoint of dyspnoea improvement • increased SET	• no significant differences in primary endpoints • significant dyspnea reduction in 83% of eligible patients	• VAS AUC scale dyspnea improvement • fewer deaths at day 180	• failed to meet primary endpoints (180-day cardiovascular death and worsening heart failure through day-5)
Observed adverse events	• no difference in adverse effect rate compared to placebo	• adverse effect on dyspnea in 17% of ineligible patients (prohibited intravenous medications)	• infrequent hypotensive events	• no serious adverse events

Abbreviations: AHF, acute heart failure; VAS AUC, visual analogue scale area under the curve.

These results follow a course that has become familiar in this area of cardiovascular medical research in recent years—ingenious and scientifically plausible novel agents show often considerable promise in pre-clinical evaluations; that promise is carried forward into Phase I trials in humans and sometimes into Phase 2 trials in patients but pivotal or definitive Phase 3 trials interventions disappoint expectations and deliver no evidence of benefit on the nominated primary endpoint(s) or on clinically-relevant outcomes such as longer-term survival. Other authors offer similar tabulations and reach similar conclusions [2,3]. In advanced heart failure (AdHF) a recent update on the field had a conspicuous focus on developments in transplantation medicine and mechanical ventricular assist devices but was strikingly silent on the topic of medical innovations [4].

In a commentary published in 2014 reasons were identified that have contributed to this frustrating state of affairs [5]. Five years on and with the situation in many ways no better, it seems timely to re-visit this issue and to ask if the latest crop of negative clinical trials would trigger a reform of heart failure-targeted clinical research. We consider a root-and-branch reform to be essential if we are to break out of the pattern intimated in Table 1 and reinvigorate a therapeutic pipeline that with few exceptions has been painfully threadbare and unproductive for several decades.

The main obstacles to progress already identified in that 2014 essay merit brief re-examination:

(1) The therapeutic field is complicated, the definitions of AHF and AdHF are not straightforward, with many aetiologies and various, often quickly evolving manifestations. Moreover, there is still a debate not only on the definition but also on the existence of some heart failure syndromes, for example, heart failure with mid-range ejection fraction [6] (HFmrEF). The combination of a broad-spectrum pathophysiology with vague definitions based on few parameters may preclude identifying meaningful group of patients benefitting of one particular drug instead of another.

(2) The barrier to new entrants is set very high by the fact that regulatory clinical trials in AHF are targeted at demonstrating a reduction in longer-term mortality from drugs intended to be used as short-term interventions. Most trials are configured to evaluate the candidate drug as an addition to standard-of-care medications—that makes it very difficult to demonstrate significant and meaningful increases in survival (or indeed in lesser outcomes such as relief of dyspnoea) [7,8]. Hence, in order to deliver convincing findings, regulatory studies need to be both large and lengthy, leading to erosion of patent life. Additional complications relate to the regulatory requirements of populous emerging markets. The need to undertake both pivotal (often international) clinical trials but increasingly also locally-conducted single-country trials to secure marketing approval in some large national markets implies a duplication of funding and other resources, all of which add to the total costs of development and weaken the business case.

(3) The use of many traditional therapies with low levels of evidence to keep patients alive and to overcome the acute decompensation (e.g., generic intravenous vasodilators, diuretics, inotropes and vasopressors) makes it very difficult for new entrants to demonstrate a persuasive risk-benefit profile when the regulatory clinical studies must be conducted versus a placebo group that mandates use of extensive "standard of care" (SoC) therapy.

All these factors may discourage the sort of ambitious investment that might produce durable innovation and progress; other therapeutic areas may appear less risky or more rewarding to pharmaceutical companies considering where to place their research and development (R&D) effort. From a commercially-focussed perspective heart failure in all its manifestations, including AHF and AdHF, is a complex condition in which "there can be no realistic expectation of a blockbuster .... .and where it is wrong (both morally and commercially) to encourage hopes that such a drug is just around the corner [5]." As a corollary of this, the emergence of an era of personalized therapies implies both an opportunity and also an obligation to focus drug research in heart failure towards specific and precisely-defined sub-pathologies and to abandon, as irrational and futile, a search for a panacea.

With no substantive additions to the therapeutic repertoire in recent times and the world of medicine (and indeed the world in general) poised for unprecedented changes in the nature, scale and accessibility of data, the argument for a complete revision of the theory, philosophy and practice of research in heart failure drug design is, we suggest, compelling. One early casualty of such a revision may be the end of almost any reliance on left ventricular ejection fraction (LVEF) as a primary metric in the characterization of heart failure.

2. A Systematic Analysis of the Past 20 Years

In order to understand better the field of drug development in the acute and advanced presentation of heart failure in the latest 20 years we performed an artificial intelligence (AI)-mediated search for all regulatory trials of Phase 3 on new chemical entities (NCE) aimed to validate the benefits of drugs developed for short-term treatment of AHF (including the wording "acutely decompensated heart failure") and/or AdHF published after the year 2000. Clinical trials were searched using full-text search against studies' descriptions with the NCE and the therapy area names. Using semantic similarity, studies implying semantic similarity of less than 30% with "heart failure" were filtered out. Reports exhibiting excessive semantic similarity with "kidney disease" or "addiction" were penalized to filter out studies focused principally on these topics and only mentioning heart diseases in passing (this condition applied for example, for studies involving dopamine). Comparator classes, first posting date of the study and patient enrolment were added to the data set. Finally, the results were checked independently by two researchers for their consistency.

We identified 36 regulatory clinical trials in the past 20 years which were classified as Phase III (Figure 1). Those studies were aimed to test the hypothesis of clinical benefits of 16 different NCE (mainly exerting hemodynamic effects such as inotropy, vasodilation, diuresis), only few of which were finally approved in the U.S.A. or in Europe for use in AHF. By plotting the studies in chronological order, it can be seen that the density of Phase III trials publications has been consistently low in the past two decades (Figure 2). To be noticed is that, among the few trials in which the hypothesis was statistically proven, three (LIDO, RUSSLAN and REVIVE) tested the effect of levosimendan in AHF.

The total number of patients included in the 36 clinical trial was circa 38,000, notwithstanding that our search did not include either the Phase I and II trials or any Phase IV study. The fact that so many patients have been enrolled in this long series of inconclusive or negative studies should be considered of significance.

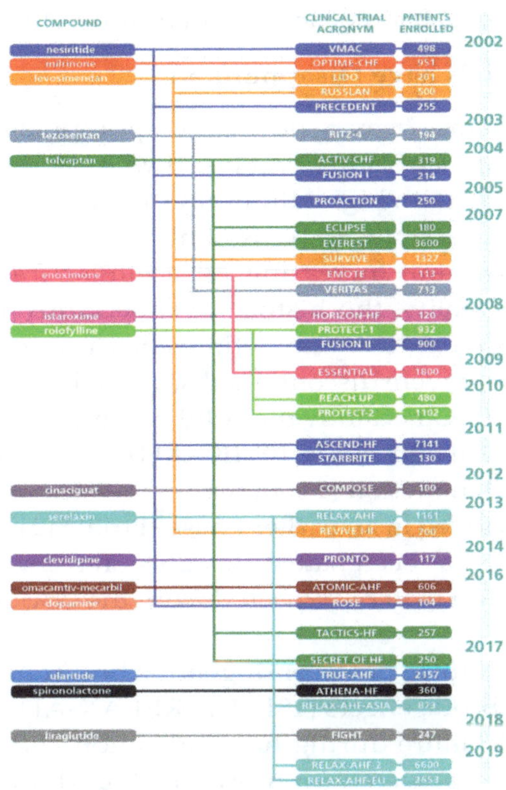

Figure 1. Regulatory clinical trials of Phase III for drugs meant for short-term treatment of acute heart failure (AHF) and/or advanced heart failure (AdHF), published in the past 20 years. For each study, the year of publication of the main report, the first author and the PMID are the following—VMAC, 2002, VMAC investigators, 11911755; OPTIME-CHF, 2002, Cuffe MS, 11911756; LIDO, 2002, Follath F, 12133653; RUSSLAN 2002 Moiseyev VS 12208222; PRECEDENT, 2002, Burger AJ, 12486437; RITZ-4, 2003, O'Connor CM, 12742280; ACTIV-CHF, 2004, M. Gheorghiade, 15113814; FUSION I, 2004, Yancy CW, 15342289; PROACTION, 2005, Peacock WF, 15915407; EVEREST, 2007, Konstam MA, 17384437; ECLIPSE, 2007, Udelison JE, published as abstract; SURVIVE, 2007, Mabazaa A, 17473298; EMOTE, 2007, Feldman AM, 17967591; VERITAS, 2007, McMurray JJ, 17986694; HORIZON-HF, 2008, Gheorghiade M, 18534276; PROTECT-1, 2008, Cotter G, 18926433; ESSENTIAL, 2009, Metra M, 19700774; FUSION II, 2008, Yancy CW, 19808265; REACH UP, 2010, Gottlieb SS, 20797594; PROTECT-2, 2010, Massie BM, 20925544; ASCEND-HF, 2011, O'Connor, 21732835; STARBRITE, 2011, Sha MR, 21807321; COMPOSE, 2012, Gheorghiade M, 22713287; RELAX-AHF, 2013, Teerlink JR, 23141816; REVIVE I-II, 2013, Packer M, 24621834; PRONTO, 2014, Peacock WF, 24655702; ATOMIC-AHF, 2016, Teerlink JR, 27012405; ROSE, 2016, Wan SH, 27512103; ROSE, 2016, Wan SH, 27512103; TACTICS-HF, 2016, Felker GM, 27654854; RELAX-AHF-ASIA, 2017, Sato N, 27825893; SECRET OF HF, 2017, Konstam MA, 28302292; TRUE-AHF, 2017, Packer M, 28402745; ATHENA-HF, 2017, Butler J, 28700781; FIGHT, 2018, Sharma A, 30120812; RELAX-AHF-EU, 2019, Maggioni AP, 30604559; RELAX-AHF-2, 2019, Metra M, 31433919.

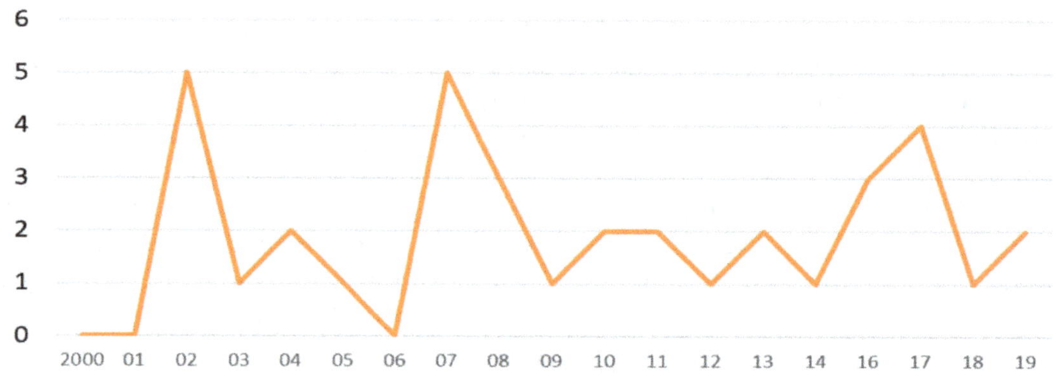

Figure 2. Amount of regulatory clinical trials of Phase III for drugs meant for short-term treatment of AHF and/or AdHF per year of publication in the period 2000–2019.

3. Also the Recent Clinical Trials have Disappointed

Before addressing these themes in more detail, it is appropriate to look briefly at some experiences in recent decades in the development of intravenous (i.v.) drug therapies.

Omecamtiv mecarbil binds with high affinity to the catalytic domain of myosin, increasing the number of myosin heads available to cross-link with actin. In theory, this augments cardiomyocyte contractility without increasing intracellular free ionic calcium or cardiomyocyte oxygen consumption [1]. In reality, the history of omecamtiv mecarbil might be seen rather as a demonstration that the pharma industry sometimes has a short memory. Candidate drugs which prolong the contractility transient were discontinued several decades ago because of their potential for harm in ischaemic conditions [9]. Omecamtiv mecarbil – at least at high plasma concentrations—shares some of these characteristics [10] and the ATOMIC-AHF trial produced a biomarker signal similar to that seen during myocardial infarction [11] (a higher median plasma troponin level) that might be related to cardiac ischemia described in an earlier Phase II trial [12]. The regulatory clinical programme for omecamtiv mecarbil in AHF has been halted. Insights on the safety and efficacy of oral omecamtiv mecarbil for chronic heart failure may be expected from the GALACTIC-HF study, due to complete in 2021.

Serelaxin is a recombinant form of the endogenous hormone relaxin-2 and exerts vasodilatory, anti-inflammatory and anti-fibrotic effects [13]. The RELAX-AHF trial produced evidence of lower incidence of worsening heart failure during hospitalization [14] but the later RELAX-AHF-2 trial, which unlike RELAX-AHF, was powered for mortality, found no impact on 180-day cardiovascular mortality and a numerical but not statistically significant effect on worsening heart failure [15]. The challenge of deciding which of these sets of findings is most relevant to the treatment of AHF patients is evident. Further illustrations of the complexities and challenges of assigning weight to the results of clinical trials is provided by the demonstration that patients in RELAX-AHF were substantially unrepresentative of patients with AHF in the United States, Latin America or Asia-Pacific [16] and by the report that the RELAX-AHF-EU trial, yielded results similar to and supportive of RELAX-AHF [17] in the context of open-label drug administration.

Ularitide, a synthetic form of the human natriuretic peptide urodilatin, exerts vasodilator, diuretic and natriuretic effects via the natriuretic peptide receptor/particulate guanylate cyclase/cyclic guanosine monophosphate pathway and displayed beneficial effects such as symptom relief and vasodilation in animal models of heart failure as well as early-phase clinical studies in heart failure patients, In a Phase 3 trial (TRUE-AHF) in patients with acute heart failure, however, short-term ularitide treatment did not affect a clinical composite end point or reduce long-term cardiovascular mortality despite various nominally favourable physiological effects (and without affecting cardiac troponin levels) [18].

The early promise of istaroxime, which promotes the activity of sarco(endo)plasmic reticulum $Ca(2^{+})$-ATPase 2 (SERCA2) and thereby promotes expulsion of free intracellular ionic calcium through transmembrane sodium/calcium channels appears not to been sustained since the publication of the findings of the HORIZON study [19–21] and the results of the CUPID-HF study suggest that gene transfer of the SERCA2 gene is not yet a proven intervention [22].

Two studies of the nitroxyl (HNO) moiety (NCT01096043 and NCT10192325), commenced in 2010 appear to remain incomplete and unreported while evaluation of a follow-up molecule designated a BMS-986231 (previously CXL-1427) are in only preliminary stages [23]. The list of set-backs continues with tezosentan, nesiritide, tolvaptan, milrinone, enoximone, rolofylline, clevidipine, SLV320, cinaciguat, dopamine, liraglutide and high-dose spironolactone (see Figure 1).

4. Levosimendan—A Rare Case

Levosimendan, an inodilator that promotes contractility by binding to calcium saturated troponin C and vasodilatory and cardioprotective effects through the opening of adenosine triphosphate-dependent potassium (K_{ATP}) channels is one of few agents of recent decades to establish itself in the medical repertoire for AHF and AdHF for its sustained hemodynamic, neurohormonal and symptomatic effects [24,25]. This status rests on findings from a series of Phase II and III studies published in the early 2000s. Two large post-approval clinical trials (SURVIVE and REVIVE) did not substantiate an indication of long-term effects but both a meta-analysis involving data from more than 6000 patients and a real-world registry involving over 5000 patients (ALARM-HF) were strongly indicative of long term survival benefit [26,27] – at a minimum to the extent that levosimendan use has never been associated with increased mortality, whereas the use of adrenergic/calcium mobilizing inotropes such as dobutamine has. At this regard, it is worth reminding that several authors in the past recognized a correlation between the effects of cardiovascular drugs on intracellular calcium and on long-term survival in heart failure, to the advantage of drugs which do not elevate either calcium transient or mitochondrial calcium, such as levosimendan [28–30].

Finally, since no attenuation of the hemodynamic effect of levosimendan is apparent in patients treated with beta-blockers [31,32] – now a substantial proportion of the overall heart failure population – the drug has been favoured for use in such patients in the most recent edition of ESC guidelines [33].

Levosimendan has also been evaluated in randomized controlled trials in advanced heart failure (Levo-Rep (NCT01065194), LION-Heart (NCT01536132) and LAICA (NCT00988806)) [34–36]. Observations in those trials are indicative of clinical benefits including reduction in NT-pro-BNP levels and trends towards reductions in heart failure readmissions and heart failure-related mortality. Those trends were corroborated in metanalyses where statistically significant reductions in long-term mortality and re-hospitalization were demonstrated [37,38] and subsequently in the RELEVANT-HF study, in which the addition of intermittent levosimendan therapy at 3-4 week intervals was associated over the course of 6 months with a substantially lower percentage of days in hospital (2.8 ± 6.6% vs. 9.4 ± 8.2%; $p < 0.0001$) and in the cumulative number and length of HF-related admissions (both $p < 0.0001$ vs. control), plus a marked but non-significant improvement in 1-year survival free from death/need for implantation of a ventricular assist device or urgent transplantation (86% vs. 78%) [39].

5. Even the Established Drugs May Not "Work."

Very recently, at the European Society of Cardiology Congress, the GALACTIC trial reported that early intensive vasodilation using personalized high doses of nitrates, oral hydralazine and rapid up-titration of ACE inhibitors or angiotensin II receptor blockers did not improve 180-day mortality in a cohort of 781 acute heart failure patients [40]. This trial is notable, among other things, for the fact that short-term use of conventional "tried and tested" (and extremely cheap) vasodilators, administered in an intensive regime and at high dose was just as ineffectual at influencing longer-term mortality as novel agents such as ularitide and serelaxin. The inability to demonstrate survival benefit even from drugs that are established as part of the therapeutic armamentarium for AHF highlights some fundamental issues contributing to the paucity of new drug therapies in recent decades—for example, are we targeting the wrong pathological processes in our drug development programmes or are we privileging inappropriate endpoints in clinical trials and thus hampering the regulatory approval of useful new agents?

The general lack of evidence for an ongoing survival benefit from acute-phase treatments for AHF requires some reflection. While perhaps not fully subscribing to its philosophical outlook we find much to agree with in the views of McCullough [41], who has argued that AHF (and by extension AdHF) is a situation often long in the making and that to expect any therapy administered for ≤48 h to make a robust difference to survival or rehospitalization many months after the index admission is to misunderstand the pathophysiology of these conditions.

6. Where Next and How to Get There?

Readers looking for a way forward from this seeming impasse may find encouragement in a recent review by Triposkiadis and colleagues [42]. We consider that publication to be a most significant contribution to this arena of cardiovascular research for the manner in which it articulates and crystallizes lines of critical thinking that have been apparent for some years but which, through advances in technology, are now poised to transform both the conception of heart failure and its modes of treatment.

A central premise of this work is that describing heart failure in terms of LVEF, while useful in its time, has become counter-productive and increasingly is obscuring the pathophysiological realities of heart failure, with adverse consequences for the evolution of therapy [43,44]. We concur with Triposkiadis et al. [42] that heart failure is "a heterogeneous syndrome in which functional and structural biomarkers change dynamically during disease progression in a patient-specific fashion" and that the condition as a whole may usefully be portrayed as a spectrum in which, depending on their proximity within that spectrum, individual presentations may or may not have overlapping phenotypes and shared underlying pathologies. Features of heart failure identified by Triposkiadis et al. [42] as occurring across the heart failure spectrum include:

1. Bidirectional transitions of LVEF due to disease treatment and progression
2. Endothelial dysfunction, cardiomyocyte dysfunction and cardiomyocyte injury
3. Systolic and diastolic left ventricular dysfunction
4. Left atrial dysfunction
5. Myocardial fibrosis
6. Skeletal myopathy
7. Heart failure serum markers
8. Neurohumoral activation

From that starting position Triposkiadis et al. [42] advocate the development of a wholly new classification of heart failure based on ultra-detailed phenotyping of the sort now made possible by advances in biological technologies and computing. This process, illustrated in Figure 3, proves a basis both for the better application of existing therapies and to shape the development of new agents. Two pathways of stratification are identified by this reasoning – one is hypothesis-driven, based for example on disease aetiology or mechanism or shaped by known pharmacological pathways of action; the other is hypothesis-free approach driven by the modern capacity to acquire unprecedented volumes of phenotype data and to analyse that data at unprecedented speeds and granularity, so identifying characteristics (or "signatures") that differentiate sub-sets of patients with different heart failure phenotypes, different outcomes and different responses to various therapies.

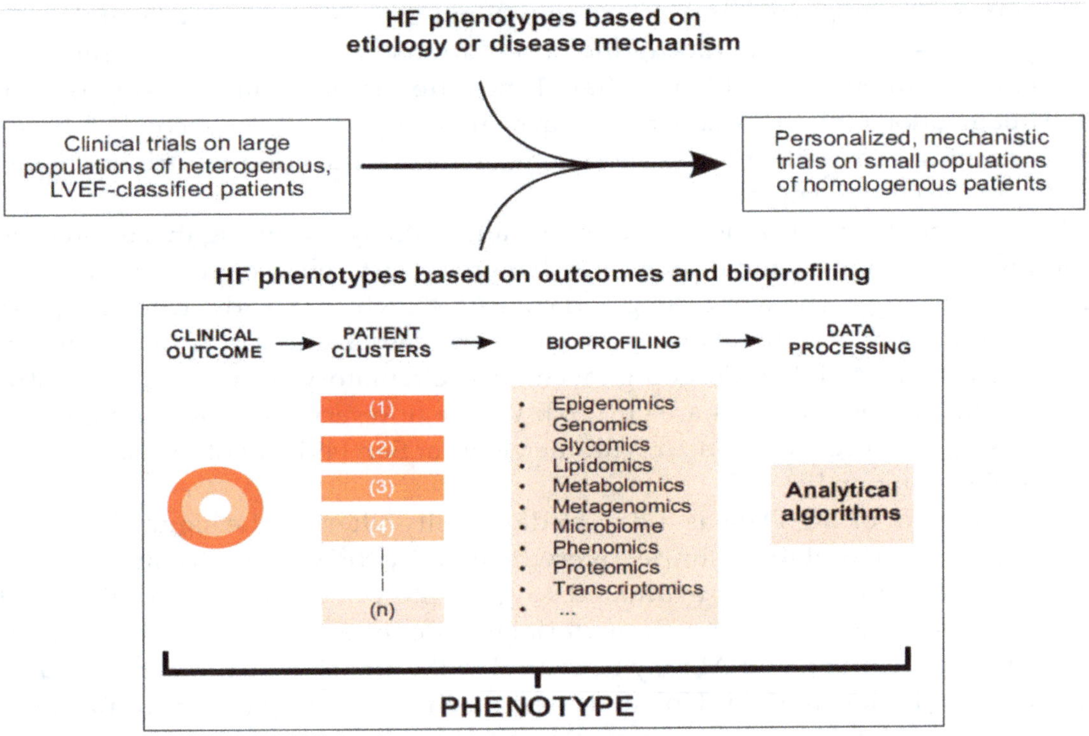

Figure 3. Advances in information and data-processing technology have created a base from which heart failure research can be re-configured towards highly defied phenotypes in ways that will facilitate both the optimal use of current therapies and the identification of new agents specifically tailored to a particular pathophysiology. See text for further discussion. Freely from Triposkiadis et al [42].

Finally, in order to stratify HF patients, it should be mandatory to consider systematically the functions of other organs such as lung, kidney, liver, brain, hematopoietic system and so on, as proposed recently [45].

7. Invasive versus Non-Invasive Monitoring

When comparing the measures suggested for the diagnosis of AHF in the most recent European guidelines [33] with previous versions, an obvious trend to avoid invasive diagnostic measures (like using a pulmonary artery catheter) in AHF can be noticed. It would be wrong to rely primarily on simple clinical signs for assessing the severity and the type of failure in AHF—its complex manifestations and haemodynamic profile cannot be adequately diagnosed and differentiated by bedside assessment. Additionally, not any single word within 85 pages of the guidelines can be found on monitoring the systemic oxygen consumption and delivery by determination of mixed or at least central venous oxygen saturation; despite heart failure is classically defined as the inability of the heart, to maintain an adequate oxygen supply to the tissues. One may argue that the lack of progress in clinical development of new agents for treatment of AHF may be also explained by the inappropriate diagnostic measures and monitoring modalities recommended by the current guidelines and that even the best drugs will fail if they are inappropriately used within the multiple manifestations of heart failure. We should also consider alternatives to the Swan Ganz catheter, as recently reviewed by a large panel of experts [46].

8. Will the Data Revolution Break the Logjam?

These proposals may be seen in the wider context of an explosion in personal data accessible for analysis and the rapidly evolving science of AI. Timely recent reviews of these themes have been published, identifying both the opportunities and the many challenges that these new technologies present [47–50]. As non-experts in those fields we are constrained in what we might say with authority about these developments but concur with Sim [49] on several aspects of the use of mobile data-reporting devices in health, including the observations that "Tracking and reporting data are a mean to an end not an end in itself" and that "Innovation in electronic sensing is in many ways outpacing the imagination for how these sensors can be used clinically." The second of those sentiments may be seen a warning to expect some developments in data acquisition to turn out to be diversions (or blind alleys) in the clinical context.

Beyond these thoughts is the much more significant challenge of sifting this unprecedented mass of data to identify signs, signals and biomarkers that are robust, reliable, meaningful and capable of being used to guide therapy. The work Deng and colleagues, who have advocated for pre-procedural gene expression profiles of peripheral blood mononuclear cells as indicative of longer-term survival prospects in patients with AdHF undergoing mechanical circulatory support, is an illustration of the immense and exciting potential in this area [51,52]. We are unreservedly positive for the longer-term prospects in this area but once more concur with the views of Sim [49] and others, about the challenges of successful implementation [53–55].

In the imminent era of Big Data as a day-to-day reality filtering the signal from the noise will be essential if clinicians are not to be simply overwhelmed by the volumes of information suddenly at their disposal. The USA alone is estimated to generate per annum 14 petabytes of data just from echocardiography results, a volume of material that defies exhaustive analysis by conventional methods [47]. Machine learning and AI may be central to the effective identification and analysis and orderly presentation of relevant data. Unsupervised machine learning (when computers are tasked to identify underlying relationships in a dataset) combined with 'pan-omic' analysis (i.e., genomics, proteomics, transcriptomics, metabolomics, etc.) from high throughput molecular profiling may provide a practical foundation for the sort of precision phenotyping aspired to by Triposkiadis et al. [42] and for 'hyper-local analytics' [47]. Deep learning, based on neural networks, is another aspect of the machine learning and AI revolution likely to find applications in cardiology [56,57].

The challenges of bringing machine learning and AI effectively into the practice of cardiology and more specifically into the management of heart failure are not to be underestimated (see Shameer et al. [47] and Johnson et al. [48] for excellent commentary on current methodologies and some of their pitfalls and limitations, including some observations on the cost barriers that may be encountered in acquiring biomedical data) but seem likely to be overcome within a short span of years. There are ample reasons for optimism in this area but confident prediction of what will become available and when and to what effect is beyond the powers of these authors.

9. Trials Design—Time for a Change?

Research into new therapies for AHF and AdHF in recent decades has come to resemble the definition of insanity ascribed to Einstein—doing the same thing over and over again and hoping for a different result. One emerging therapy after another is added to the SoC repertoire in a Phase 3 trial and in that context each in turn fails to meet the prespecified endpoints for meaningful efficacy.

We may have reached a stage where the broad-spectrum pathophysiology of HF, with different signs, symptoms and manifestations, different aetiologies and different patient co-morbidities, explored against a background of SoC medication, may preclude identifying meaningful incremental clinical benefits using traditional trial methodology.

One response to this situation may lie in the adoption of a composite clinical endpoint evaluated in a hierarchical manner. The methodology ensures that all trial participants contribute to the overall outcome analysis through one or more of the specified outcomes; this has helpful practical implications for the number of patients needed and the length of follow-up required to generate endpoint data. Highly affirmative initial results have emerged from the ATTR-ACT study, which used this methodology to evaluate tafamidis in transthyretin amyloid cardiomyopathy [58] and the LeoDOR study (NCT03437226) is currently using a similar approach to outcome assessment in AdHF patients receiving intermittent cycles of levosimendan therapy [59,60].

More radical ways forward may include the adoption of Bayesian adaptive trial design, which facilitates the study of multiple treatment approaches and therapies in multiple patient phenotypes within a single trial, while maintaining a reasonable sample size [61]. Another possibility is the adoption of the group-sequential multi-arm multi-stage (MAMS) trial. The relative strengths and limitations of these methods have been reviewed in detail [62,63]. Overarching these methods is the concept of the "platform" trial, a clinical study with a single master protocol in which multiple treatments are evaluated simultaneously. This offers flexibilities such as dropping treatments for futility or adding new treatments during the course of a trial. Platform trials have the attraction of being able to deliver robust results with fewer patients and less time than a traditional two-arm trial [64].

Some cautionary comments are appropriate at this point. These emergent trial methods may be attractive for their statistical and methodological properties but their implementation in practice can be very highly resource-intensive, even by usual standards and especially when they include biomarkers. Essential preparation for Bayesian adaptive platform trials includes extensive stakeholder consultations, in-depth statistical modelling and definition of both the best outcome measures and intra-study endpoints. Morrell et al. [65], Hague and colleagues [66] and Schiavone et al. [67] have recently offered some observations on the practicalities of conducting platform trials, based on first-hand experience and enquiry. One aspect of note is that "the biomarker-stratified trial has the effect of making staff in the trial office aware of specific patients in a unique way compared to non-stratified trials," despite anonymization" [65]. This represents a profound alteration to the human environment of clinical trials' conduct, which may be amplified by the emergence of 'decentralized' clinical trials that are conducted via mobile health or telemedicine platforms and involve virtual recruitment, delivery of trial products direct to the participants' homes and smartphone-assisted outcome assessment [49].

10. Some Views for the Future

The various trends and opportunities we have identified in this review outline a future for the development of treatments for acute or advanced heart failure perhaps very different from those of the past 20 years. Significantly, however, we might re-write that sentence to give an important different emphasis—*"The various trends and opportunities we have identified in this review outline a future for the treatment of acute or advanced heart failure perhaps very different from those of the past 20 years."* Readers will note that this second description emphasizes changes in the usage of drugs over the development of new drugs.

Our views in this regard are shaped by two notable recent publications [2,68], both of which have argued that what matters to patients who are hospitalized with a decompensation event is that they avoid further such hospitalizations and avoid the increase in mortality that occurs during the recovery phase. Viewed from that perspective the clinical stabilization achieved during the acute phase of hospital admission may be a secondary objective and to a substantial degree disconnected from the longer-term outcomes that patients prize. As Hamo and colleagues have pointed out [2], the physiological changes that lead to hospitalization take place days or weeks before hospitalization whereas the major adverse outcomes of death or rehospitalization mostly occur post-discharge. That temporal difference, combined with the now extensive evidence that acute-phase symptom relief with available therapies does not reliably improve long-term outcomes strongly suggests that either (a) relief of symptoms may be dissociated from central pathophysiological mechanisms; or (b) any pathophysiological pathway that is targeted by an acute-phase intervention is not going to be fully rectified by such short-term therapy. Conceivably both of these considerations may apply simultaneously.

Further, it is difficult to distinguish between patients suffering from the heart failure syndrome who still have cardiac reserve and respond to short-term therapy with stabilization and those who display a similar a clinical picture but show little benefit and poor outcome due to a totally worn out heart.

The need, as Hamo et al. [2] express it, to assign the right drug to the right patients at the right time to deliver meaningful benefit to AHF or AdHF patients is likely to be facilitated to a quite extraordinary degree by the developments in data acquisition and analysis we have acknowledged and the hyper-detailed phenotyping anticipated by Triposkiadis et al. [42]. That pathway of evolution in patient profiling might indeed provide insights and a firmer basis for the development of effective and successful new intravenous therapies. One possible outcome from this transformation is that the SoC repertoire that has dominated since the 1980s is finally superseded. The disappointing experience in clinical trials during the past 20 years of adding of new agents to SoC has created an impression that SoC rather than providing a foundation for further advances has acted as a glass ceiling through which newer agents struggle to break. With hyperdetailed insights into the pathophysiology of individual patients the way may finally be open to new agents precisely targeted to specific pathophysiological processes while the population-wide application of, say, ACE inhibitors and/or beta-blockers may come to be seen as too imprecise to be justifiable.

It is not less plausible, however, that the data revolution might re-shape clinical strategy around AHF and AdHF into a very different course in which an incident of decompensation is seen as a cue to intensify and optimise out-patient management with the express purpose of preventing future re-hospitalizations. We note in this context recent encouraging results using machine learning algorithms for the early detection of acute cardiac decompensation [69,70] or estimation of a patient's risk for early re-admission after an index event [71] plus descriptions of the use of machine learning and telemedicine to predict and monitor patients' treatment adherence [49,72]. Similar technologies might also be deployed to optimise the functioning and performance of specialist AdHF units such as that recently described by Kreusser and colleagues [73]. The success of the TIM-HF2 (NCT01878630) trial of telemedical interventional management in reducing unplanned cardiovascular hospital admissions and all-cause mortality is also highly pertinent in this context [74,75].

In such a scenario the emphasis in the development of overall effective medical therapy for AHF and AdHF may well be towards drugs that can be accommodated in the outpatient repertoire (and therefore probably given orally) rather than towards drugs (probably given parenterally) that are intended for the management of a decompensation crisis. Repurposing of existing agents, including drugs with no current cardiology indication, guided by new in-depth knowledge of pathophysiology is another possible line of development [76]. An ultimate goal for such a pathway would be to develop patient monitoring to such a degree of immediacy and accuracy ("ecological momentary assessment [49]") that decompensations are wholly avoided by prompt, appropriate clinical responses. Such a programme, if successfully implemented, might render the concept of "acute-phase intervention" substantially redundant by eliminating episodes of decompensation. A review of notable ongoing research in this area has recently appeared in this Journal [77].

As regards drug discovery and translational science in the field of acute cardiac care, the translational committee of the ESC-HFA issued some scientific bases [78] designed to pave the way towards the development of new agents but the preclinical field remains scarcely populated, with just some notable exceptions such as the calcium sensitizer/PDE inhibitor ORM-3819 [79,80].

11. Implications for Drug Development

Commercial and societal responses to this new world of ultra-detailed patient characterization and real-time monitoring must be considered. In an era of hyper-detailed patient profiling it may transpire that fitting the right drug to the right patient translates in practice to each new drug being appropriate for a small, even tiny, number of patients. "Heart failure" might be transformed into a myriad of orphan drug indications. The implications on the 'evidence based medicine' predilection for large trials is evident. The implications for commercial profitability and/or drug acquisition costs is even more prominent.

Some pertinent and sharply framed observations that have recently emerged on the possibility of a not-for-profit model of antibiotic development might conceivably also come to apply to drug design in heart failure [81]. We take no position on whether such a shift would be inherently a good or bad thing but certainly it would mark a profound departure from the current model of drug discovery and development. (See Dungen et al. [82] for another perspective on this issue.)

These financial pressures will not be confined to cardiology – medicine as a whole faces similar pressures and opportunities. To that extent we anticipate, therefore, that new arrangements for the funding of medical treatments will address these tensions—but we are not equipped to speculate about the form these new arrangements may take or any unintended consequences they may create.

12. Conclusions

Hospitalization for heart failure, whether as a presentation of AHF or a decompensation in the context of AdHF, results in a down-shift in the trajectory of the syndrome that is associated with worsening outcomes and patient quality of life and increased costs of care. Medical progress to address these challenges has substantially stalled in the past 20 years but advances in data technology and analytics, along with developments in clinical trials design now offer opportunities to re-envision heart failure as a complex pathophysiological continuum in ways that may help to bring a new generation of therapies into clinical use. Meanwhile it would be advisable for the clinicians to evaluate if the nearly total absence of evidence of benefit with some of the traditional i.v. drugs used in AHF and AdHF (such as the catecholamines or the phosphodiesterase inhibitors) warrants their elimination from routine use in favour of treatments where such evidence has been accrued (e.g., for levosimendan).

Author Contributions: P.P. sketched the working hypotheses of the review. P.P. and Z.P. guided, monitored and corrected the AI-driven search. All authors contributed to the discussion and approved the final version of the manuscript.

Acknowledgments: We thank Eemil Väisänen, Reaktor Group Oy, Helsinki, Finland, for invaluable help with setting up the AI-driven search and Shrestha Roy and Johanna Kuusisto, Orion Pharma Oyj, Espoo, Finland, for the graphic solutions. We acknowledge Hughes associates, Oxford, UK, for editorial assistance in the preparation of the manuscript.

References

1. Machaj, F.; Dembowska, E.; Rosik, J.; Szostak, B.; Mazurek-Mochol, M.; Pawlik, A. New therapies for the treatment of heart failure: A summary of recent accomplishments. *Clin. Risk Manag.* **2019**, *15*, 147–155. [CrossRef] [PubMed]
2. Hamo, C.E.; Butler, J.; Gheorghiade, M.; Chioncel, O. The bumpy road to drug development for acute heart failure. *Eur. Heart J. Suppl.* **2016**, *18*, G19–G32. [CrossRef]
3. Tamargo, J.; Caballero, R.; Delpón, E. New drugs in preclinical and early stage clinical development in the treatment of heart failure. *Expert Opin. Investig. Drugs* **2019**, *28*, 51–71. [CrossRef] [PubMed]
4. Rame, J.E. Introduction to topical collection on updates in advanced heart failure. *Curr. Heart Fail. Rep.* **2019**. [CrossRef]
5. Pollesello, P. Drug discovery and development for acute heart failure drugs: Are expectations too high? *Int. J. Cardiol.* **2014**, *172*, 11–13. [CrossRef]
6. Farmakis, D.; Simitsis, P.; Bistola, V.; Triposkiadis, F.; Ikonomidis, I.; Katsanos, S.; Bakosis, G.; Hatziagelaki, E.; Lekakis, J.; Mebazaa, A.; et al. Acute heart failure with mid-range left ventricular ejection fraction: Clinical profile, in-hospital management, and short-term outcome. *Clin. Res. Cardiol.* **2017**, *106*, 359–368. [CrossRef]
7. Packer, M.; Colucci, W.; Fisher, L.; Massie, B.M.; Teerlink, J.R.; Young, J.; Padley, R.J.; Thakkar, R.; Delgado-Herrera, L.; Salon, J.; et al. Effect of levosimendan on the short-term clinical course of patients with acutely decompensated heart failure. *JACC Heart Fail.* **2013**, *1*, 103–111. [CrossRef]
8. Metra, M.; Teerlink, J.R.; Felker, G.M.; Greenberg, B.H.; Filippatos, G.; Ponikowski, P.; Teichman, S.L.; Unemori, E.; Voors, A.A.; Weatherley, B.D.; et al. Dyspnoea and worsening heart failure in patients with acute heart failure: results from the Pre-RELAX-AHF study. *Eur. J. Heart Fail.* **2010**, *12*, 1130–1139. [CrossRef]

9. Haikala, H.; Pollesello, P. Calcium sensitivity enhancers. *IDrugs* **2000**, *3*, 1199–1205.
10. Malik, F.I.; Hartman, J.J.; Elias, K.A.; Morgan, B.P.; Rodriguez, H.; Brejc, K.; Anderson, R.L.; Sueoka, S.H.; Lee, K.H.; Finer, J.T.; et al. Cardiac myosin activation: A potential therapeutic approach for systolic heart failure. *Science* **2011**, *331*, 1439–1443. [CrossRef]
11. Teerlink, J.R.; Felker, G.M.; McMurray, J.J.V.; Ponikowski, P.; Metra, M.; Filippatos, G.S.; Ezekowitz, J.A.; Dickstein, K.; Cleland, J.G.F.; Kim, J.B.; et al. Acute treatment with omecamtiv mecarbil to increase contractility in acute heart failure. *J. Am. Coll. Cardiol.* **2016**, *67*, 1444–1455. [CrossRef] [PubMed]
12. Cleland, J.G.; Teerlink, J.R.; Senior, R.; Nifontov, E.M.; Mc Murray, J.J.; Lang, C.C.; Tsyrlin, V.A.; Greenberg, B.H.; Mayet, J.; Francis, D.P.; et al. The effects of the cardiac myosin activator, omecamtiv mecarbil, on cardiac function in systolic heart failure: A double-blind, placebo-controlled, crossover, dose-ranging phase 2 trial. *Lancet* **2011**, *378*, 676–683. [CrossRef]
13. Gouda, P.; Ezekowitz, J.A. Update on the diagnosis and management of acute heart failure. *Curr. Opin. Cardiol.* **2019**, *34*, 202–206. [CrossRef] [PubMed]
14. Teerlink, J.R.; Cotter, G.; Davison, B.A.; Felker, G.M.; Filippatos, G.; Greenberg, B.H.; Ponikowski, P.; Unemori, E.; Voors, A.A.; Adams, K.F.; et al. Serelaxin, recombinant human relaxin-2, for treatment of acute heart failure (RELAX-AHF): A randomised, placebo-controlled trial. *Lancet* **2013**, *381*, 29–39. [CrossRef]
15. Metra, M.; Teerlink, J.R.; Cotter, G.; Davison, B.A.; Felker, G.M.; Filippatos, G.; Greenberg, B.H.; Pang, P.S.; Ponikowski, P.; Voors, A.A.; et al. Effects of serelaxin in patients with acute heart failure. *N. Engl. J. Med.* **2019**, *381*, 716–726. [CrossRef]
16. Wang, T.S.; Hellkamp, A.S.; Patel, C.B.; Ezekowitz, J.A.; Fonarow, G.C.; Hernandez, A.F. Representativeness of RELAX-AHF clinical trial population in acute heart failure. *Circ. Cardiovasc. Qual. Outcomes* **2014**, *7*, 259–268. [CrossRef]
17. Maggioni, A.P.; López-Sendón, J.; Nielsen, O.W.; Hallén, J.; Aalamian-Mattheis, M.; Wang, Y.; Ertl, G. Efficacy and safety of serelaxin when added to standard of care in patients with acute heart failure: Results from a PROBE study, RELAX-AHF-EU. *Eur. J. Heart Fail.* **2019**, *21*, 322–333. [CrossRef]
18. Packer, M.; O'Connor, C.; McMurray, J.J.V.; Wittes, J.; Abraham, W.T.; Anker, S.D.; Dickstein, K.; Filippatos, G.; Holcomb, R.; Krum, H.; et al. Effect of ularitide on cardiovascular mortality in acute heart failure. *N. Engl. J. Med.* **2017**, *376*, 1956–1964. [CrossRef]
19. Khan, H.; Metra, M.; Blair, J.E.A.; Vogel, M.; Harinstein, M.E.; Filippatos, G.S.; Sabbah, H.N.; Porchet, H.; Valentini, G.; Gheorghiade, M. Istaroxime, a first in class new chemical entity exhibiting SERCA-2 activation and Na–K-ATPase inhibition: A new promising treatment for acute heart failure syndromes? *Heart Fail. Rev.* **2009**, *14*, 277–287. [CrossRef]
20. Gheorghiade, M.; Blair, J.E.A.; Filippatos, G.S.; Macarie, C.; Ruzyllo, W.; Korewicki, J.; Bubenek-Turconi, S.I.; Ceracchi, M.; Bianchetti, M.; Carminati, P.; et al. Hemodynamic, echocardiographic, and neurohormonal effects of istaroxime, a novel intravenous inotropic and lusitropic agent. *J. Am. Coll. Cardiol.* **2008**, *51*, 2276–2285. [CrossRef]
21. NCT00616161, U.S. National Library of Medicine. Available online: https://clinicaltrials.gov/ct2/show/NCT00616161 (accessed on 6 September 2019).
22. Greenberg, B.; Butler, J.; Felker, G.M.; Ponikowski, P.; Voors, A.A.; Desai, A.S.; Barnard, D.; Bouchard, A.; Jaski, B.; Lyon, A.R.; et al. Calcium upregulation by percutaneous administration of gene therapy in patients with cardiac disease (CUPID 2): A randomised, multinational, double-blind, placebo-controlled, phase 2b trial. *Lancet* **2016**, *387*, 1178–1186. [CrossRef]
23. U.S. National Library of Medicine. Available online: https://clinicaltrials.gov (accessed on 1 September 2019).
24. Papp, Z.; Édes, I.; Fruhwald, S.; De Hert, SG.; Salmenperä, M.; Leppikangas, H.; Mebazaa, A.; Landoni, G.; Grossini, E.; Caimmi, P.; et al. Levosimendan: Molecular mechanisms and clinical implications: Consensus of experts on the mechanisms of action of levosimendan. *Int. J. Cardiol.* **2012**, *159*, 82–87. [CrossRef] [PubMed]
25. Farmakis, D.; Alvarez, J.; Gal, T.B.; Brito, D.; Fedele, F.; Fonseca, C.; Gordon, A.C.; Gotsman, I.; Grossini, E.; Guarracino, F.; et al. Levosimendan beyond inotropy and acute heart failure: Evidence of pleiotropic effects on the heart and other organs: An expert panel position paper. *Int. J. Cardiol.* **2016**, *222*, 303–312. [CrossRef] [PubMed]
26. Mebazaa, A.; Parissis, J.; Porcher, R.; Gayat, E.; Nikolaou, M.; Boas, F.V.; Delgado, J.F.; Follath, F. Short-term survival by treatment among patients hospitalized with acute heart failure: The global

ALARM-HF registry using propensity scoring methods. *Intensive Care Med.* **2011**, *37*, 290–301. [CrossRef] [PubMed]

27. Pollesello, P.; Parissis, J.; Kivikko, M.; Harjola, V.-P. Levosimendan meta-analyses: Is there a pattern in the effect on mortality? *Int. J. Cardiol.* **2016**, *209*, 77–83. [CrossRef] [PubMed]
28. Hasenfuss, G.; Pieske, B.; Castell, M.; Kretschmann, B.; Maier, L.S.; Just, H. Influence of the novel inotropic agent levosimendan on isometric tension and calcium cycling in failing human myocardium. *Circulation* **1998**, *98*, 2141–2147. [CrossRef] [PubMed]
29. Nagy, L.; Pollesello, P.; Papp, Z. Inotropes and inodilators for acute heart failure: Sarcomere active drugs in focus. *J. Cardiovasc. Pharmacol.* **2014**, *64*, 199–208. [CrossRef]
30. Pollesello, P.; Papp, Z.; Papp, J.G. Calcium sensitizers: What have we learned over the last 25 years? *Int. J. Cardiol.* **2016**, *203*, 543–548. [CrossRef]
31. Mebazaa, A.; Nieminen, M.S.; Filippatos, G.S.; Cleland, J.G.; Salon, J.E.; Thakkar, R.; Padley, R.J.; Huang, B.; Cohen-Solal, A. Levosimendan vs. dobutamine: Outcomes for acute heart failure patients on β-blockers in SURVIVE. *Eur. J. Heart Fail.* **2009**, *11*, 304–311. [CrossRef]
32. Bergh, C.-H.; Andersson, B.; Dahlström, U.; Forfang, K.; Kivikko, M.; Sarapohja, T.; Ullman, B.; Wikström, G. Intravenous levosimendan vs. dobutamine in acute decompensated heart failure patients on beta-blockers. *Eur. J. Heart Fail.* **2010**, *12*, 404–410. [CrossRef]
33. Ponikowski, P.; Voors, A.A.; Anker, S.D.; Bueno, H.; Cleland, J.G.F.; Coats, A.J.S.; Falk, V.; González-Juanatey, J.R.; Harjola, V.-P.; Jankowska, E.A.; et al. 2016 ESC Guidelines for the diagnosis and treatment of acute and chronic heart failure: The Task Force for the diagnosis and treatment of acute and chronic heart failure of the European Society of Cardiology (ESC) Developed with the special contribution of the Heart Failure Association (HFA) of the ESC. *Eur. Heart J.* **2016**, *37*, 2129–2200. [PubMed]
34. Altenberger, J.; Parissis, J.T.; Ulmer, H.; Poelzl, G.; LevoRep Investigators. Rationale and design of the multicentre randomized trial investigating the efficacy and safety of pulsed infusions of levosimendan in outpatients with advanced heart failure (LevoRep study). *Eur. J. Heart Fail.* **2010**, *12*, 186–192. [CrossRef] [PubMed]
35. Comín-Colet, J.; Manito, N.; Segovia-Cubero, J.; Delgado, J.; García Pinilla, J.M.; Almenar, L.; Crespo-Leiro, M.G.; Sionis, A.; Blasco, T.; Pascual-Figal, D.; et al. Efficacy and safety of intermittent intravenous outpatient administration of levosimendan in patients with advanced heart failure: The LION-HEART multicentre randomised trial: Levosimendan in advanced HF: The LION-HEART trial. *Eur. J. Heart Fail.* **2018**, *20*, 1128–1136. [CrossRef] [PubMed]
36. García-González, M.J.; LAICA Study Investigators. Efficacy and security of intermittent repeated levosimendan administration in patients with advanced heart failure: A randomized, double-blind, placebo controlled multicenter trial: LAICA study. In Proceedings of the European Society of Cardiology—Heart Failure Association Congress, Florence, Italy, 21 May 2016.
37. Silvetti, S.; Nieminen, M.S. Repeated or intermittent levosimendan treatment in advanced heart failure: An updated meta-analysis. *Int. J. Cardiol.* **2016**, *202*, 138–143. [CrossRef]
38. Silvetti, S.; Belletti, A.; Fontana, A.; Pollesello, P. Rehospitalization after intermittent levosimendan treatment in advanced heart failure patients: A meta-analysis of randomized trials: Repeated levosimendan in AdHF and rehospitalization. *ESC Heart Fail.* **2017**, *4*, 595–604. [CrossRef]
39. Oliva, F.; Perna, E.; Marini, M.; Nassiacos, D.; Cirò, A.; Malfatto, G.; Morandi, F.; Caico, I.; Perna, G.; Meloni, S.; et al. Scheduled intermittent inotropes for ambulatory advanced heart failure. The RELEVANT-HF multicentre collaboration. *Int. J. Cardiol.* **2018**, *272*, 255–259. [CrossRef]
40. Müller, C.E. GALACTIC—Goal-Directed AfterLoad Reduction in Acute Congestive Cardiac Decompensation. ESC Congress 2019, Paris, France. Hot Line Session 3. Available online: https://esc365.escardio.org/Congress/ESC-CONGRESS-2019/Hot-Line-Session-3/202174-galactic-goal-directed-afterload-reduction-in-acute-congestive-cardiac-decompensation-a-randomized-controlled-trial#video (accessed on 3 October 2019).
41. McCullough, P.A. How trialists and pharmaceutical sponsors have failed us by thinking that acute heart failure Is a 48-hour illness. *Am. J. Cardiol.* **2017**, *120*, 505–508. [CrossRef]
42. Triposkiadis, F.; Butler, J.; Abboud, F.M.; Armstrong, P.W.; Adamopoulos, S.; Atherton, J.J.; Backs, J.; Bauersachs, J.; Burkhoff, D.; Bonow, R.O.; et al. The continuous heart failure spectrum: Moving beyond an ejection fraction classification. *Eur. Heart. J.* **2019**, *40*, 2155–2163. [CrossRef]

43. Severino, P.; Mariani, M.V.; Fedele, F. Futility in cardiology: The need for a change in perspectives. *Eur. J. Heart Fail.* **2019**. [CrossRef]
44. Fedele, F.; Mancone, M.; Adamo, F.; Severino, P. Heart failure with preserved, mid-range, and reduced ejection fraction: The misleading definition of the new guidelines. *Cardiol. Rev.* **2017**, *25*, 4–5. [CrossRef]
45. Fedele, F.; Severino, P.; Calcagno, S.; Mancone, M. Heart failure: TNM-like classification. *J. Am. Coll. Cardiol.* **2014**, *63*, 1959–1960. [CrossRef] [PubMed]
46. De Backer, D.; Bakker, J.; Cecconi, M.; Hajjar, L.; Liu, D.W.; Lobo, S.; Monnet, X.; Morelli, A.; Myatra, S.N.; Perel, A.; et al. Alternatives to the Swan–Ganz catheter. *Intensive Care Med.* **2018**, *44*, 730–741. [CrossRef] [PubMed]
47. Shameer, K.; Johnson, K.W.; Glicksberg, B.S.; Dudley, J.T.; Sengupta, P.P. Machine learning in cardiovascular medicine: Are we there yet? *Heart* **2018**, *104*, 1156–1164. [CrossRef] [PubMed]
48. Johnson, K.W.; Torres Soto, J.; Glicksberg, B.S.; Shameer, K.; Miotto, R.; Ali, M.; Ashley, E.; Dudley, J.T. Artificial Intelligence in Cardiology. *J. Am. Coll. Cardiol.* **2018**, *71*, 2668–2679. [CrossRef] [PubMed]
49. Sim, I. Mobile Devices and Health. *N. Engl. J. Med.* **2019**, *381*, 956–968. [CrossRef]
50. Eurlings, C.G.M.J.; Boyne, J.J.; de Boer, R.A.; Brunner-La Rocca, H.P. Telemedicine in heart failure—more than nice to have? *Neth. Heart J.* **2019**, *27*, 5–15. [CrossRef]
51. Bondar, G.; Togashi, R.; Cadeiras, M.; Schaenman, J.; Cheng, R.K.; Masukawa, L.; Hai, J.; Bao, T.-M.; Chu, D.; Chang, E.; et al. Association between preoperative peripheral blood mononuclear cell gene expression profiles, early postoperative organ function recovery potential and long-term survival in advanced heart failure patients undergoing mechanical circulatory support. *PLoS ONE* **2017**, *12*, e0189420. [CrossRef]
52. Deng, M.C. A peripheral blood transcriptome biomarker test to diagnose functional recovery potential in advanced heart failure. *Biomark. Med.* **2018**, *12*, 619–635. [CrossRef]
53. Krittanawong, C.; Namath, A.; Lanfear, D.E.; Tang, W.H.W. Practical pharmacogenomic approaches to heart failure therapeutics. *Curr. Treat. Options Cardiovasc. Med.* **2016**, *18*, 60. [CrossRef]
54. Gensini, G.F.; Alderighi, C.; Rasoini, R.; Mazzanti, M.; Casolo, G. Value of telemonitoring and telemedicine in heart failure management. *Card. Fail. Rev.* **2017**, *3*, 116–121. [CrossRef]
55. Hemingway, H.; Asselbergs, F.W.; Danesh, J.; Dobson, R.; Maniadakis, N.; Maggioni, A.; van Thiel, G.J.M.; Cronin, M.; Brobert, G.; Vardas, P.; et al. Big data from electronic health records for early and late translational cardiovascular research: Challenges and potential. *Eur. Heart J.* **2018**, *39*, 1481–1495. [CrossRef] [PubMed]
56. Narula, S.; Shameer, K.; Salem Omar, A.M.; Dudley, J.T.; Sengupta, P.P. Machine-learning algorithms to automate morphological and functional assessments in 2D echocardiography. *J. Am. Coll. Cardiol.* **2016**, *68*, 2287–2295. [CrossRef] [PubMed]
57. Maragatham, G.; Devi, S. LSTM model for prediction of heart failure in big data. *J. Med. Syst.* **2019**, *43*, 111. [CrossRef] [PubMed]
58. Safety and Efficacy of Tafamidis in Patients with Transthyretin Cardimyopathy (ATTR-ACT). Available online: https://clinicaltrials.gov/ct2/show/results/NCT01994889?term=NCT01994889.&rank=1 (accessed on 11 September 2019).
59. Pölzl, G.; Allipour Birgani, S.; Comín-Colet, J.; Delgado, J.F.; Fedele, F.; García-Gonzáles, M.J.; Gustafsson, F.; Masip, J.; Papp, Z.; Störk, S.; et al. Repetitive levosimendan infusions for patients with advanced Chronic heart failure in the vulnerable post-discharge period: Rationale and design of the LeoDOR Trial. *Esc. Heart Fail.* **2019**, *6*, 174–181. [CrossRef] [PubMed]
60. Pölzl, G.; Altenberger, J.; Baholli, L.; Beltrán, P.; Borbély, A.; Comin-Colet, J.; Delgado, J.F.; Fedele, F.; Fontana, A.; Fruhwald, F.; et al. Repetitive use of levosimendan in advanced heart failure: Need for stronger evidence in a field in dire need of a useful therapy. *Int. J. Cardiol.* **2017**, *243*, 389–395. [CrossRef] [PubMed]
61. Collins, S.P.; Lindsell, C.J.; Pang, P.S.; Storrow, A.B.; Peacock, W.F.; Levy, P.; Rahbar, M.H.; Del Junco, D.; Gheorghiade, M.; Berry, D.A. Bayesian adaptive trial design in acute heart failure syndromes: Moving beyond the mega trial. *Am. Heart J.* **2012**, *164*, 138–145. [CrossRef] [PubMed]
62. Lin, J.; Bunn, V. Comparison of multi-arm multi-stage design and adaptive randomization in platform clinical trials. *Contemp. Clin. Trials* **2017**, *54*, 48–59. [CrossRef]
63. Wason, J.M.S.; Trippa, L. A comparison of Bayesian adaptive randomization and multi-stage designs for multi-arm clinical trials. *Stat. Med.* **2014**, *33*, 2206–2221. [CrossRef]
64. Saville, B.R.; Berry, S.M. Efficiencies of platform clinical trials: A vision of the future. *Clin. Trials* **2016**, *13*, 358–366. [CrossRef]

65. Morrell, L.; Hordern, J.; Brown, L.; Sydes, M.R.; Amos, C.L.; Kaplan, R.S.; Parmar, M.K.B.; Maughan, T.S. Mind the gap? The platform trial as a working environment. *Trials* **2019**, *20*, 297. [CrossRef]

66. Hague, D.; Townsend, S.; Masters, L.; Rauchenberger, M.; Van Looy, N.; Diaz-Montana, C.; Gannon, M.; James, N.; Maughan, T.; Parmar, M.K.B.; et al. Changing platforms without stopping the train: Experiences of data management and data management systems when adapting platform protocols by adding and closing comparisons. *Trials* **2019**, *20*, 294. [CrossRef] [PubMed]

67. Schiavone, F.; Bathia, R.; Letchemanan, K.; Masters, L.; Amos, C.; Bara, A.; Brown, L.; Gilson, C.; Pugh, C.; Atako, N.; et al. This is a platform alteration: A trial management perspective on the operational aspects of adaptive and platform and umbrella protocols. *Trials* **2019**, *20*, 264. [CrossRef] [PubMed]

68. Packer, M. Why are physicians so confused about acute heart failure? *N. Engl. J. Med.* **2019**, *381*, 776–777. [CrossRef] [PubMed]

69. Blecker, S.; Sontag, D.; Horwitz, L.I.; Kuperman, G.; Park, H.; Reyentovich, A.; Katz, S.D. Early identification of patients with acute decompensated heart failure. *J. Card. Fail.* **2018**, *24*, 357–362. [CrossRef]

70. Blecker, S.; Katz, S.D.; Horwitz, L.I.; Kuperman, G.; Park, H.; Gold, A.; Sontag, D. Comparison of approaches for heart failure case identification from electronic health record data. *JAMA Cardiol.* **2016**, *1*, 1014. [CrossRef]

71. Golas, S.B.; Shibahara, T.; Agboola, S.; Otaki, H.; Sato, J.; Nakae, T.; Hisamitsu, T.; Kojima, G.; Felsted, J.; Kakarmath, S.; et al. A machine learning model to predict the risk of 30-day readmissions in patients with heart failure: A retrospective analysis of electronic medical records data. *BMC Med. Inf. Decis. Mak.* **2018**, *18*, 44. [CrossRef]

72. Karanasiou, G.S.; Tripoliti, E.E.; Papadopoulos, T.G.; Kalatzis, F.G.; Goletsis, Y.; Naka, K.K.; Bechlioulis, A.; Errachid, A.; Fotiadis, D.I. Predicting adherence of patients with HF through machine learning techniques. *Healthc. Technol. Lett.* **2016**, *3*, 165–170. [CrossRef]

73. Kreusser, M.M.; Tschierschke, R.; Beckendorf, J.; Baxmann, T.; Frankenstein, L.; Dösch, A.O.; Schultz, J.-H.; Giannitsis, E.; Pleger, S.T.; Ruhparwar, A.; et al. The need for dedicated advanced heart failure units to optimize heart failure care: Impact of optimized advanced heart failure unit care on heart transplant outcome in high-risk patients: The need for dedicated AHFUs to optimize HF care. *ESC Heart Fail.* **2018**, *5*, 1108–1117. [CrossRef]

74. Koehler, F.; Koehler, K.; Deckwart, O.; Prescher, S.; Wegscheider, K.; Kirwan, B.-A.; Winkler, S.; Vettorazzi, E.; Bruch, L.; Oeff, M.; et al. Efficacy of telemedical interventional management in patients with heart failure (TIM-HF2): A randomised, controlled, parallel-group, unmasked trial. *Lancet* **2018**, *392*, 1047–1057. [CrossRef]

75. Möckel, M.; Koehler, K.; Anker, S.D.; Vollert, J.; Moeller, V.; Koehler, M.; Gehrig, S.; Wiemer, J.C.; Haehling, S.; Koehler, F. Biomarker guidance allows a more personalized allocation of patients for remote patient management in heart failure: Results from the TIM-HF2 trial. *Eur. J. Heart Fail.* **2019**. [CrossRef]

76. Matsumura, T.; Matsui, M.; Iwata, Y.; Asakura, M.; Saito, T.; Fujimura, H.; Sakoda, S. A Pilot Study of Tranilast for Cardiomyopathy of Muscular Dystrophy. *Intern. Med.* **2018**, *57*, 311–318. [CrossRef] [PubMed]

77. Andrès, E.; Talha, S.; Zulfiqar, A.-A.; Hajjam, M.; Ervé, S.; Hajjam, J.; Gény, B.; Hajjam El Hassani, A. Current research and new perspectives of telemedicine in chronic heart failure: Narrative review and points of interest for the clinician. *J. Clin. Med.* **2018**, *7*, 544. [CrossRef] [PubMed]

78. Maack, C.; Eschenhagen, T.; Hamdani, N.; Heinzel, F.R.; Lyon, A.R.; Manstein, D.J.; Metzger, J.; Papp, Z.; Tocchetti, C.G.; Yilmaz, M.B.; et al. Treatments targeting inotropy. *Eur. Heart J.* **2018**. [CrossRef] [PubMed]

79. Nagy, L.; Pollesello, P.; Haikala, H.; Végh, Á.; Sorsa, T.; Levijoki, J.; Szilágyi, S.; Édes, I.; Tóth, A.; Papp, Z.; et al. ORM-3819 promotes cardiac contractility through Ca2+ sensitization in combination with selective PDE III inhibition, a novel approach to inotropy. *Eur. J. Pharm.* **2016**, *775*, 120–129. [CrossRef] [PubMed]

80. Márton, Z.; Pataricza, J.; Pollesello, P.; Varró, A.; Papp, J.G. The Novel inodilator ORM-3819 relaxes isolated porcine coronary arteries: Role of voltage-gated potassium channel activation. *J. Cardiovasc. Pharm.* **2019**, *74*, 218–224. [CrossRef] [PubMed]

81. Nielsen, T.B.; Brass, E.P.; Gilbert, D.N.; Bartlett, J.G.; Spellberg, B. Sustainable discovery and development of antibiotics—Is a nonprofit approach the future? *N. Engl. J. Med.* **2019**, *381*, 503–505. [CrossRef]

82. Dungen, H.-D.; Petroni, R.; Correale, M.; Coiro, S.; Monitillo, F.; Triggiani, M.; Leone, M.; Antohi, E.-L.; Ishihara, S.; Sarwar, C.M.S.; et al. A new educational program in heart failure drug development: The Brescia international master program. *J. Cardiovasc. Med.* **2018**, *19*, 411–421. [CrossRef]

14

Hypertension, Thrombosis, Kidney Failure and Diabetes: Is COVID-19 an Endothelial Disease? A Comprehensive Evaluation of Clinical and Basic Evidence

Celestino Sardu [1,2,†], Jessica Gambardella [3,4,†], Marco Bruno Morelli [4,5,†], Xujun Wang [4], Raffaele Marfella [1] and Gaetano Santulli [3,4,5,*]

1 Department of Advanced Medical and Surgical Sciences, University of Campania "Luigi Vanvitelli", 80100 Naples, Italy; drsarducele@gmail.com (C.S.); raffaele.marfella@unicampania.it (R.M.)
2 Department of Medical Sciences, International University of Health and Medical Sciences "Saint Camillus", 00131 Rome, Italy
3 Department of Advanced Biomedical Sciences, International Translational Research and Medical Education Academic Research Unit (ITME), "Federico II" University, 80131 Naples, Italy; jessica.gambardella@einsteinmed.org
4 Department of Medicine, Division of Cardiology, Albert Einstein College of Medicine, Wilf Family Cardiovascular Research Institute, New York, NY 10461, USA; marco.morelli@einstein.yu.edu (M.B.M.); xujun.wang@einsteinmed.org (X.W.)
5 Department of Molecular Pharmacology, Fleischer Institute for Diabetes and Metabolism (FIDAM), Montefiore University Hospital, New York, NY 10461, USA
* Correspondence: gaetano.santulli@einsteinmed.org
† These authors equally contributed to this work.

Abstract: The symptoms most commonly reported by patients affected by coronavirus disease (COVID-19) include cough, fever, and shortness of breath. However, other major events usually observed in COVID-19 patients (e.g., high blood pressure, arterial and venous thromboembolism, kidney disease, neurologic disorders, and diabetes mellitus) indicate that the virus is targeting the endothelium, one of the largest organs in the human body. Herein, we report a systematic and comprehensive evaluation of both clinical and preclinical evidence supporting the hypothesis that the endothelium is a key target organ in COVID-19, providing a mechanistic rationale behind its systemic manifestations.

Keywords: ACE2, acute kidney injury; blood pressure; catepsin; coronavirus; COVID; cytokine storm; endothelium; heparin; Kawasaki disease

---

1. Introduction

Coronavirus disease (COVID-19) represents a public health crisis of global proportions [1]. Caused by the *severe acute respiratory syndrome corona virus 2* (SARS-CoV-2), COVID-19 was first announced in December 2019 in Wuhan, the capital of China's Hubei province [2,3].

The symptoms most commonly reported include cough, fever, and shortness of breath. The pathophysiology of the disease explains why respiratory symptoms are so common: indeed, the virus accesses host cells via the protein angiotensin-converting enzyme 2 (ACE2) [4,5], which is very abundant in the lungs [6].

Nevertheless, ACE2 is also expressed by endothelial cells [7,8], and other major clinical events usually observed in COVID-19 patients (e.g., high blood pressure [9–13], thrombosis [14–16] kidney disease [17,18], pulmonary embolism [19,20], cerebrovascular and neurologic disorders [21,22]) indicate that the virus is targeting the endothelium [23], one of the largest organs in the human body [24–26]. The cases of Kawasaki disease reported in young COVID-19 patients [27] support our view of a systemic vasculitis caused by SARS-CoV-2.

2. Pathogenesis of COVID-19

To access host cells, SARS-CoV-2 uses a surface glycoprotein (peplomer) known as spike; ACE2 has been shown to be a co-receptor for coronavirus entry [28–30]. Therefore, the density of ACE2 in each tissue may correlate with the severity of the disease in that tissue [31–36]. Other receptors on the surface of human cells have been suggested to mediate the entry of SARS-CoV-2 [5], including transmembrane serine protease 2 (TMPRSS2) [37,38], sialic acid receptors [39,40], and extracellular matrix metalloproteinase inducer (CD147, also known as basigin) [41]. Additionally, catepsin B and L have been shown to be critical entry factors in the pathogenesis of COVID-19 [38,42].

Intriguingly, all of these factors involved in the entry of SARS-CoV-2 in the host cell are known to be expressed by endothelial cells [43–49] (Figure 1).

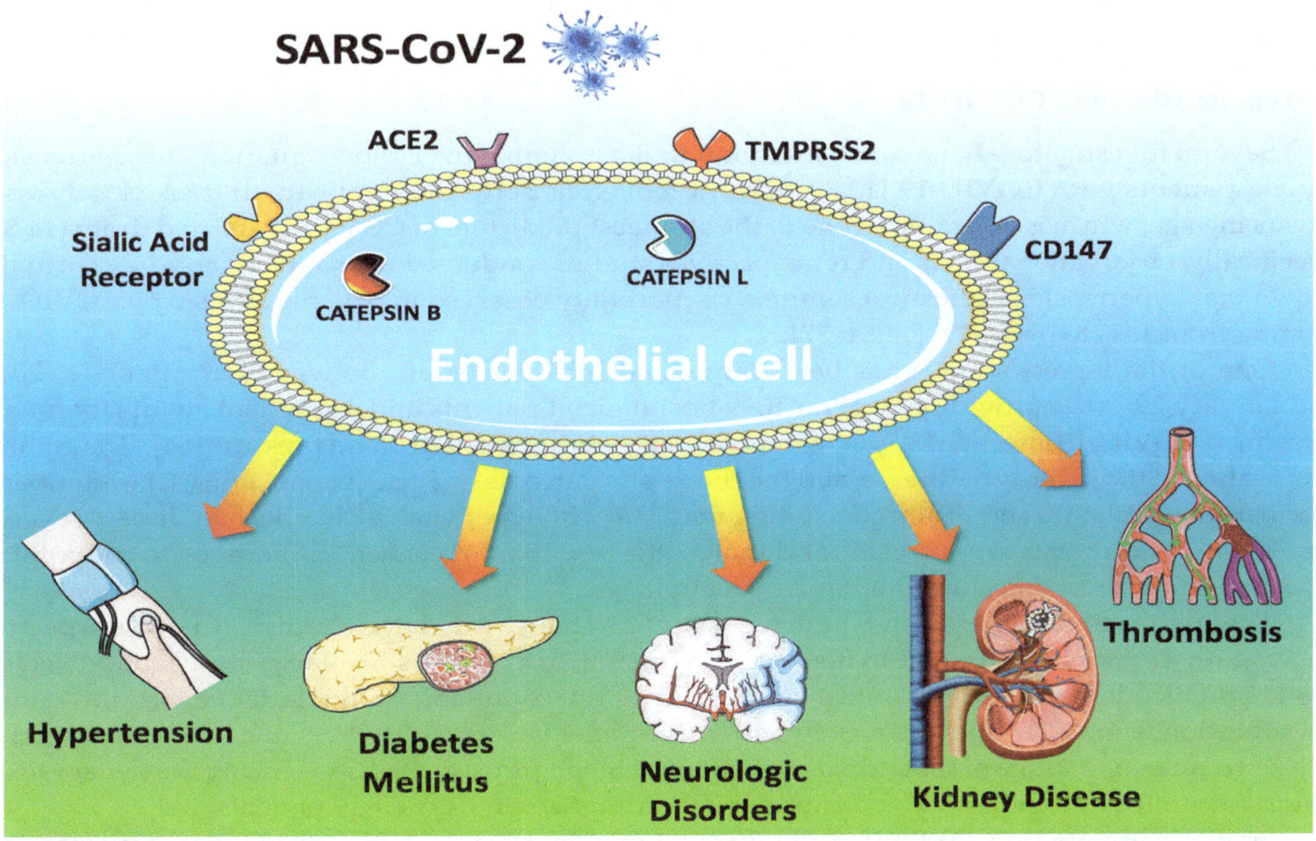

Figure 1. Endothelial dysfunction is a major determinant of COVID-19. The SARS-CoV-2 coronavirus accesses host cells via the binding of its spike glycoprotein to angiotensin-converting enzyme 2 (ACE2), sialic acid receptor, transmembrane serine protease 2 (TMPRSS2), and extracellular matrix metalloproteinase inducer (CD147); catepsin B and L also participate in virus entry. All of these factors are expressed in endothelial cells. Endothelial dysfunction is a common feature of the clinical manifestations observed in COVID-19 patients. All of the drugs proposed as a potential therapeutic strategy to treat COVID-19 patients have been shown to improve endothelial function, including tocilizumab, colchicine, chloroquine/hydroxychloroquine, azithromycin, and famotidine (see text for details and references).

ACE2 remains the most studied of these receptors [34,50–54]: for instance, its genetic inactivation has been shown to cause severe lung injury in H5N1-challenged mice [55], whereas administration of recombinant human ACE2 ameliorates H5N1 virus-induced lung injury in mice [55].

ACE2 is currently at the center of a heated debate among physicians [56–59], and there are concerns that medical management of hypertension, including the use of inhibitors of the renin-angiotensin-aldosterone system (RAAS), may contribute to the adverse health outcomes observed [34,60,61]; TMPRSS2 binds the viral spike glycoprotein [37]; recent structural assays have suggested that coronaviruses can bind sialic acid receptors [39]; CD147 has been shown to be essential for the entry of cytomegalovirus into endothelial cells [46]; both catepsin B [47] and L [49] are present in endothelial cells (Figure 1).

The endothelium prevents blood clotting by providing an antithrombotic surface, maintained by heparan sulphate present in the matrix surrounding the cells [62,63], by the expression of tissue factor inhibitor [64], thrombomodulin [65], and by the production of tissue-type plasminogen activator that promotes fibrinolysis [66,67].

Endothelial dysfunction refers to a systemic condition in which the endothelium loses its physiological properties, including the tendency to promote vasodilation, fibrinolysis, and anti-aggregation [68–72]; moreover, endothelial dysfunction appears to be a consistent finding in patients with diabetes [69,73–78]. Here we will discuss clinical and preclinical findings supporting our hypothesis [79] that COVID-19 impairs endothelial function (Figure 1).

3. Hypertension and COVID-19

Several investigators have called attention to the potential over-representation of hypertension among patients with COVID-19 [13,80–82]. Moreover, hypertension appears to track closely with advancing age, which is emerging as one of the strongest predictors of COVID-19–related death [14,83]. Specifically, observational trials and retrospectives studies conducted near Wuhan area have actually shown that hypertension is the most common co-morbidity observed in patients affected by COVID-19, ranging from 15% to over 30% [14,84–87].

One of the largest studies has been conducted by Guan et al. between December 11, 2019, and January 29, 2020, providing data on 1099 hospitalized patients and outpatients with laboratory-confirmed COVID-19 infection [84]; in this cohort, 165 (~15%) had high blood pressure [84]. The authors also evaluated the severity of disease, and the composite outcome of intensive care unit (ICU) admission, mechanical ventilation and death, concluding that 23.7% of hypertensive patients had disease severity (vs. 13.4% of normotensive subjects), and that 35.8% (vs. 13.7%) reached the composite endpoint of ICU admission, mechanical ventilation and death [84].

The high rate of hypertensive patients with COVID-19 was later confirmed in a prospective analysis on 41 patients admitted to hospital in Wuhan [85] as well as in a large study conducted on 138 hospitalized patients with confirmed COVID-19 infection [86]. In the latter report, the rate of hypertension was 31.2%, and 58.3% of hypertensive patients with COVID-19 infection were admitted to ICU compared to 21.6% of individuals with normal blood pressure [86], evidencing the hypertensive state as a common co-morbidity and cause of ICU admission in COVID-19 patients [86].

Similarly, among 191 COVID-19 patients from Jinyintan Hospital and Wuhan Pulmonary Hospital, 58 (30%) had hypertension, and 26 (48%) did not survive COVID-19, whereas 32 (23%) were survivors [14]. The 30% rate of hypertensive patients was further confirmed in an analysis based on the severity of COVID-19 conducted on 140 patients in Wuhan: 58 patients were classified as severe vs. 82 patients classified as not severe: hypertensive patients represented 37.9% of severe vs. 24.4% of not severe COVID-19 patients [87]. In a cohort of 1590 patients from 575 hospitals, underlying hypertension was independently associated with severe COVID-19 (hazard ratio 1.58, 95% CI: 1.07–2.32) [13]. Overall, these findings confirm a dual aspect of hypertension during COVID-19 pandemic: first, hypertension is the most common co-morbidity observed in COVID-19 patients; second, hypertension is evidenced in patients with worse prognosis and higher rate of death.

These studies also raise numerous questions regarding the association between hypertension and COVID-19. Indeed, hypertension is known to be one of most common diseases and co-morbidities worldwide, considered a silent killer for the worldwide population [88]. We speculate that the higher rate of hypertension and the worse prognosis in patients with COVID-19 infection could be seen as the spy of a cause-effect mechanism, more than as a casual pre-existing association between these two different diseases.

4. ACE2 and Anti-Hypertensive Drugs: What Do We Know?

ACE inhibitors (ACEi) and angiotensin II receptor blockers (ARB) represent very effective strategies for the treatment of hypertension [88]. These drugs reduce the effects of renin-angiotensin axis by inhibiting ACE (ACEi) or by blocking the angiotensin receptors (ARB), as shown in Figure 2. A growing question for the scientific community and physicians is to understand whether ACEi/ARB could affect the prognosis of hypertensive COVID-19 patients [34,89–91].

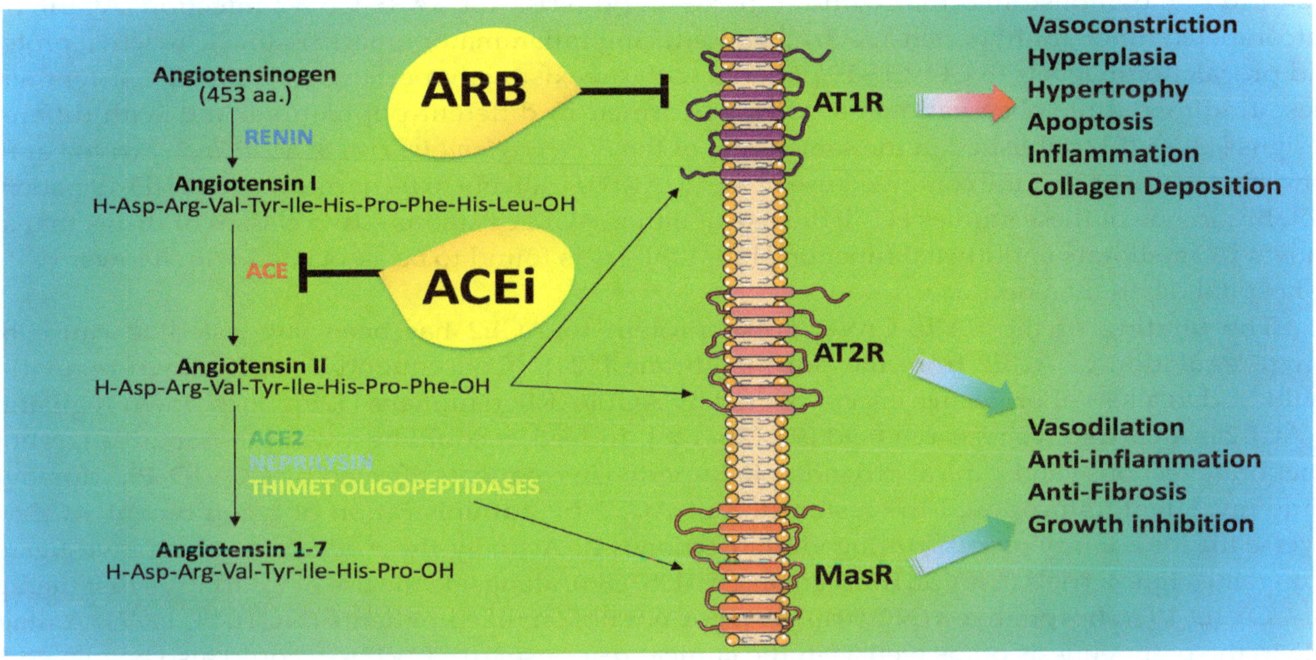

Figure 2. Angiotensin-converting enzyme inhibitors (ACEi) and blockers of the angiotensin receptor 1 (ARB). Angiotensin II and Angiotensin 1–7 binds heptahelical receptors; namely, angiotensin II can activate AT1R (type 1 angiotensin II receptor) and AT2R (type 2 angiotensin II receptor), whereas angiotensin 1–7 binds the Mas Receptor (MasR). The actions mediated by these receptors are depicted in the figure.

The exact role of ACEi/ARB in the control of ACE2 molecular pathways is controversial: indeed, preclinical studies evidenced that the selective blockade of either angiotensin II synthesis or activity in rats induces increases in ACE2 gene expression and activity [92–96]; similarly, treating infarcted rats with ARB increased plasma concentration of angiotensin 1–7 and ACE2 [97]. In mice, ARB treatment augmented ACE2 mRNA and protein levels [98,99] and prevented the decrease in ACE2 protein levels induced by Angiotensin II [100]. Equally important, mineralocorticoid receptor blockers prevented aldosterone-induced reduction in cardiac ACE2 mRNA expression in rat cardiomyocytes [101] and increased ACE2 expression and activity in murine hearts and in monocyte-derived macrophages obtained from ten patients with heart failure [102].

Nevertheless, there is no clinical evidence that ACEi could directly affect molecular pathways linked to ACE2 activity. For instance, urinary ACE2 levels were reported to be higher in patients treated with olmesartan vs. untreated controls, but this finding was not observed in patients treated with other ARB or enalapril [103]; instead, another study reported no difference in ACE2 activity in patients who were taking ACEi or ARB vs. untreated patients [89]. Of note, ACE2, which functions as a carboxypeptidase [104] is not inhibited by clinically prescribed ACEi.

In particular, ACE2 acts to counterbalance the effect of ACE [105]; indeed, whereas ACE generates angiotensin II from angiotensin I, ACE2 converts angiotensin II into an active heptapeptide (angiotensin 1-7), which binds the Mas receptor (MasR), triggering vasodilative, anti-oxidant, and anti-inflammatory properties [106–109] (Figure 2).

Some media sources have recently called for the discontinuation of ACEi and ARB, both prophylactically and in the context of suspected COVID-19 [110]. However, several associations have recommended not to suspend these therapies [61,111–114], and these recommendations have been confirmed by three recent studies: the first one performed on 362 hypertensive patients showed that ACEIs/ARBs are not associated with the severity or mortality of COVID-19 [91]; the second one verified the effects of ACEI/ARB on 1128 hypertensive COVID-19 patients, showing that the use of ACEI/ARB was associated with lower risk of all-cause mortality compared with ACEI/ARB non-users [115]; the third one demonstrated that without increasing the risk for SARS-CoV-2 infection, ACEI/ARB outcompeted other antihypertensive drugs in reducing inflammatory markers like C-reactive protein and procalcitonin levels in COVID-19 patients with preexisting hypertension [116]. Consistent with these findings, three observational studies performed in different populations and with different designs [117–119] (published in the same issue of the *New England Journal of Medicine*), arrived at the consistent message that the continued use of ACEI/ARB is unlikely to be harmful in COVID-19 patients. Notably, in one of these studies [117], the use of either ACEI or statins—two classes of drugs that are known to ameliorate endothelial function [120–123]—was found to be associated with a lower risk of in-hospital death than non-use.

The binding of the SARS-CoV-2 spike protein to ACE2 has been suggested to cause the down-regulation of ACE2 from the cell membrane [124]. Consequently, ACE2 down-regulation could lead to a loss of protective effects exerted by ACEi/ARB in humans [125]. Such down-regulation of ACE2 is an attractive research field [95,126–128]. Indeed, it could be a valid therapeutic target to ameliorate response and clinical prognosis in hypertensive patients affected by COVID-19. Moreover, some investigators proposed the restoration of ACE2 by administration of recombinant ACE2 to reverse the lung-injury process during viral infections [4]. Actually, these effects are being investigated in ongoing clinical trials (ClinicalTrials.gov NCT04287686), alongside the use of losartan as first therapy for COVID-19 in hospitalized (NCT04312009) or not hospitalized patients (NCT04311177). A major role in the pathogenesis of (as well as in the clinical response to) COVID-19 could also be played by ACE2 polymorphisms, which are relatively under-investigated if compared to ACE [129,130].

Finally, we have to consider the higher rate of cardiac injury and adverse outcomes in hypertensive patients during the COVID-19 pandemic [131–133]. Therefore, ACEi/ARB chronic therapy should not be discontinued in hypertensive patients with COVID-19. Indeed, the loss of their pneumo- and cardio-protective effects could be detrimental [88]. In addition, in the absence of adequate follow-up visits, switching from ACEi/ARB to another anti-hypertensive therapy could cause a suboptimal control of blood pressure.

Thus, as suggested by several medical associations [110], in the absence of definitive clinical studies and without clear evidence, hypertensive patients should avoid discontinuation and/or therapeutic switching during COVID-19 infection.

Another noteworthy feature of COVID-19 for cardiologists is the significant decrease in the rates of hospital admissions for acute coronary syndromes which has been reported both in Italy [134] and US [135] during the COVID-19 outbreak, and despite being initially attributed to reduced air pollution, better adherence to treatment, or absence of occupational stress during lockdown, this phenomenon seems to be most likely due to the fear of going to the hospital and/or seeking medical attention during a pandemic. Unfortunately, the current decline in hospitalization for acute coronary syndromes will trigger an increase in cases of heart failure in the near future.

5. Kidney Disease in COVID-19

Acute kidney injury (AKI) has been reported in > 20% of critically ill or deceased COVID-19 patients, a percentage that is consistent in studies from China [136], Italy [137] and United States [10]. It is important to note that AKI, proteinuria, and hematuria have been independently associated with a higher risk of death in COVID-19 patients [138]. Furthermore, in a meta-analysis including 1389 COVID-19 patients [139], the prevalence of underlying chronic kidney disease was significantly more frequent among those with a severe COVID-19 disease (3.3% vs. 0.4%; odds ratio 3.03, 95% CI: 1.09–8.47).

According to immunohistochemistry assays [140], ACE2 seems not to be expressed in renal endothelial cells; however, a study based on single-cell analysis has confirmed the expression of ACE2 and TMPRSS2 in human renal endothelial cells [141], and most recently the presence of viral particles was confirmed by electron microscopy in endothelial cells of the glomerular capillary loops of a COVID-19 patient [142]. Besides, endothelial damage was a common finding in renal histopathological analyses of 26 COVID-19 patients, in the absence of interstitial inflammatory infiltrates [143].

6. Diabetes and COVID-19

Diabetes mellitus is a frequent co-morbidity and a cause of worse prognosis in COVID-19 patients [12,144–148]. Indeed, evaluating pneumonia cases of unknown causes reported in Wuhan and in patients with history of exposure to Huanan seafood market before Jan 1, 2020, 20% had diabetes [85]. Similarly, among 1099 COVID-19 patients analyzed by Guan and colleagues, 7.4% had diabetes: this percentage goes up to 16.2% among patients with severe disease (vs. 5.7% in patients with non-severe disease) [84]; furthermore, 35.8% of patients experiencing the composite endpoint of ICU admission, mechanical ventilation and death, had diabetes (vs. 13.7% of patients that did not experience such endpoint) [84]. Data from Italy show that more than two-thirds of COVID-19 patients that did not survive had diabetes [149]. In summary, diabetes is a frequent co-morbidity, a risk factor, and an independent prognostic factor in COVID-19 patients. A strong evidence of the negative effects of diabetes in COVID-19 patients is also corroborated by two meta-analyses [150,151].

The worse prognosis in patients with diabetes and COVID-19 could be attributed to the fact that the pneumonia evolves towards clinical stages more refractory to medical therapies, oxygen administration and mechanical ventilation, with necessity of ICU care. These data have been investigated in a previous study conducted in patients with SARS [152], in which the relationship between a known history of diabetes and fasting plasma glucose (FPG) levels with death and morbidity rate was assessed, showing that the percentage of patients with diabetes was significantly higher in deceased vs. survivors (21.5% vs. 3.9%, $p < 0.01$) [152]. Moreover, diabetic subjects with hypoxemia ($SaO_2 < 93\%$) had higher FPG levels and FPG was independently associated with an increased hazard ratio of mortality (1.1, 95% CI: 1.0–1.1) and hypoxia (1.1, 95% CI: 1.0–1.1) after controlling for age and gender [152]; the authors concluded that both diabetes (3.0, 95% CI: 1.4–6.3) and FPG > or = 7.0 mmol/l (3.3, 95% CI: 1.4–7.7) were independent predictors of death [152].

In COVID-19 patients, the incidence of diabetes is two times higher in ICU/severe vs. non-ICU/severe cases [151]. Indeed, the diagnosis of diabetes in a cohort of patients with COVID-19 infection evidenced a sub-group of patients with a 2.26-fold higher risk of experiencing adverse disease outcome analyses [150]. Additionally, patients with obesity and/or glucose intolerance seem to be particularly vulnerable to COVID-19 [10,148,153,154]. Unfortunately, no data are hitherto available on anti-diabetic medications and glucose homeostasis in COVID-19 patients. This aspect is really limiting, because diabetes and altered glucose homeostasis during a condition of severe pneumonia with SARS are reported as main factors of worse prognosis and death [152]. COVID-19 could also induce new onset diabetes, by augmenting insulin resistance and/or by a direct action [155] on the islets of Langerhans; supporting this view, previous studies have shown that ACE2 can be a therapeutic target to ameliorate microcirculation in the islets [156], and ACE2 is known to be expressed by pancreatic beta cells [157–162].

Moreover, frequent cases of ketoacidosis in COVID-19 patients have been reported [163]. Therefore, the investigation of anti-diabetic medications and glucose homeostasis could be harnessed to evaluate patients with higher risk of experiencing worse prognosis and death by COVID-19. We speculate that the amelioration of glucose homeostasis in diabetic COVID-19 patients by specific hypoglycemic drugs could result in the amelioration of clinical outcomes with death reduction. However, these data are not reported in trials on COVID-19, and they need to be investigated in further studies [164].

7. Thromboembolism and COVID-19

Patients with COVID19 often show clotting disorders, with organ dysfunction and coagulopathy, resulting in higher mortality [15,165,166]. Critical data came from the analysis of coagulation tests including prothrombin time (PT), activated partial thromboplastin time (APTT), antithrombin activity (AT), fibrinogen, fibrin degradation product (FDP), and D-dimer, in samples collected on admission and during the hospital stay of COVID-19 patients [167]. Non-survivors had significantly higher D-dimer and FDP levels, and longer PT vs. survivors on admission [167]. Moreover, significant reduction and lowering of fibrinogen and AT levels were observed in non-survivors during late stages of hospitalization, which is compatible with a clinical diagnosis of disseminated intravascular coagulation (DIC) [167,168]. Specifically, among 191 COVID-19 patients seen at two hospitals in Wuhan, D-dimer levels over 1 μg/L at admission predicted an 18-fold increase in odds of dying before discharge [14]. Of note, when DIC is caused by a systemic infection, it features an acute systemic over-inflammatory response, strictly linked to endothelial dysfunction [169].

Most recently a case of a COVID-19 patient with an increase of Factor VIII clotting activity and a massive elevation of von Willebrand Factor (vWF) has been reported [170], further supporting our theory: indeed, vWF can be seen as a marker of endothelial damage, since it is normally stored in Weibel-Palade bodies within endothelial cells [171]. Equally important, angiotensin II level in the plasma of COVID-19 patients was markedly elevated and linearly associated to viral load and lung injury [172]; notably, angiotensin II is known to increase microvascular permeability [173,174], to induce the transcription of tissue factor in endothelial cells [175–177], and to activate platelets [178–180]. Additionally, angiotensin II can trigger the release of several components of the complement system from endothelial cells [181–187], further corroborating the key role of endothelium in the pathogenesis of venous and arterial thrombosis in COVID-19 patients [188,189].

A dysregulated immune response, as observed in COVID-19, especially in the late stages of the disease, plays a decisive role in endothelial dysfunction and thrombosis [190,191], and microvascular permeability is crucial in viral infections [192]. Indeed, pulmonary endothelium represent a fundamental barrier between the blood and interstitium and have vital regulatory functions; specifically, endothelial cells represent one-third of the cell population of the lung [193], and pulmonary endothelial damage is considered the hallmark of acute respiratory distress syndrome (ARDS) [194]. Animal models of coronavirus-induced severe ARDS have shown that reduced ACE2 activity and loss of ACE2 in the lungs is mirrored by enhanced vascular permeability, and exacerbated pulmonary edema [108]. The functional role of endothelium in pulmonary disease is also suggested by previous reports [195,196]; for instance, the H3N2 influenza virus has been shown to infect endothelial cells in vitro and to trigger endothelial cell apoptosis, which is known to enhance platelet adhesion [197]: endothelial cell death would cause exposure of the extracellular matrix to circulating blood, favoring platelet binding; similarly, the endothelium has been shown to contribute to the development of severe disease during H5N1 influenza infection [198].

Deep vein thrombosis and/or pulmonary embolism have been previously described in patients with SARS [199–202] and cases of thrombosis complicating influenza-associated pneumonia have also been reported [203–205]. Excessive activation of the immune system in response to pathogens can lead to pathological inflammatory consequences. In the case of highly virulent 1918 and avian H5N1 influenza virus infections, the recruitment of inflammatory leukocytes followed by excessive cytokine responses is considered to be the key contributor to morbidity and mortality of the infection [206,207].

Cytokine storm syndromes (CSS) are a group of disorders representing a variety of inflammatory etiologies with the final result of overwhelming systemic inflammation, hemodynamic instability, multiple organ dysfunction, and potentially death [208,209]. Specifically, macrophage activation syndrome [210] and hemophagocytic lymphohistiocytosis (HLH) [211] represent two clinically similar CSS with an unknown degree of etiopathogenic overlap [208]. The interaction between endothelial and immune cells could play a crucial role in COVID-19, especially in severe cases and in the late stages of the disease [212]. For instance, the cytokine storm might lead to an abrupt deterioration of the inflammatory response and hyper-coagulation; the increased vulnerability of patients with cardiovascular diseases and/or diabetes might therefore simply reflect the impact of the underlying chronic inflammation and its response during SARS-CoV-2 infection. If this is the case, endothelial alterations could just be seen as an epiphenomenon.

However, according to numerous investigators, the inflammatory response observed in COVID-19 patients can be considered mild if compared to the one observed in typical ARDS and in cytokine-release syndrome [212–215]: indeed, in ARDS patients, levels of interleukin-1β and interleukin-6 have been shown to be 10 to 60 fold higher than in COVID-19 [216,217]. Therefore, other mechanisms have to be involved in order to explain the systemic manifestations reported in COVID-19 patients, and endothelial cells, known orchestrators of cytokine amplification during viral infections [218], seem to be one of the best candidates in this sense. Further supporting our view, catecholamines are considered an essential component of the cytokine release syndrome [215] and we have demonstrated that endothelial cells are able to synthetize and release catecholamines [219].

Acute pulmonary embolism, reported in COVID-19 patients [20,220–222], has been shown to be a cause of clinical deterioration in viral pneumonias [205,223]. Endothelial dysfunction is known to be a key determinant in hypertension, thrombosis, and DIC [72,224–227]. Henceforth, it is important to select COVID-19 patients at higher risk of pulmonary embolism, and practice computed tomography pulmonary angiography for the diagnosis of pulmonary thromboembolism especially in case of significant increase of D-dimer values. Anticoagulation could be a necessary therapy to control and reduce pro-thrombotic events, as well as to prevent pulmonary embolism [228].

8. Anticoagulation as a Key Therapy for COVID-19

The clinical course of COVID-19 consists of two main phases: viral infection and immune/inflammatory response (Figure 3), which require distinct therapeutic approaches. Strikingly, several drugs suggested as a potential therapeutic strategy for COVID-19 [229–231] have been shown to ameliorate endothelial function, including interleukin 6 (IL-6) receptor antagonists (e.g., tocilizumab [232]), colchicine [233], azithromycin [234], and famotidine [235].

Even the antimalaric agents chloroquine and hydroxychloroquine, initially proposed as a therapy for COVID-19 based on anecdotal data [229,236], have been shown to improve endothelial function [237,238]. If our theory is correct [239], other drugs that might be effective in treating COVID-19 patients through their beneficial effects on endothelial cells include $\alpha1$ adrenergic receptor blockers (e.g., doxazosin) [240], modulators of Sigma receptors [241–243], metformin [244], indomethacin [245], and endothelin receptor antagonists (e.g., bosentan) [246]. However, data from randomized trials confirming the actual efficacy of these drugs are not (yet) available.

As discussed before, COVID-19 infection could cause endothelial dysfunction and a hyper-coagulation state. This condition is aggravated by hypoxia, which augments thrombosis by both increasing blood viscosity and hypoxia-inducible transcription factor-dependent signaling pathway [247]. Consequently, these phenomena could result in pulmonary embolism with occlusion and micro-thrombosis in pulmonary small vessels, as observed in critical COVID-19 patients [248]. Apart from cases of pulmonary embolism, COVID-19 can cause a sepsis-associated DIC, which is defined as "sepsis-induced coagulopathy" (SIC) [169]. Thus, there is an increasing interest in anticoagulant therapy to treat COVID-19 [249].

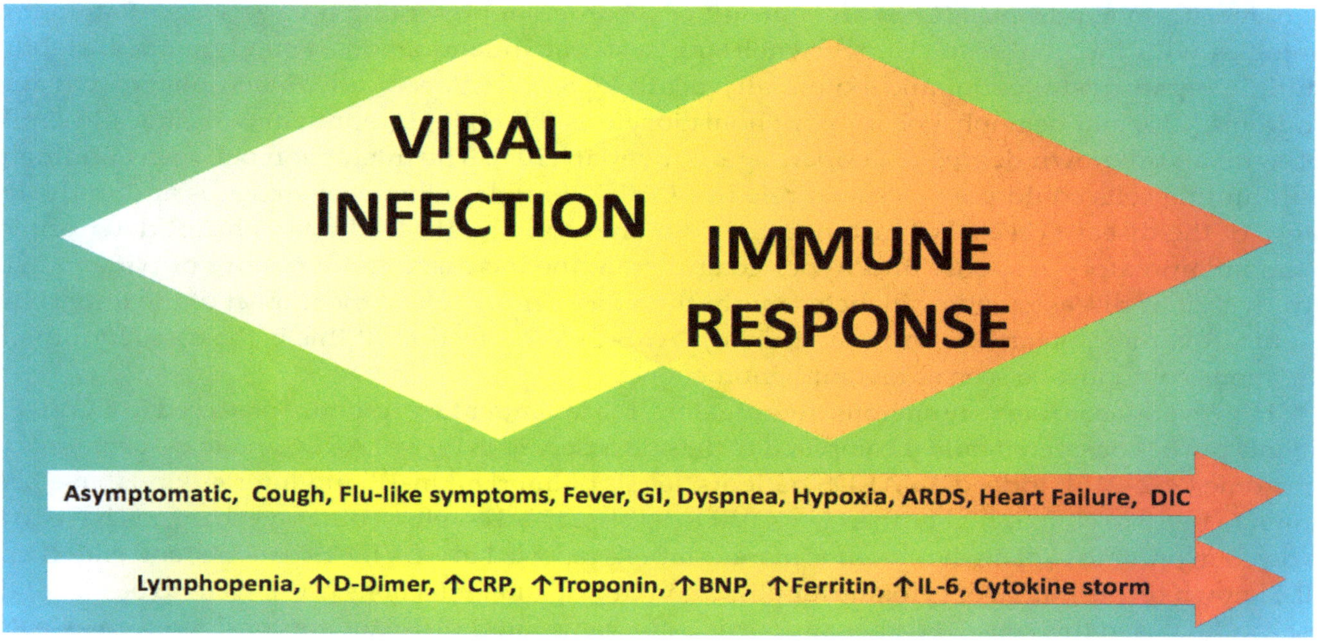

Figure 3. Clinical course of COVID-19 patients. Two main overlapping phases constitute the key pathogenic events in COVID-19: the acute phase represented by viral infection, followed by the immune/inflammatory response. Common clinical and laboratory findings are reported within the arrows at the bottom of the figure.

In a retrospective analysis conducted at Tongji Hospital of Huazhong University of Science and Technology in Wuhan, the authors examined 449 patients affected by severe COVID-19 [228]. The diagnosis of severe COVID-19 disease was made by evidence of respiratory rate ≥ 30 breaths/min, arterial oxygen saturation ≤ 93% at rest and $PaO_2/FiO_2 \leq 300$ mmHg [228]. In these patients, they reviewed and compared the parameters of coagulation tests and clinical characteristics between survivors and non-survivors to evaluate the effects of heparin therapy [228]: 94 patients received low molecular weight heparin (LMWH, 40–60 mg enoxaparin/day) and 5 received unfractionated heparin (UFH, 10000–15000 U/day), without other anti-coagulants [228]. Heparin therapy significantly reduced mortality in patients with SIC score ≥4 (40.0% vs. 64.2%, $p < 0.05$), but not in those with SIC score < 4 (29.0% vs. 22.6%, $p > 0.05$) [228]. D-dimer, PT, and age were positively, while platelet count was negatively, correlated with 28-day mortality [228]. In addition, stratifying by D-dimer values the study population, the authors reported in heparin non-users a rise of mortality linked to the rising D-dimer, and 20% reduction of mortality for patients under heparin with D-dimer exceeding 3.0 μg/mL [228]. Therefore, heparin treatment appears to be associated with better prognosis in severe COVID-19 patients with coagulopathy. The beneficial effects of heparin-based therapies are also supported by the structural analogies between heparin and heparan-sulphate, which according to some investigators may confer heparin with antiviral properties [250–254]. In absence of contraindications, we suggest the use of enoxaparin 40 mg/day in all COVID-19 patients, to be raised up to 1 mg/kg every 12 h in case of D-dimer > 3.0 μg/mL; apixaban (5 mg every 12 h) could represent a useful alternative.

Of course, the full clinical evaluation of patients with COVID-19 infection cannot leave aside the analysis of laboratory and imaging data. We believe that PT/PTT, fibrinogen, and D-Dimer should be monitored daily and anticoagulation therapy should be recommended for COVID-19 patients when the D-Dimer value is four times higher than the normal upper limit, except for patients with anticoagulant contraindications. The confirmed diagnosis of severe COVID-19 disease in patients with hypercoagulation and organ failure could evidence an early stage of sepsis-induced DIC. On the other hand, anticoagulant may not benefit unselected patients. Consequently, further prospective studies are needed to confirm these findings in COVID-19 patients, also testing other anti-aggregants and anti-coagulants (at different doses).

Author Contributions: Conceptualization, G.S.; data curation, C.S., J.G., M.B.M., X.W., R.M. and G.S. and S.R.; writing—original draft preparation, C.S., J.G. and G.S.; writing—review and editing, J.G., M.B.M. and G.S.; visualization, M.B.M. and G.S.; supervision, G.S.; funding acquisition, G.S. and J.G. A preprint version of the manuscript was sent to preprints.org by on 9 April 2020: *Preprints* 2020, 2020040204 (doi:10.20944/preprints202004.0204.v1). All authors have read and agreed to the published version of the manuscript.

References

1. Fauci, A.S.; Lane, H.C.; Redfield, R.R. Covid-19—Navigating the Uncharted. *N. Engl. J. Med.* **2020**, *382*, 1268–1269. [CrossRef] [PubMed]
2. Paules, C.I.; Marston, H.D.; Fauci, A.S. Coronavirus Infections-More Than Just the Common Cold. *JAMA* **2020**, *323*, 707. [CrossRef] [PubMed]
3. Hui, D.S.; Azhar, E.E.; Madani, T.A.; Ntoumi, F.; Kock, R.; Dar, O.; Ippolito, G.; McHugh, T.D.; Memish, Z.A.; Drosten, C.; et al. The continuing 2019-nCoV epidemic threat of novel coronaviruses to global health—The latest 2019 novel coronavirus outbreak in Wuhan, China. *Int. J. Infect. Dis.* **2020**, *91*, 264–266. [CrossRef] [PubMed]
4. Zhang, H.; Penninger, J.M.; Li, Y.; Zhong, N.; Slutsky, A.S. Angiotensin-converting enzyme 2 (ACE2) as a SARS-CoV-2 receptor: Molecular mechanisms and potential therapeutic target. *Intensive Care Med.* **2020**, *46*, 586–590. [CrossRef] [PubMed]
5. Zhou, P.; Yang, X.L.; Wang, X.G.; Hu, B.; Zhang, L.; Zhang, W.; Si, H.R.; Zhu, Y.; Li, B.; Huang, C.L.; et al. A pneumonia outbreak associated with a new coronavirus of probable bat origin. *Nature* **2020**, *579*, 270–273. [CrossRef]
6. Hamming, I.; Timens, W.; Bulthuis, M.L.; Lely, A.T.; Navis, G.; van Goor, H. Tissue distribution of ACE2 protein, the functional receptor for SARS coronavirus. A first step in understanding SARS pathogenesis. *J. Pathol.* **2004**, *203*, 631–637. [CrossRef]
7. Lovren, F.; Pan, Y.; Quan, A.; Teoh, H.; Wang, G.; Shukla, P.C.; Levitt, K.S.; Oudit, G.Y.; Al-Omran, M.; Stewart, D.J.; et al. Angiotensin converting enzyme-2 confers endothelial protection and attenuates atherosclerosis. *Am. J. Physiol. Circ. Physiol.* **2008**, *295*, H1377–H1384. [CrossRef]
8. Sluimer, J.C.; Gasc, J.M.; Hamming, I.; van Goor, H.; Michaud, A.; van den Akker, L.H.; Jutten, B.; Cleutjens, J.; Bijnens, A.P.; Corvol, P.; et al. Angiotensin-converting enzyme 2 (ACE2) expression and activity in human carotid atherosclerotic lesions. *J. Pathol.* **2008**, *215*, 273–279. [CrossRef]
9. Schiffrin, E.L.; Flack, J.; Ito, S.; Muntner, P.; Webb, C. Hypertension and COVID-19. *Am. J. Hypertens.* **2020**, *33*, 33–373. [CrossRef]
10. Richardson, S.; Hirsch, J.S.; Narasimhan, M.; Crawford, J.M.; McGinn, T.; Davidson, K.W. The Northwell COVID-19 Research Consortium. Presenting Characteristics, Comorbidities, and Outcomes among 5700 Patients Hospitalized With COVID-19 in the New York City Area. *JAMA* **2020**. [CrossRef]
11. Chen, T.; Wu, D.; Chen, H.; Yan, W.; Yang, D.; Chen, G.; Ma, K.; Xu, D.; Yu, H.; Wang, H.; et al. Clinical characteristics of 113 deceased patients with coronavirus disease 2019: Retrospective study. *BMJ* **2020**, *368*, m1091. [CrossRef] [PubMed]
12. Myers, L.C.; Parodi, S.M.; Escobar, G.J.; Liu, V.X. Characteristics of Hospitalized Adults With COVID-19 in an Integrated Health Care System in California. *JAMA* **2020**. [CrossRef] [PubMed]
13. Guan, W.J.; Liang, W.H.; Zhao, Y.; Liang, H.R.; Chen, Z.S.; Li, Y.M.; Liu, X.Q.; Chen, R.C.; Tang, C.L.; Wang, T.; et al. Comorbidity and its impact on 1590 patients with Covid-19 in China: A Nationwide Analysis. *Eur. Respir. J.* **2020**, 2000547. [CrossRef] [PubMed]

14. Zhou, F.; Yu, T.; Du, R.; Fan, G.; Liu, Y.; Liu, Z.; Xiang, J.; Wang, Y.; Song, B.; Gu, X.; et al. Clinical course and risk factors for mortality of adult inpatients with COVID-19 in Wuhan, China: A retrospective cohort study. *Lancet* **2020**, *395*, 1054–1062. [CrossRef]
15. Bikdeli, B.; Madhavan, M.V.; Jimenez, D.; Chuich, T.; Dreyfus, I.; Driggin, E.; Nigoghossian, C.; Ageno, W.; Madjid, M.; Guo, Y.; et al. Lip GYH. COVID-19 and Thrombotic or Thromboembolic Disease: Implications for Prevention, Antithrombotic Therapy, and Follow-up. *J. Am. Coll. Cardiol.* **2020**. [CrossRef]
16. Klok, F.A.; Kruip, M.; van der Meer, N.J.M.; Arbous, M.S.; Gommers, D.; Kant, K.M.; Kaptein, F.H.J.; van Paassen, J.; Stals, M.A.M.; Huisman, M.V.; et al. Incidence of thrombotic complications in critically ill ICU patients with COVID-19. *Thromb. Res.* **2020**. [CrossRef]
17. Durvasula, R.; Wellington, T.; McNamara, E.; Watnick, S. COVID-19 and Kidney Failure in the Acute Care Setting: Our Experience From Seattle. *Am. J. Kidney Dis.* **2020**. [CrossRef]
18. Ronco, C.; Reis, T. Kidney involvement in COVID-19 and rationale for extracorporeal therapies. *Nat. Rev. Nephrol.* **2020**, 1–3. [CrossRef]
19. Rotzinger, D.C.; Beigelman-Aubry, C.; von Garnier, C.; Qanadli, S.D. Pulmonary embolism in patients with COVID-19: Time to change the paradigm of computed tomography. *Thromb. Res.* **2020**, *190*, 58–59. [CrossRef]
20. Poissy, J.; Goutay, J.; Caplan, M.; Parmentier, E.; Duburcq, T.; Lassalle, F.; Jeanpierre, E.; Rauch, A.; Labreuche, J.; Susen, S. Pulmonary Embolism in COVID-19 Patients: Awareness of an Increased Prevalence. *Circulation* **2020**. [CrossRef]
21. Aggarwal, G.; Lippi, G.; Michael Henry, B. Cerebrovascular disease is associated with an increased disease severity in patients with Coronavirus Disease 2019 (COVID-19): A pooled analysis of published literature. *Int. J. Stroke* **2020**, 1747493020921664. [CrossRef] [PubMed]
22. Mao, L.; Jin, H.; Wang, M.; Hu, Y.; Chen, S.; He, Q.; Chang, J.; Hong, C.; Zhou, Y.; Wang, D.; et al. Neurologic Manifestations of Hospitalized Patients With Coronavirus Disease 2019 in Wuhan, China. *JAMA Neurol.* **2020**. [CrossRef] [PubMed]
23. Santulli, G.; Morelli, M.; Gambardella, J. Is Endothelial Dysfunction the Concealed Cornerstone of COVID-19? *BMJ* **2020**, in press.
24. Cooke, J.P. The endothelium: A new target for therapy. *Vasc. Med.* **2000**, *5*, 49–53. [CrossRef] [PubMed]
25. Aird, W.C. Endothelium as an organ system. *Crit. Care Med.* **2004**, *32*, S271–S279. [CrossRef] [PubMed]
26. Inagami, T.; Naruse, M.; Hoover, R. Endothelium as an endocrine organ. *Annu. Rev. Physiol.* **1995**, *57*, 171–189. [CrossRef] [PubMed]
27. Riphagen, S.; Gomez, R.; Gonzalez-Martinez, C.; Wilkinson, N.; Theocharis, P. Hyperinflammatory shock in children during COVID-19 pandemic. *Lancet* **2020**, in press. [CrossRef]
28. Letko, M.; Marzi, A.; Munster, V. Functional assessment of cell entry and receptor usage for SARS-CoV-2 and other lineage B betacoronaviruses. *Nat. Microbiol.* **2020**, *5*, 562–569. [CrossRef]
29. Wang, Q.; Zhang, Y.; Wu, L.; Niu, S.; Song, C.; Zhang, Z.; Lu, G.; Qiao, C.; Hu, Y.; Yuen, K.Y.; et al. Structural and Functional Basis of SARS-CoV-2 Entry by Using Human ACE2. *Cell* **2020**. [CrossRef]
30. Guzzi, P.H.; Mercatelli, D.; Ceraolo, C.; Giorgi, F.M. Master Regulator Analysis of the SARS-CoV-2/Human Interactome. *J. Clin. Med.* **2020**, *9*, 982. [CrossRef]
31. Xu, H.; Zhong, L.; Deng, J.; Peng, J.; Dan, H.; Zeng, X.; Li, T.; Chen, Q. High expression of ACE2 receptor of 2019-nCoV on the epithelial cells of oral mucosa. *Int. J. Oral Sci.* **2020**, *12*, 8. [CrossRef] [PubMed]
32. Jia, H.P.; Look, D.C.; Shi, L.; Hickey, M.; Pewe, L.; Netland, J.; Farzan, M.; Wohlford-Lenane, C.; Perlman, S.; McCray, P.B., Jr. ACE2 receptor expression and severe acute respiratory syndrome coronavirus infection depend on differentiation of human airway epithelia. *J. Virol.* **2005**, *79*, 14614–14621. [CrossRef] [PubMed]
33. Perico, L.; Benigni, A.; Remuzzi, G. Should COVID-19 Concern Nephrologists? Why and to What Extent? The Emerging Impasse of Angiotensin Blockade. *Nephron* **2020**, 1–9. [CrossRef] [PubMed]
34. Gheblawi, M.; Wang, K.; Viveiros, A.; Nguyen, Q.; Zhong, J.; Turner, A.T.; Raizada, M.K.; Grant, M.B.; Oudit, G.Y. Angiotensin Converting Enzyme 2: SARS-CoV-2 Receptor and Regulator of the Renin-Angiotensin System. *Circ. Res.* **2020**, *126*. [CrossRef] [PubMed]
35. Li, M.; Chen, L.; Zhang, J.; Xiong, C.; Li, X. The SARS-CoV-2 receptor ACE2 expression of maternal-fetal interface and fetal organs by single-cell transcriptome study. *PLoS ONE* **2020**, *15*, e0230295. [CrossRef]
36. Gallagher, T.M.; Buchmeier, M.J. Coronavirus spike proteins in viral entry and pathogenesis. *Virology* **2001**, *279*, 371–374. [CrossRef]

37. Matsuyama, S.; Nao, N.; Shirato, K.; Kawase, M.; Saito, S.; Takayama, I.; Nagata, N.; Sekizuka, T.; Katoh, H.; Kato, F.; et al. Enhanced isolation of SARS-CoV-2 by TMPRSS2-expressing cells. *Proc. Natl. Acad. Sci. USA* **2020**, *117*, 7001–7003. [CrossRef]
38. Sungnak, W.; Huang, N.; Becavin, C.; Berg, M.; Queen, R.; Litvinukova, M.; Talavera-Lopez, C.; Maatz, H.; Reichart, D.; Sampaziotis, F.; et al. SARS-CoV-2 entry factors are highly expressed in nasal epithelial cells together with innate immune genes. *Nat. Med.* **2020**. [CrossRef]
39. Tortorici, M.A.; Walls, A.C.; Lang, Y.; Wang, C.; Li, Z.; Koerhuis, D.; Boons, G.-J.; Bosch, B.-J.; Rey, F.A.; De Groot, R.J.; et al. Structural basis for human coronavirus attachment to sialic acid receptors. *Nat. Struct. Mol. Biol.* **2019**, *26*, 481–489. [CrossRef]
40. Hulswit, R.; Lang, Y.; Bakkers, M.J.G.; Li, W.; Li, Z.; Schouten, A.; Ophorst, B.; Van Kuppeveld, F.J.M.; Boons, G.-J.; Bosch, B.-J.; et al. Human coronaviruses OC43 and HKU1 bind to 9-O-acetylated sialic acids via a conserved receptor-binding site in spike protein domain A. *Proc. Natl. Acad. Sci. USA* **2019**, *116*, 2681–2690. [CrossRef]
41. Chen, Z.; Mi, L.; Xu, J.; Yu, J.; Wang, X.; Jiang, J.; Xing, J.; Shang, P.; Qian, A.; Li, Y.; et al. Function of HAb18G/CD147 in invasion of host cells by severe acute respiratory syndrome coronavirus. *J. Infect. Dis.* **2005**, *191*, 755–760. [CrossRef] [PubMed]
42. Ou, X.; Liu, Y.; Lei, X.; Li, P.; Mi, D.; Ren, L.; Guo, L.; Guo, R.; Chen, T.; Hu, J.; et al. Characterization of spike glycoprotein of SARS-CoV-2 on virus entry and its immune cross-reactivity with SARS-CoV. *Nat. Commun.* **2020**, *11*, 1620. [CrossRef] [PubMed]
43. Yang, J.; Feng, X.; Zhou, Q.; Cheng, W.; Shang, C.; Han, P.; Lin, C.-H.; Chen, H.-S.V.; Quertermous, T.; Chang, C.-P. Pathological Ace2-to-Ace enzyme switch in the stressed heart is transcriptionally controlled by the endothelial Brg1-FoxM1 complex. *Proc. Natl. Acad. Sci. USA* **2016**, *113*, E5628–E5635. [CrossRef] [PubMed]
44. Aimes, R.; Zijlstra, A.; Hooper, J.; Ogbourne, S.; Sit, M.-L.; Fuchs, S.; Gotley, D.; Quigley, J.P.; Antalis, T. Endothelial cell serine proteases expressed during vascular morphogenesis and angiogenesis. *Thromb. Haemost.* **2003**, *89*, 561–572. [CrossRef] [PubMed]
45. Huang, D.T.-N.; Lu, C.-Y.; Chi, Y.; Li, W.-L.; Chang, L.-Y.; Lai, M.-J.; Chen, J.-S.; Hsu, W.-M.; Huang, L.-M. Adaptation of influenza A (H7N9) virus in primary human airway epithelial cells. *Sci. Rep.* **2017**, *7*, 11300. [CrossRef]
46. Vanarsdall, A.L.; Pritchard, S.R.; Wisner, T.W.; Liu, J.; Jardetzky, T.S.; Johnson, D.C. CD147 Promotes Entry of Pentamer-Expressing Human Cytomegalovirus into Epithelial and Endothelial Cells. *mBio* **2018**, *9*, e00781-18. [CrossRef]
47. Im, E.; Venkatakrishnan, A.; Kazlauskas, A. Cathepsin B regulates the intrinsic angiogenic threshold of endothelial cells. *Mol. Biol. Cell.* **2005**, *16*, 3488–3500. [CrossRef]
48. Platt, M.O.; Shockey, W.A. Endothelial cells and cathepsins: Biochemical and biomechanical regulation. *Biochimie* **2016**, *122*, 314–323. [CrossRef]
49. Cai, J.; Zhong, H.; Wu, J.; Chen, R.-F.; Yang, H.; Al-Abed, Y.; Li, Y.; Li, X.; Jiang, W.; Montenegro, M.F.; et al. Cathepsin L promotes Vascular Intimal Hyperplasia after Arterial Injury. *Mol. Med.* **2017**, *23*, 92–100. [CrossRef]
50. Rivellese, F.; Prediletto, E. ACE2 at the centre of COVID-19 from paucisymptomatic infections to severe pneumonia. *Autoimmun. Rev.* **2020**, 102536. [CrossRef]
51. Touyz, R.M.; Li, H.; Delles, C. ACE2 the Janus-faced protein—From cardiovascular protection to severe acute respiratory syndrome-coronavirus and COVID-19. *Clin. Sci. (Lond.)* **2020**, *134*, 747–750. [CrossRef]
52. Leng, Z.; Zhu, R.; Hou, W.; Fengchun, Z.; Yangyang, Z.; Luchan, D.; Shan, G.; Meng, F.; Du, D.; Wang, S.; et al. Transplantation of ACE2(-) Mesenchymal Stem Cells Improves the Outcome of Patients with COVID-19 Pneumonia. *Aging Dis.* **2020**, *11*, 216–228. [CrossRef] [PubMed]
53. Brake, S.; Barnsley, K.; Lu, W.; McAlinden, K.; Eapen, M.S.; Sohal, S.S. Smoking Upregulates Angiotensin-Converting Enzyme-2 Receptor: A Potential Adhesion Site for Novel Coronavirus SARS-CoV-2 (Covid-19). *J. Clin. Med.* **2020**, *9*, 841. [CrossRef] [PubMed]
54. Jakovac, H. COVID-19-is the ACE2 just a foe? *Am. J. Physiol. Cell. Mol. Physiol.* **2020**. [CrossRef] [PubMed]
55. Zou, Z.; Yan, Y.; Shu, Y.; Gao, R.; Sun, Y.; Li, X.; Ju, X.; Liang, Z.; Liu, Q.; Zhao, Y.; et al. Angiotensin-converting enzyme 2 protects from lethal avian influenza A H5N1 infections. *Nat. Commun.* **2014**, *5*, 3594. [CrossRef] [PubMed]

56. Guo, J.; Huang, Z.; Lin, L.; Lv, J. Coronavirus Disease 2019 (COVID-19) and Cardiovascular Disease: A Viewpoint on the Potential Influence of Angiotensin-Converting Enzyme Inhibitors/Angiotensin Receptor Blockers on Onset and Severity of Severe Acute Respiratory Syndrome Coronavirus 2 Infection. *J. Am. Heart Assoc.* **2020**, *9*, e016219. [PubMed]
57. Mourad, J.-J.; Levy, B.I. Interaction between RAAS inhibitors and ACE2 in the context of COVID-19. *Nat. Rev. Cardiol.* **2020**, *17*, 313. [CrossRef]
58. South, A.M.; Diz, D.; Chappell, M.C. COVID-19, ACE2 and the Cardiovascular Consequences. *Am. J. Physiol. Heart Circ. Physiol.* **2020**. [CrossRef]
59. Chen, L.; Li, X.; Chen, M.; Feng, Y.; Xiong, C. The ACE2 expression in human heart indicates new potential mechanism of heart injury among patients infected with SARS-CoV-2. *Cardiovasc. Res.* **2020**, *116*, 1097–1100. [CrossRef]
60. Sommerstein, R.; Kochen, M.M.; Messerli, F.H.; Grani, C. Coronavirus Disease 2019 (COVID-19): Do Angiotensin-Converting Enzyme Inhibitors/Angiotensin Receptor Blockers Have a Biphasic Effect? *J. Am. Heart Assoc.* **2020**, *9*, e016509. [CrossRef]
61. Danser, A.J.; Epstein, M.; Batlle, D. Renin-Angiotensin System Blockers and the COVID-19 Pandemic: At Present There Is No Evidence to Abandon Renin-Angiotensin System Blockers. *Hypertension* **2020**, 12015082. [CrossRef] [PubMed]
62. Wang, M.; Hao, H.; Leeper, N.J.; Zhu, L. Thrombotic Regulation from the Endothelial Cell Perspectives. *Arter. Thromb. Vasc. Biol.* **2018**, *38*, e90–e95. [CrossRef] [PubMed]
63. Bernfield, M.; Götte, M.; Park, P.W.; Reizes, O.; Fitzgerald, M.L.; Lincecum, J.; Zako, M. Functions of cell surface heparan sulfate proteoglycans. *Annu. Rev. Biochem.* **1999**, *68*, 729–777. [CrossRef] [PubMed]
64. Mast, A.E. Tissue Factor Pathway Inhibitor: Multiple Anticoagulant Activities for a Single Protein. *Arter. Thromb. Vasc. Biol.* **2016**, *36*, 9–14. [CrossRef]
65. Martin, F.A.; Murphy, R.P.; Cummins, P.M. Thrombomodulin and the vascular endothelium: Insights into functional, regulatory, and therapeutic aspects. *Am. J. Physiol. Circ. Physiol.* **2013**, *304*, H1585–H1597. [CrossRef]
66. Oliver, J.; Webb, D.J.; Newby, D.E. Stimulated tissue plasminogen activator release as a marker of endothelial function in humans. *Arter. Thromb. Vasc. Biol.* **2005**, *25*, 2470–2479. [CrossRef]
67. Huber, D.; Cramer, E.M.; Kaufmann, J.E.; Meda, P.; Massé, J.-M.; Kruithof, E.K.O.; Vischer, U.M. Tissue-type plasminogen activator (t-PA) is stored in Weibel-Palade bodies in human endothelial cells both in vitro and in vivo. *Blood* **2002**, *99*, 3637–3645. [CrossRef]
68. Godo, S.; Shimokawa, H. Endothelial Functions. *Arter. Thromb. Vasc Biol.* **2017**, *37*, e108–e114. [CrossRef]
69. Vanhoutte, P.M.; Shimokawa, H.; Tang, E.H.; Feletou, M. Endothelial dysfunction and vascular disease. *Acta Physiol.* **2009**, *196*, 193–222. [CrossRef]
70. Boyce, S.; Lwaleed, B.; Kazmi, R. Homeostasis of Hemostasis: The Role of Endothelium. *Semin. Thromb. Hemost.* **2015**, *41*, 549–555. [CrossRef]
71. Loscalzo, J. Oxidative stress in endothelial cell dysfunction and thrombosis. *Pathophysiol. Haemost. Thromb.* **2002**, *32*, 359–360. [CrossRef] [PubMed]
72. Santulli, G. Endothelial cells: The heart attack of the Clones. *Sci. Transl. Med.* **2018**, *10*, eaar7529. [CrossRef] [PubMed]
73. Avogaro, A.; Albiero, M.; Menegazzo, L.; De Kreutzenberg, S.; Fadini, G.P. Endothelial dysfunction in diabetes: The role of reparatory mechanisms. *Diabetes Care* **2011**, *34* (Suppl. 2), S285–S290. [CrossRef] [PubMed]
74. Goligorsky, M.S. Vascular endothelium in diabetes. *Am. J. Physiol. Physiol.* **2017**, *312*, F266–F275. [CrossRef] [PubMed]
75. Kaur, R.; Kaur, M.; Singh, J. Endothelial dysfunction and platelet hyperactivity in type 2 diabetes mellitus: Molecular insights and therapeutic strategies. *Cardiovasc. Diabetol.* **2018**, *17*, 121. [CrossRef]
76. Maamoun, H.; Abdelsalam, S.S.; Zeidan, A.; Korashy, H.M.; Agouni, A. Endoplasmic Reticulum Stress: A Critical Molecular Driver of Endothelial Dysfunction and Cardiovascular Disturbances Associated with Diabetes. *Int. J. Mol. Sci.* **2019**, *20*, 1658. [CrossRef]
77. Eringa, E.C.; Serné, E.H.; Meijer, R.I.; Schalkwijk, C.G.; Houben, A.J.H.M.; Stehouwer, C.D.A.; Smulders, Y.M.; Van Hinsbergh, V.W.M. Endothelial dysfunction in (pre)diabetes: Characteristics, causative mechanisms and pathogenic role in type 2 diabetes. *Rev. Endocr. Metab. Disord.* **2013**, *14*, 39–48. [CrossRef]

78. Jansson, P.A. Endothelial dysfunction in insulin resistance and type 2 diabetes. *J. Intern. Med.* **2007**, *262*, 173–183. [CrossRef]
79. Gambardella, J.; Sardu, C.; Santulli, G. COVID-19 and endothelial dysfunction. *JAMA* **2020**, in press.
80. Esler, M.; Esler, D. Can angiotensin receptor-blocking drugs perhaps be harmful in the COVID-19 pandemic? *J. Hypertens.* **2020**, *38*, 781–782. [CrossRef]
81. Fang, L.; Karakiulakis, G.; Roth, M. Are patients with hypertension and diabetes mellitus at increased risk for COVID-19 infection? *Lancet Respir. Med.* **2020**, *8*, e21. [CrossRef]
82. Nascimento, I.J.B.D.; Cacic, N.; Abdulazeem, H.M.; Von Groote, T.; Jayarajah, U.; Weerasekara, I.; Esfahani, M.A.; Civile, V.T.; Marusic, A.; Jeroncic, A.; et al. Novel Coronavirus Infection (COVID-19) in Humans: A Scoping Review and Meta-Analysis. *Clin. Med.* **2020**, *9*, 941. [CrossRef] [PubMed]
83. Wu, J.T.; Leung, K.; Bushman, M.; Kishore, N.; Niehus, R.; De Salazar, P.M.; Cowling, B.J.; Lipsitch, M.; Leung, G.M. Estimating clinical severity of COVID-19 from the transmission dynamics in Wuhan, China. *Nat. Med.* **2020**, *26*, 506–510. [CrossRef] [PubMed]
84. Guan, W.-J.; Ni, Z.-Y.; Hu, Y.; Liang, W.-H.; Ou, C.-Q.; He, J.-X.; Liu, L.; Shan, H.; Lei, C.-L.; Hui, D.S.; et al. Clinical Characteristics of Coronavirus Disease 2019 in China. *N. Engl. J. Med.* **2020**, *382*, 1708–1720. [CrossRef] [PubMed]
85. Huang, C.; Wang, Y.; Li, X.; Ren, L.; Zhao, J.; Hu, Y.; Zhang, L.; Fan, G.; Xu, J.; Gu, X.; et al. Clinical features of patients infected with 2019 novel coronavirus in Wuhan, China. *Lancet* **2020**, *395*, 497–506. [CrossRef]
86. Wang, D.; Hu, B.; Hu, C.; Zhu, F.; Liu, X.; Zhang, J.; Wang, B.; Xiang, H.; Cheng, Z.; Xiong, Y.; et al. Clinical Characteristics of 138 Hospitalized Patients With 2019 Novel Coronavirus-Infected Pneumonia in Wuhan, China. *JAMA* **2020**, *323*, 1061. [CrossRef]
87. Zhang, J.-J.; Dong, X.; Cao, Y.-Y.; Yuan, Y.-D.; Yang, Y.-B.; Yan, Y.-Q.; Akdis, C.A.; Gao, Y.-D. Clinical characteristics of 140 patients infected with SARS-CoV-2 in Wuhan, China. *Allergy* **2020**. [CrossRef]
88. Williams, B.; Mancia, G.; Spiering, W.; Rosei, E.A.; Azizi, M.; Burnier, M.; Clement, D.L.; Coca, A.; De Simone, G.; Dominiczak, A.F.; et al. 2018 ESC/ESH Guidelines for the management of arterial hypertension. *Eur. Heart J.* **2018**, *39*, 3021–3104. [CrossRef]
89. Vaduganathan, M.; Vardeny, O.; Michel, T.; McMurray, J.J.V.; Pfeffer, M.A.; Solomon, S. Renin-Angiotensin-Aldosterone System Inhibitors in Patients with Covid-19. *N. Engl. J. Med.* **2020**, *382*, 1653–1659. [CrossRef]
90. Gurwitz, D. Angiotensin receptor blockers as tentative SARS-CoV-2 therapeutics. *Drug Dev. Res.* **2020**. [CrossRef]
91. Li, J.; Wang, X.; Chen, J.; Zhang, H.; Deng, A. Association of Renin-Angiotensin System Inhibitors With Severity or Risk of Death in Patients With Hypertension Hospitalized for Coronavirus Disease 2019 (COVID-19) Infection in Wuhan, China. *JAMA Cardiol.* **2020**. [CrossRef] [PubMed]
92. Ferrario, C.M.; Jessup, J.; Chappell, M.; Averill, D.B.; Brosnihan, K.B.; Tallant, E.A.; Diz, D.I.; Gallagher, P.E. Effect of angiotensin-converting enzyme inhibition and angiotensin II receptor blockers on cardiac angiotensin-converting enzyme 2. *Circulation* **2005**, *111*, 2605–2610. [CrossRef] [PubMed]
93. Jessup, J.A.; Gallagher, P.E.; Averill, D.B.; Brosnihan, K.B.; Tallant, E.A.; Chappell, M.C.; Ferrario, C.M. Effect of angiotensin II blockade on a new congenic model of hypertension derived from transgenic Ren-2 rats. *Am. J. Physiol. Circ. Physiol.* **2006**, *291*, H2166–H2172. [CrossRef] [PubMed]
94. Igase, M.; Strawn, W.B.; Gallagher, P.E.; Geary, R.L.; Ferrario, C.M. Angiotensin II AT1 receptors regulate ACE2 and angiotensin-(1-7) expression in the aorta of spontaneously hypertensive rats. *Am. J. Physiol. Circ. Physiol.* **2005**, *289*, H1013–H1019. [CrossRef]
95. South, A.M.; Tomlinson, L.; Edmonston, D.; Hiremath, S.; Sparks, M.A. Controversies of renin-angiotensin system inhibition during the COVID-19 pandemic. *Nat. Rev. Nephrol.* **2020**. [CrossRef]
96. Ferrario, C.M.; Ahmad, S.; Groban, L. Mechanisms by which angiotensin-receptor blockers increase ACE2 levels. *Nat. Rev. Cardiol.* **2020**. [CrossRef]
97. Ishiyama, Y.; Gallagher, P.E.; Averill, D.B.; Tallant, E.A.; Brosnihan, K.B.; Ferrario, C.M. Upregulation of angiotensin-converting enzyme 2 after myocardial infarction by blockade of angiotensin II receptors. *Hypertension* **2004**, *43*, 970–976. [CrossRef]
98. Jin, H.-Y.; Song, B.; Oudit, G.Y.; Davidge, S.T.; Yu, H.-M.; Jiang, Y.-Y.; Gao, P.-J.; Zhu, D.-L.; Ning, G.; Kassiri, Z.; et al. ACE2 deficiency enhances angiotensin II-mediated aortic profilin-1 expression, inflammation and peroxynitrite production. *PLoS ONE* **2012**, *7*, e38502. [CrossRef]

99. Soler, M.J.; Ye, M.; Wysocki, J.; William, J.; Lloveras, J.; Batlle, D. Localization of ACE2 in the renal vasculature: Amplification by angiotensin II type 1 receptor blockade using telmisartan. *Am. J. Physiol. Physiol.* **2009**, *296*, F398–F405. [CrossRef]
100. Patel, V.B.; Clarke, N.; Wang, Z.; Fan, D.; Parajuli, N.; Basu, R.; Putko, B.; Kassiri, Z.; Turner, A.J.; Oudit, G.Y. Angiotensin II induced proteolytic cleavage of myocardial ACE2 is mediated by TACE/ADAM-17: A positive feedback mechanism in the RAS. *J. Mol. Cell. Cardiol.* **2014**, *66*, 167–176. [CrossRef]
101. Yamamuro, M.; Yoshimura, M.; Nakayama, M.; Abe, K.; Sumida, H.; Sugiyama, S.; Saito, Y.; Nakao, K.; Yasue, H.; Ogawa, H. Aldosterone, but not angiotensin II, reduces angiotensin converting enzyme 2 gene expression levels in cultured neonatal rat cardiomyocytes. *Circ. J.* **2008**, *72*, 1346–1350. [CrossRef] [PubMed]
102. Keidar, S.; Gamliel-Lazarovich, A.; Kaplan, M.; Pavlotzky, E.; Hamoud, S.; Hayek, T.; Karry, R.; Abassi, Z. Mineralocorticoid Receptor Blocker Increases Angiotensin-Converting Enzyme 2 Activity in Congestive Heart Failure Patients. *Circ. Res.* **2005**, *97*, 946–953. [CrossRef] [PubMed]
103. Furuhashi, M.; Moniwa, N.; Mita, T.; Fuseya, T.; Ishimura, S.; Ohno, K.; Shibata, S.; Tanaka, M.; Watanabe, Y.; Akasaka, H.; et al. Urinary angiotensin-converting enzyme 2 in hypertensive patients may be increased by olmesartan, an angiotensin II receptor blocker. *Am. J. Hypertens.* **2015**, *28*, 15–21. [CrossRef] [PubMed]
104. Rice, G.I.; Thomas, D.A.; Grant, P.J.; Turner, A.J.; Hooper, N.M. Evaluation of angiotensin-converting enzyme (ACE), its homologue ACE2 and neprilysin in angiotensin peptide metabolism. *Biochem. J.* **2004**, *383*, 45–51. [CrossRef] [PubMed]
105. Nicholls, J.; Peiris, M. Good ACE, bad ACE do battle in lung injury, SARS. *Nat. Med.* **2005**, *11*, 821–822. [CrossRef] [PubMed]
106. Santos, R.A. Angiotensin-(1-7). *Hypertension* **2014**, *63*, 1138–1147. [CrossRef] [PubMed]
107. El-Hashim, A.Z.; Renno, W.M.; Raghupathy, R.; Abduo, H.T.; Akhtar, S.; Benter, I.F. Angiotensin-(1-7) inhibits allergic inflammation, via the MAS1 receptor, through suppression of ERK1/2- and NF-kappaB-dependent pathways. *Br. J. Pharmacol.* **2012**, *166*, 1964–1976. [CrossRef]
108. Kuba, K.; Imai, Y.; Rao, S.; Gao, H.; Guo, F.; Guan, B.; Huan, Y.; Yang, P.; Zhang, Y.; Deng, W.; et al. A crucial role of angiotensin converting enzyme 2 (ACE2) in SARS coronavirus-induced lung injury. *Nat. Med.* **2005**, *11*, 875–879. [CrossRef]
109. Povlsen, A.L.; Grimm, D.; Wehland, M.; Infanger, M.; Kruger, M. The Vasoactive Mas Receptor in Essential Hypertension. *J. Clin. Med.* **2020**, *9*, 267. [CrossRef]
110. Patel, A.B.; Verma, A. COVID-19 and Angiotensin-Converting Enzyme Inhibitors and Angiotensin Receptor Blockers: What Is the Evidence? *JAMA* **2020**. [CrossRef]
111. de Simone, G.; Mancusi, C. Speculation is not evidence: Antihypertensive therapy and COVID-19. *Eur. Heart J. Cardiovasc. Pharm.* **2020**. [CrossRef] [PubMed]
112. Iaccarino, G.; Borghi, C.; Cicero, A.F.G.; Ferri, C.; Minuz, P.; Muiesan, M.L.; Mulatero, P.; Mule, G.; Pucci, G.; Salvetti, M.; et al. Renin-Angiotensin System Inhibition in Cardiovascular Patients at the Time of COVID19: Much Ado for Nothing? A Statement of Activity from the Directors of the Board and the Scientific Directors of the Italian Society of Hypertension. *High Blood Press. Cardiovasc. Prev.* **2020**, *27*, 105–108. [CrossRef] [PubMed]
113. Sultana, J.; Trotta, F.; Addis, A.; Brown, J.S.; Gil, M.; Menniti-Ippolito, F.; Milozzi, F.; Suissa, S.; Trifiro, G. Healthcare Database Networks for Drug Regulatory Policies: International Workshop on the Canadian, US and Spanish Experience and Future Steps for Italy. *Drug Saf.* **2020**, *43*, 1–5. [CrossRef] [PubMed]
114. Talreja, H.; Tan, J.; Dawes, M.; Supershad, S.; Rabindranath, K.; Fisher, J.; Valappil, S.; van der Merwe, V.; Wong, L.; van der Merwe, W.; et al. A consensus statement on the use of angiotensin receptor blockers and angiotensin converting enzyme inhibitors in relation to COVID-19 (corona virus disease 2019). *N. Z. Med. J.* **2020**, *133*, 85–87.
115. Zhang, P.; Zhu, L.; Cai, J.; Lei, F.; Qin, J.J.; Xie, J.; Liu, Y.M.; Zhao, Y.C.; Huang, X.; Lin, L.; et al. Association of Inpatient Use of Angiotensin Converting Enzyme Inhibitors and Angiotensin II Receptor Blockers with Mortality Among Patients With Hypertension Hospitalized With COVID-19. *Circ. Res.* **2020**. [CrossRef]
116. Yang, G.; Tan, Z.; Zhou, L.; Yang, M.; Peng, L.; Liu, J.; Cai, J.; Yang, R.; Han, J.; Huang, Y.; et al. Effects Of ARBs And ACEIs On Virus Infection, Inflammatory Status And Clinical Outcomes In COVID-19 Patients With Hypertension: A Single Center Retrospective Study. *Hypertension* **2020**. [CrossRef]
117. Mehra, M.; Desai, S.; Kuy, S.; Henry, T.; Patel, A. Cardiovascular Disease, Drug Therapy, and Mortality in Covid-19. *NEJM* **2019**, in press. [CrossRef]

118. Reynolds, H.; Adhikari, S.; Pulgarin, C.; Troxel, A.; Iturrate, E.; Johnson, S.; Hausvater, A.; Newman, J.; Berger, J.; Bangalore, S.; et al. Renin–Angiotensin–Aldosterone System Inhibitors and Risk of Covid-19. *NEJM* **2019**, in press. [CrossRef]
119. Mancia, G.; Rea, F.; Ludergnani, M.; Apolone, G.; Corrao, G. Renin–Angiotensin–Aldosterone System Inhibitors and Risk of Covid-19. *NEJM* **2019**, in press.
120. Rajagopalan, S.; Harrison, D.G. Reversing endothelial dysfunction with ACE inhibitors. A new trend. *Circulation* **1996**, *94*, 240–243. [CrossRef]
121. Beckman, J.A.; Creager, M.A. The nonlipid effects of statins on endothelial function. *Trends Cardiovasc. Med.* **2006**, *16*, 156–162. [CrossRef]
122. Ruszkowski, P.; Masajtis-Zagajewska, A.; Nowicki, M. Effects of combined statin and ACE inhibitor therapy on endothelial function and blood pressure in essential hypertension—A randomised double-blind, placebo controlled crossover study. *J. Renin Angiotensin Aldosterone Syst.* **2019**, *20*, 1470320319868890. [CrossRef]
123. Blum, A.; Shamburek, R. The pleiotropic effects of statins on endothelial function, vascular inflammation, immunomodulation and thrombogenesis. *Atherosclerosis* **2009**, *203*, 325–330. [CrossRef]
124. Glowacka, I.; Bertram, S.; Herzog, P.; Pfefferle, S.; Steffen, I.; Muench, M.O.; Simmons, G.; Hofmann, H.; Kuri, T.; Weber, F.; et al. Differential downregulation of ACE2 by the spike proteins of severe acute respiratory syndrome coronavirus and human coronavirus NL63. *J. Virol.* **2010**, *84*, 1198–1205. [CrossRef]
125. Luque, M.; Martin, P.; Martell, N.; Fernandez, C.; Brosnihan, K.B.; Ferrario, C.M. Effects of captopril related to increased levels of prostacyclin and angiotensin-(1-7) in essential hypertension. *J. Hypertens.* **1996**, *14*, 799–805. [CrossRef]
126. Chen, L.; Hao, G. The role of angiotensin-converting enzyme 2 in coronaviruses/influenza viruses and cardiovascular disease. *Cardiovasc. Res.* **2020**. [CrossRef]
127. Murray, E.; Tomaszewski, M.; Guzik, T.J. Binding of SARS-CoV-2 and angiotensin-converting enzyme 2: Clinical implications. *Cardiovasc. Res.* **2020**. [CrossRef]
128. Sunden-Cullberg, J. Chronic Use of Angiotensin-Converting Enzyme Inhibitors and Angiotensin II Receptor Blockers Is High Among Intensive Care Unit Patients With Non-COVID-19 Sepsis but Carry a Moderately Increased Risk of Death. *Hypertension* **2020**. [CrossRef]
129. Fan, Z.; Wu, G.; Yue, M.; Ye, J.; Chen, Y.; Xu, B.; Shu, Z.; Zhu, J.; Lu, N.; Tan, X. Hypertension and hypertensive left ventricular hypertrophy are associated with ACE2 genetic polymorphism. *Life Sci.* **2019**, *225*, 39–45. [CrossRef]
130. Pinheiro, D.S.; Santos, R.S.; Jardim, P.; Silva, E.G.; Reis, A.A.S.; Pedrino, G.R.; Ulhoa, C.J. The combination of ACE I/D and ACE2 G8790A polymorphisms revels susceptibility to hypertension: A genetic association study in Brazilian patients. *PLoS ONE* **2019**, *14*, e0221248. [CrossRef]
131. Lackland, D.T. Racial differences in hypertension: Implications for high blood pressure management. *Am. J. Med. Sci.* **2014**, *348*, 135–138. [CrossRef] [PubMed]
132. Bonow, R.O.; Fonarow, G.C.; O'Gara, P.T.; Yancy, C.W. Association of Coronavirus Disease 2019 (COVID-19) With Myocardial Injury and Mortality. *JAMA Cardiol.* **2020**. [CrossRef] [PubMed]
133. Guo, T.; Fan, Y.; Chen, M.; Wu, X.; Zhang, L.; He, T.; Wang, H.; Wan, J.; Wang, X.; Lu, Z. Cardiovascular Implications of Fatal Outcomes of Patients With Coronavirus Disease 2019 (COVID-19). *JAMA Cardiol.* **2020**. [CrossRef]
134. De Filippo, O.; D'Ascenzo, F.; Angelini, F.; Bocchino, P.P.; Conrotto, F.; Saglietto, A.; Secco, G.G.; Campo, G.; Gallone, G.; Verardi, R.; et al. Reduced Rate of Hospital Admissions for ACS during Covid-19 Outbreak in Northern Italy. *New Engl. J. Med.* **2020**. [CrossRef]
135. Garcia, S.; Albaghdadi, M.S.; Meraj, P.M.; Schmidt, C.; Garberich, R.; Jaffer, F.A.; Dixon, S.; Rade, J.J.; Tannenbaum, M.; Chambers, J.; et al. Reduction in ST-Segment Elevation Cardiac Catheterization Laboratory Activations in the United States during COVID-19 Pandemic. *J. Am. Coll Cardiol.* **2020**. [CrossRef]
136. Yang, X.; Yu, Y.; Xu, J.; Shu, H.; Xia, J.; Liu, H.; Wu, Y.; Zhang, L.; Yu, Z.; Fang, M.; et al. Clinical course and outcomes of critically ill patients with SARS-CoV-2 pneumonia in Wuhan, China: A single-centered, retrospective, observational study. *Lancet Respir. Med.* **2020**, *8*, 475–481. [CrossRef]
137. Fanelli, V.; Fiorentino, M.; Cantaluppi, V.; Gesualdo, L.; Stallone, G.; Ronco, C.; Castellano, G. Acute kidney injury in SARS-CoV-2 infected patients. *Crit. Care* **2020**, *24*, 155. [CrossRef]
138. Cheng, Y.; Luo, R.; Wang, K.; Zhang, M.; Wang, Z.; Dong, L.; Li, J.; Yao, Y.; Ge, S.; Xu, G. Kidney disease is associated with in-hospital death of patients with COVID-19. *Kidney Int.* **2020**. [CrossRef]

139. Henry, B.M.; Lippi, G. Chronic kidney disease is associated with severe coronavirus disease 2019 (COVID-19) infection. *Int. Urol. Nephrol.* **2020**. [CrossRef]
140. Ye, M.; Wysocki, J.; William, J.; Soler, M.J.; Cokic, I.; Batlle, D. Glomerular localization and expression of Angiotensin-converting enzyme 2 and Angiotensin-converting enzyme: Implications for albuminuria in diabetes. *J. Am. Soc. Nephrol.* **2006**, *17*, 3067–3075. [CrossRef] [PubMed]
141. Han, L.; We, X.; Liu, C.; Volpe, G.; Wang, Z. Single-cell atlas of a non-human primate reveals new pathogenic mechanisms of COVID-19. *bioRXiv* **2020**. [CrossRef]
142. Varga, Z.; Flammer, A.J.; Steiger, P.; Haberecker, M.; Andermatt, R.; Zinkernagel, A.S.; Mehra, M.R.; Schuepbach, R.A.; Ruschitzka, F.; Moch, H. Endothelial cell infection and endotheliitis in COVID-19. *Lancet* **2020**, *395*, 1417–1418. [CrossRef]
143. Su, H.; Yang, M.; Wan, C.; Yi, L.X.; Tang, F.; Zhu, H.Y.; Yi, F.; Yang, H.C.; Fogo, A.B.; Nie, X.; et al. Renal histopathological analysis of 26 postmortem findings of patients with COVID-19 in China. *Kidney Int.* **2020**. [CrossRef] [PubMed]
144. Gentile, S.; Strollo, F.; Ceriello, A. COVID-19 Infection in italian people with diabetes: Lessons learned for our future (an experience to be used). *Diabetes Res. Clin. Pract.* **2020**, 108137. [CrossRef] [PubMed]
145. Ma, R.C.W.; Holt, R.I.G. COVID-19 and diabetes. *Diabet. Med.* **2020**, *37*, 723–725. [CrossRef] [PubMed]
146. Muniyappa, R.; Gubbi, S. COVID-19 Pandemic, Corona Viruses, and Diabetes Mellitus. *Am. J. Physiol. Endocrinol. Metab.* **2020**. [CrossRef]
147. Arentz, M.; Yim, E.; Klaff, L.; Lokhandwala, S.; Riedo, F.X.; Chong, M.; Lee, M. Characteristics and Outcomes of 21 Critically Ill Patients With COVID-19 in Washington State. *JAMA* **2020**, *323*, 1612. [CrossRef]
148. Bornstein, S.R.; Dalan, R.; Hopkins, D.; Mingrone, G.; Boehm, B.O. Endocrine and metabolic link to coronavirus infection. *Nat. Rev. Endocrinol.* **2020**. [CrossRef]
149. Remuzzi, A.; Remuzzi, G. COVID-19 and Italy: What next? *Lancet* **2020**, *395*, 1225–1228. [CrossRef]
150. Fadini, G.P.; Morieri, M.L.; Longato, E.; Avogaro, A. Prevalence and impact of diabetes among people infected with SARS-CoV-2. *J. Endocrinol. Investig.* **2020**. [CrossRef]
151. Li, B.; Yang, J.; Zhao, F.; Zhi, L.; Wang, X.; Liu, L.; Bi, Z.; Zhao, Y. Prevalence and impact of cardiovascular metabolic diseases on COVID-19 in China. *Clin. Res. Cardiol.* **2020**, *109*, 531–538. [CrossRef] [PubMed]
152. Yang, J.K.; Feng, Y.; Yuan, M.Y.; Yuan, S.Y.; Fu, H.J.; Wu, B.Y.; Sun, G.Z.; Yang, G.R.; Zhang, X.L.; Wang, L.; et al. Plasma glucose levels and diabetes are independent predictors for mortality and morbidity in patients with SARS. *Diabet. Med.* **2006**, *23*, 623–628. [CrossRef] [PubMed]
153. Simonnet, A.; Chetboun, M.; Poissy, J.; Raverdy, V.; Noulette, J.; Duhamel, A.; Labreuche, J.; Mathieu, D.; Pattou, F.; Jourdain, M. High prevalence of obesity in severe acute respiratory syndrome coronavirus-2 (SARS-CoV-2) requiring invasive mechanical ventilation. *Obesity (Silver Spring)* **2020**. [CrossRef] [PubMed]
154. Wang, A.; Zhao, W.; Xu, Z.; Gu, J. Timely blood glucose management for the outbreak of 2019 novel coronavirus disease (COVID-19) is urgently needed. *Diabetes Res. Clin. Pract.* **2020**, *162*, 108118. [CrossRef] [PubMed]
155. Yang, J.K.; Lin, S.S.; Ji, X.J.; Guo, L.M. Binding of SARS coronavirus to its receptor damages islets and causes acute diabetes. *Acta Diabetol.* **2010**, *47*, 193–199. [CrossRef] [PubMed]
156. Lu, C.L.; Wang, Y.; Yuan, L.; Li, Y.; Li, X.Y. The angiotensin-converting enzyme 2/angiotensin (1-7)/Mas axis protects the function of pancreatic beta cells by improving the function of islet microvascular endothelial cells. *Int. J. Mol. Med.* **2014**, *34*, 1293–1300. [CrossRef]
157. Xuan, X.; Gao, F.; Ma, X.; Huang, C.; Wang, Y.; Deng, H.; Wang, S.; Li, W.; Yuan, L. Activation of ACE2/angiotensin (1-7) attenuates pancreatic beta cell dedifferentiation in a high-fat-diet mouse model. *Metabolism* **2018**, *81*, 83–96. [CrossRef]
158. Shoemaker, R.; Yiannikouris, F.; Thatcher, S.; Cassis, L. ACE2 deficiency reduces beta-cell mass and impairs beta-cell proliferation in obese C57BL/6 mice. *Am. J. Physiol. Endocrinol. Metab.* **2015**, *309*, E621–E631. [CrossRef]
159. Bindom, S.M.; Lazartigues, E. The sweeter side of ACE2: Physiological evidence for a role in diabetes. *Mol. Cell Endocrinol.* **2009**, *302*, 193–202. [CrossRef]
160. Roca-Ho, H.; Riera, M.; Palau, V.; Pascual, J.; Soler, M.J. Characterization of ACE and ACE2 Expression within Different Organs of the NOD Mouse. *Int. J. Mol. Sci.* **2017**, *18*, 563. [CrossRef]

161. Blodgett, D.M.; Nowosielska, A.; Afik, S.; Pechhold, S.; Cura, A.J.; Kennedy, N.J.; Kim, S.; Kucukural, A.; Davis, R.J.; Kent, S.C.; et al. Novel Observations From Next-Generation RNA Sequencing of Highly Purified Human Adult and Fetal Islet Cell Subsets. *Diabetes* **2015**, *64*, 3172–3181. [CrossRef] [PubMed]
162. Wang, H.; Bender, A.; Wang, P.; Karakose, E.; Inabnet, W.B.; Libutti, S.K.; Arnold, A.; Lambertini, L.; Stang, M.; Chen, H.; et al. Insights into beta cell regeneration for diabetes via integration of molecular landscapes in human insulinomas. *Nat. Commun.* **2017**, *8*, 767. [CrossRef] [PubMed]
163. Li, J.; Wang, X.; Chen, J.; Zuo, X.; Zhang, H.; Deng, A. COVID-19 infection may cause ketosis and ketoacidosis. *Diabetes Obes. Metab.* **2020**. [CrossRef] [PubMed]
164. Stoian, A.P.; Banerjee, Y.; Rizvi, A.A.; Rizzo, M. Diabetes and the COVID-19 Pandemic: How Insights from Recent Experience Might Guide Future Management. *Metab. Syndr. Relat. Disord.* **2020**. [CrossRef] [PubMed]
165. Zhang, M.D.; Xiao, M.; Zhang, S.; Xia, P.; Caio, W.; Jiang, W. Coagulopathy and Antiphospholipid Antibodies in Patients with Covid-19. *NEJM* **2020**, *382*, e38. [CrossRef] [PubMed]
166. Zhou, B.; She, J.; Wang, Y.; Ma, X. Venous thrombosis and arteriosclerosis obliterans of lower extremities in a very severe patient with 2019 novel coronavirus disease: A case report. *J. Thromb. Thrombolysis* **2020**. [CrossRef]
167. Tang, N.; Li, D.; Wang, X.; Sun, Z. Abnormal coagulation parameters are associated with poor prognosis in patients with novel coronavirus pneumonia. *J. Thromb. Haemost.* **2020**, *18*, 844–847. [CrossRef]
168. Lin, L.; Lu, L.; Cao, W.; Li, T. Hypothesis for potential pathogenesis of SARS-CoV-2 infection-a review of immune changes in patients with viral pneumonia. *Emerg. Microbes Infect.* **2020**, *9*, 727–732. [CrossRef]
169. Iba, T.; Levy, J.H.; Warkentin, T.E.; Thachil, J.; van der Poll, T.; Levi, M. Scientific, Standardization Committee on DIC, the S, Standardization Committee on P, Critical Care of the International Society on T and Haemostasis. Diagnosis and management of sepsis-induced coagulopathy and disseminated intravascular coagulation. *J. Thromb. Haemost.* **2019**, *17*, 1989–1994. [CrossRef]
170. Escher, R.; Breakey, N.; Lammle, B. Severe COVID-19 infection associated with endothelial activation. *Thromb. Res.* **2020**, *190*, 62. [CrossRef]
171. McCormack, J.J.; Lopes da Silva, M.; Ferraro, F.; Patella, F.; Cutler, D.F. Weibel-Palade bodies at a glance. *J. Cell Sci.* **2017**, *130*, 3611–3617. [CrossRef] [PubMed]
172. Liu, Y.; Yang, Y.; Zhang, C.; Huang, F.; Wang, F.; Yuan, J.; Wang, Z.; Li, J.; Li, J.; Feng, C.; et al. Clinical and biochemical indexes from 2019-nCoV infected patients linked to viral loads and lung injury. *Sci. China Life Sci.* **2020**, *63*, 364–374. [CrossRef] [PubMed]
173. Williams, B.; Baker, A.Q.; Gallacher, B.; Lodwick, D. Angiotensin II increases vascular permeability factor gene expression by human vascular smooth muscle cells. *Hypertension* **1995**, *25*, 913–917. [CrossRef] [PubMed]
174. Victorino, G.P.; Newton, C.R.; Curran, B. Effect of angiotensin II on microvascular permeability. *J. Surg. Res.* **2002**, *104*, 77–81. [CrossRef] [PubMed]
175. Dielis, A.W.; Smid, M.; Spronk, H.M.; Hamulyak, K.; Kroon, A.A.; ten Cate, H.; de Leeuw, P.W. The prothrombotic paradox of hypertension: Role of the renin-angiotensin and kallikrein-kinin systems. *Hypertension* **2005**, *46*, 1236–1242. [CrossRef]
176. Watanabe, T.; Barker, T.A.; Berk, B.C. Angiotensin II and the endothelium: Diverse signals and effects. *Hypertension* **2005**, *45*, 163–169. [CrossRef]
177. Celi, A.; Cianchetti, S.; Dell'Omo, G.; Pedrinelli, R. Angiotensin II, tissue factor and the thrombotic paradox of hypertension. *Expert Rev. Cardiovasc. Ther.* **2010**, *8*, 1723–1729. [CrossRef]
178. Jagroop, I.A.; Mikhailidis, D.P. Angiotensin II can induce and potentiate shape change in human platelets: Effect of losartan. *J. Hum. Hypertens.* **2000**, *14*, 581–585. [CrossRef]
179. Ding, Y.A.; MacIntyre, D.E.; Kenyon, C.J.; Semple, P.F. Angiotensin II effects on platelet function. *J. Hypertens. Suppl.* **1985**, *3*, S251–S253. [CrossRef]
180. Larsson, P.T.; Schwieler, J.H.; Wallen, N.H. Platelet activation during angiotensin II infusion in healthy volunteers. *Blood Coagul. Fibrinolysis* **2000**, *11*, 61–69. [CrossRef]
181. Langeggen, H.; Berge, K.E.; Macor, P.; Fischetti, F.; Tedesco, F.; Hetland, G.; Berg, K.; Johnson, E. Detection of mRNA for the terminal complement components C5, C6, C8 and C9 in human umbilical vein endothelial cells in vitro. *Apmis* **2001**, *109*, 73–78. [CrossRef] [PubMed]
182. Langeggen, H.; Pausa, M.; Johnson, E.; Casarsa, C.; Tedesco, F. The endothelium is an extrahepatic site of synthesis of the seventh component of the complement system. *Clin. Exp. Immunol.* **2000**, *121*, 69–76. [CrossRef] [PubMed]

183. Dauchel, H.; Julen, N.; Lemercier, C.; Daveau, M.; Ozanne, D.; Fontaine, M.; Ripoche, J. Expression of complement alternative pathway proteins by endothelial cells. Differential regulation by interleukin 1 and glucocorticoids. *Eur. J. Immunol.* **1990**, *20*, 1669–1675. [CrossRef] [PubMed]
184. Warren, H.B.; Pantazis, P.; Davies, P.F. The third component of complement is transcribed and secreted by cultured human endothelial cells. *Am. J. Pathol.* **1987**, *129*, 9–13. [PubMed]
185. Johnson, E.; Hetland, G. Human umbilical vein endothelial cells synthesize functional C3, C5, C6, C8 and C9 in vitro. *Scand J. Immunol.* **1991**, *33*, 667–671. [CrossRef] [PubMed]
186. Shagdarsuren, E.; Wellner, M.; Braesen, J.H.; Park, J.K.; Fiebeler, A.; Henke, N.; Dechend, R.; Gratze, P.; Luft, F.C.; Muller, D.N. Complement activation in angiotensin II-induced organ damage. *Circ. Res.* **2005**, *97*, 716–724. [CrossRef]
187. Ruan, C.C.; Gao, P.J. Role of Complement-Related Inflammation and Vascular Dysfunction in Hypertension. *Hypertension* **2019**, *73*, 965–971. [CrossRef]
188. Fischetti, F.; Tedesco, F. Cross-talk between the complement system and endothelial cells in physiologic conditions and in vascular diseases. *Autoimmunity* **2006**, *39*, 417–428. [CrossRef]
189. Risitano, A.M.; Mastellos, D.C.; Huber-Lang, M.; Yancopoulou, D.; Garlanda, C.; Ciceri, F.; Lambris, J.D. Complement as a target in COVID-19? *Nat. Rev. Immunol.* **2020**. [CrossRef]
190. Schulz, C.; Engelmann, B.; Massberg, S. Crossroads of coagulation and innate immunity: The case of deep vein thrombosis. *J. Thromb. Haemost.* **2013**, *11* (Suppl. 1), 233–241. [CrossRef]
191. abret, N.; Britton, G.J.; Gruber, C.; Hegde, S.; Kim, J.; Kuksin, M.; Levantovsky, R.; Malle, L.; Moreira, A.; Park, M.D.; et al. The Sinai Immunology Review Project. Immunology of COVID-19: Current state of the science. *Immunity* **2020**. [CrossRef]
192. Steinberg, B.E.; Goldenberg, N.M.; Lee, W.L. Do viral infections mimic bacterial sepsis? The role of microvascular permeability: A review of mechanisms and methods. *Antiviral. Res.* **2012**, *93*, 2–15. [CrossRef] [PubMed]
193. Zeng, H.; Pappas, C.; Belser, J.A.; Houser, K.V.; Zhong, W.; Wadford, D.A.; Stevens, T.; Balczon, R.; Katz, J.M.; Tumpey, T.M. Human pulmonary microvascular endothelial cells support productive replication of highly pathogenic avian influenza viruses: Possible involvement in the pathogenesis of human H5N1 virus infection. *J. Virol.* **2012**, *86*, 667–678. [CrossRef] [PubMed]
194. Maniatis, N.A.; Orfanos, S.E. The endothelium in acute lung injury/acute respiratory distress syndrome. *Curr. Opin. Crit. Care* **2008**, *14*, 22–30. [CrossRef] [PubMed]
195. Polverino, F.; Celli, B.R.; Owen, C.A. COPD as an endothelial disorder: Endothelial injury linking lesions in the lungs and other organs? (2017 Grover Conference Series). *Pulm. Circ.* **2018**, *8*, 2045894018758528. [CrossRef] [PubMed]
196. Millar, F.R.; Summers, C.; Griffiths, M.J.; Toshner, M.R.; Proudfoot, A.G. The pulmonary endothelium in acute respiratory distress syndrome: Insights and therapeutic opportunities. *Thorax* **2016**, *71*, 462–473. [CrossRef]
197. Armstrong, S.M.; Wang, C.; Tigdi, J.; Si, X.; Dumpit, C.; Charles, S.; Gamage, A.; Moraes, T.J.; Lee, W.L. Influenza infects lung microvascular endothelium leading to microvascular leak: Role of apoptosis and claudin-5. *PLoS ONE* **2012**, *7*, e47323. [CrossRef]
198. Chan, M.C.; Chan, R.W.; Yu, W.C.; Ho, C.C.; Chui, W.H.; Lo, C.K.; Yuen, K.M.; Guan, Y.I.; Nicholls, J.M.; Peiris, J.S. Influenza H5N1 virus infection of polarized human alveolar epithelial cells and lung microvascular endothelial cells. *Respir. Res.* **2009**, *10*, 102. [CrossRef]
199. Lee, N.; Hui, D.; Wu, A.; Chan, P.; Cameron, P.; Joynt, G.M.; Ahuja, A.; Yung, M.Y.; Leung, C.B.; To, K.F.; et al. A major outbreak of severe acute respiratory syndrome in Hong Kong. *N. Engl. J. Med.* **2003**, *348*, 1986–1994. [CrossRef]
200. Wong, R.S.; Wu, A.; To, K.F.; Lee, N.; Lam, C.W.; Wong, C.K.; Chan, P.K.; Ng, M.H.; Yu, L.M.; Hui, D.S.; et al. Haematological manifestations in patients with severe acute respiratory syndrome: Retrospective analysis. *BMJ* **2003**, *326*, 1358–1362. [CrossRef]
201. Xiang-Hua, Y.; Le-Min, W.; Ai-Bin, L.; Zhu, G.; Riquan, L.; Xu-You, Z.; Wei-Wei, R.; Ye-Nan, W. Severe acute respiratory syndrome and venous thromboembolism in multiple organs. *Am. J. Respir. Crit. Care Med.* **2010**, *182*, 436–437. [CrossRef] [PubMed]
202. de Wit, E.; van Doremalen, N.; Falzarano, D.; Munster, V.J. SARS and MERS: Recent insights into emerging coronaviruses. *Nat. Rev. Microbiol.* **2016**, *14*, 523–534. [CrossRef] [PubMed]

203. Bunce, P.E.; High, S.M.; Nadjafi, M.; Stanley, K.; Liles, W.C.; Christian, M.D. Pandemic H1N1 influenza infection and vascular thrombosis. *Clin. Infect. Dis.* **2011**, *52*, e14–e17. [CrossRef]
204. Huzmeli, C.; Saglam, M.; Arikan, A.; Doner, B.; Akinci, G.; Candan, F. Infrarenal Aorta Thrombosis Associated with H1N1 Influenza A Virus Infection. *Case Rep. Infect. Dis.* **2016**, *2016*, 9567495. [CrossRef] [PubMed]
205. Ishiguro, T.; Matsuo, K.; Fujii, S.; Takayanagi, N. Acute thrombotic vascular events complicating influenza-associated pneumonia. *Respir. Med. Case Rep.* **2019**, *28*, 100884. [CrossRef] [PubMed]
206. Iwasaki, A.; Medzhitov, R. A new shield for a cytokine storm. *Cell* **2011**, *146*, 861–862. [CrossRef]
207. Tscherne, D.M.; Garcia-Sastre, A. Virulence determinants of pandemic influenza viruses. *J. Clin. Investig.* **2011**, *121*, 6–13. [CrossRef]
208. Canna, S.W.; Behrens, E.M. Making sense of the cytokine storm: A conceptual framework for understanding, diagnosing, and treating hemophagocytic syndromes. *Pediatr. Clin. N. Am.* **2012**, *59*, 329–344. [CrossRef]
209. Chaudhry, H.; Zhou, J.; Zhong, Y.; Ali, M.M.; McGuire, F.; Nagarkatti, P.S.; Nagarkatti, M. Role of cytokines as a double-edged sword in sepsis. *In Vivo* **2013**, *27*, 669–684.
210. Bracaglia, C.; Prencipe, G.; De Benedetti, F. Macrophage Activation Syndrome: Different mechanisms leading to a one clinical syndrome. *Pediatr. Rheumatol. Online J.* **2017**, *15*, 5. [CrossRef]
211. Hayden, A.; Park, S.; Giustini, D.; Lee, A.Y.; Chen, L.Y. Hemophagocytic syndromes (HPSs) including hemophagocytic lymphohistiocytosis (HLH) in adults: A systematic scoping review. *Blood Rev.* **2016**, *30*, 411–420. [CrossRef] [PubMed]
212. Mehta, P.; McAuley, D.F.; Brown, M.; Sanchez, E.; Tattersall, R.S.; Manson, J.J.; Hlh Across Speciality Collaboration UK. COVID-19: Consider cytokine storm syndromes and immunosuppression. *Lancet* **2020**, *395*, 1033–1034. [CrossRef]
213. Gattinoni, L.; Coppola, S.; Cressoni, M.; Busana, M.; Rossi, S.; Chiumello, D. Covid-19 Does Not Lead to a "Typical" Acute Respiratory Distress Syndrome. *Am. J. Respir. Crit. Care Med.* **2020**. [CrossRef] [PubMed]
214. Pedersen, S.F.; Ho, Y.C. SARS-CoV-2: A storm is raging. *J. Clin. Investig.* **2020**, *130*, 2202–2205. [CrossRef] [PubMed]
215. Staedtke, V.; Bai, R.Y.; Kim, K.; Darvas, M.; Davila, M.L.; Riggins, G.J.; Rothman, P.B.; Papadopoulos, N.; Kinzler, K.W.; Vogelstein, B.; et al. Disruption of a self-amplifying catecholamine loop reduces cytokine release syndrome. *Nature* **2018**, *564*, 273–277. [CrossRef]
216. Sinha, P.; Delucchi, K.L.; McAuley, D.F.; O'Kane, C.M.; Matthay, M.A.; Calfee, C.S. Development and validation of parsimonious algorithms to classify acute respiratory distress syndrome phenotypes: A secondary analysis of randomised controlled trials. *Lancet Respir. Med.* **2020**, *8*, 247–257. [CrossRef]
217. Qin, C.; Zhou, L.; Hu, Z.; Zhang, S.; Yang, S.; Tao, Y.; Xie, C.; Ma, K.; Shang, K.; Wang, W.; et al. Dysregulation of immune response in patients with COVID-19 in Wuhan, China. *Clin. Infect. Dis.* **2020**. [CrossRef]
218. Teijaro, J.R.; Walsh, K.B.; Cahalan, S.; Fremgen, D.M.; Roberts, E.; Scott, F.; Martinborough, E.; Peach, R.; Oldstone, M.B.; Rosen, H. Endothelial cells are central orchestrators of cytokine amplification during influenza virus infection. *Cell* **2011**, *146*, 980–991. [CrossRef]
219. Sorriento, D.; Santulli, G.; Del Giudice, C.; Anastasio, A.; Trimarco, B.; Iaccarino, G. Endothelial cells are able to synthesize and release catecholamines both in vitro and in vivo. *Hypertension* **2012**, *60*, 129–136. [CrossRef]
220. Xie, Y.; Wang, X.; Yang, P.; Shutong, Z. COVID-19 complicated by acute pulmonary embolism. *Radiology* **2020**, *2*, e200067. [CrossRef]
221. Danzi, G.B.; Loffi, M.; Galeazzi, G.; Gherbesi, E. Acute pulmonary embolism and COVID-19 pneumonia: A random association? *Eur. Heart J.* **2020**. [CrossRef]
222. Leonard-Lorant, I.; Delabranche, X.; Severac, F.; Helms, J.; Pauzet, C.; Collange, O.; Schneider, F.; Labani, A.; Bilbault, P.; Moliere, S.; et al. Acute Pulmonary Embolism in COVID-19 Patients on CT Angiography and Relationship to D-Dimer Levels. *Radiology* **2020**, 201561. [CrossRef]
223. Jolobe, O.M.P. Similarities Between Community-Acquired Pneumonia and Pulmonary Embolism. *Am. J. Med.* **2019**, *132*, e863. [CrossRef]
224. Santulli, G. MicroRNAs and Endothelial (Dys) Function. *J. Cell Physiol.* **2016**, *231*, 1638–1644. [CrossRef] [PubMed]
225. Yuan, Q.; Yang, J.; Santulli, G.; Reiken, S.R.; Wronska, A.; Kim, M.M.; Osborne, B.W.; Lacampagne, A.; Yin, Y.; Marks, A.R. Maintenance of normal blood pressure is dependent on IP3R1-mediated regulation of eNOS. *Proc. Natl. Acad. Sci. USA* **2016**, *113*, 8532–8537. [CrossRef] [PubMed]

226. Gando, S.; Levi, M.; Toh, C.H. Disseminated intravascular coagulation. *Nat. Rev. Dis. Primers.* **2016**, *2*, 16037. [CrossRef] [PubMed]
227. Walborn, A.; Rondina, M.; Mosier, M.; Fareed, J.; Hoppensteadt, D. Endothelial Dysfunction Is Associated with Mortality and Severity of Coagulopathy in Patients with Sepsis and Disseminated Intravascular Coagulation. *Clin. Appl. Thromb. Hemost.* **2019**, *25*, 1076029619852163. [CrossRef] [PubMed]
228. Tang, N.; Bai, H.; Chen, X.; Gong, J.; Li, D.; Sun, Z. Anticoagulant treatment is associated with decreased mortality in severe coronavirus disease 2019 patients with coagulopathy. *J. Thromb. Haemost.* **2020**. [CrossRef] [PubMed]
229. Rubin, E.J.; Baden, L.R.; Morrissey, S. Audio Interview: New Research on Possible Treatments for Covid-19. *New Engl. J. Med.* **2020**, *382*, e30. [CrossRef]
230. Ahn, D.G.; Shin, H.J.; Kim, M.H.; Lee, S.; Kim, H.S.; Myoung, J.; Kim, B.T.; Kim, S.J. Current Status of Epidemiology, Diagnosis, Therapeutics, and Vaccines for Novel Coronavirus Disease 2019 (COVID-19). *J. Microbiol. Biotechnol.* **2020**, *30*, 313–324. [CrossRef]
231. Xu, X.; Han, M.; Li, T.; Sun, W.; Wang, D.; Fu, B.; Zhou, Y.; Zheng, X.; Yang, Y.; Li, X.; et al. Effective treatment of severe COVID-19 patients with tocilizumab. *Proc. Natl. Acad. Sci. USA* **2020**, 202005615. [CrossRef] [PubMed]
232. Ruiz-Limon, P.; Ortega, R.; Arias de la Rosa, I.; Abalos-Aguilera, M.D.C.; Perez-Sanchez, C.; Jimenez-Gomez, Y.; Peralbo-Santaella, E.; Font, P.; Ruiz-Vilches, D.; Ferrin, G.; et al. Tocilizumab improves the proatherothrombotic profile of rheumatoid arthritis patients modulating endothelial dysfunction, NETosis, and inflammation. *Transl. Res.* **2017**, *183*, 87–103. [CrossRef] [PubMed]
233. Kajikawa, M.; Higashi, Y.; Tomiyama, H.; Maruhashi, T.; Kurisu, S.; Kihara, Y.; Mutoh, A.; Ueda, S.I. Effect of short-term colchicine treatment on endothelial function in patients with coronary artery disease. *Int. J. Cardiol.* **2019**, *281*, 35–39. [CrossRef] [PubMed]
234. Parchure, N.; Zouridakis, E.G.; Kaski, J.C. Effect of azithromycin treatment on endothelial function in patients with coronary artery disease and evidence of Chlamydia pneumoniae infection. *Circulation* **2002**, *105*, 1298–1303. [CrossRef] [PubMed]
235. Luo, T.; Chen, B.; Zhao, Z.; He, N.; Zeng, Z.; Wu, B.; Fukushima, Y.; Dai, M.; Huang, Q.; Xu, D.; et al. Histamine H2 receptor activation exacerbates myocardial ischemia/reperfusion injury by disturbing mitochondrial and endothelial function. *Basic Res. Cardiol.* **2013**, *108*, 342. [CrossRef] [PubMed]
236. Yazdany, J.; Kim, A.H.J. Use of Hydroxychloroquine and Chloroquine During the COVID-19 Pandemic: What Every Clinician Should Know. *Ann. Intern. Med.* **2020**. [CrossRef]
237. Le, N.T.; Takei, Y.; Izawa-Ishizawa, Y.; Heo, K.S.; Lee, H.; Smrcka, A.V.; Miller, B.L.; Ko, K.A.; Ture, S.; Morrell, C.; et al. Identification of activators of ERK5 transcriptional activity by high-throughput screening and the role of endothelial ERK5 in vasoprotective effects induced by statins and antimalarial agents. *J. Immunol.* **2014**, *193*, 3803–3815. [CrossRef]
238. Rahman, R.; Murthi, P.; Singh, H.; Gurusinghe, S.; Mockler, J.C.; Lim, R.; Wallace, E.M. The effects of hydroxychloroquine on endothelial dysfunction. *Pregnancy Hypertens.* **2016**, *6*, 259–262. [CrossRef]
239. Gambardella, J.; Morelli, M.; Sardu, C.; Santulli, G. Targeting Endothelial Dysfunction in COVID-19. *Nature* **2020**, in press.
240. Ciccarelli, M.; Santulli, G.; Campanile, A.; Galasso, G.; Cervero, P.; Altobelli, G.G.; Cimini, V.; Pastore, L.; Piscione, F.; Trimarco, B.; et al. Endothelial alpha1-adrenoceptors regulate neo-angiogenesis. *Br. J. Pharmacol.* **2008**, *153*, 936–946. [CrossRef]
241. Wilbert-Lampen, U.; Seliger, C.; Zilker, T.; Arendt, R.M. Cocaine increases the endothelial release of immunoreactive endothelin and its concentrations in human plasma and urine: Reversal by coincubation with sigma-receptor antagonists. *Circulation* **1998**, *98*, 385–390. [CrossRef] [PubMed]
242. Amer, M.S.; McKeown, L.; Tumova, S.; Liu, R.; Seymour, V.A.; Wilson, L.A.; Naylor, J.; Greenhalgh, K.; Hou, B.; Majeed, Y.; et al. Inhibition of endothelial cell Ca(2)(+) entry and transient receptor potential channels by Sigma-1 receptor ligands. *Br. J. Pharmacol.* **2013**, *168*, 1445–1455. [CrossRef] [PubMed]
243. Massamiri, T.; Duckles, S.P. Sigma receptor ligands inhibit rat tail artery contractile responses by multiple mechanisms. *J. Pharmacol. Exp. Ther.* **1991**, *259*, 22–29. [PubMed]
244. Hamidi Shishavan, M.; Henning, R.H.; van Buiten, A.; Goris, M.; Deelman, L.E.; Buikema, H. Metformin Improves Endothelial Function and Reduces Blood Pressure in Diabetic Spontaneously Hypertensive Rats Independent from Glycemia Control: Comparison to Vildagliptin. *Sci. Rep.* **2017**, *7*, 10975. [CrossRef]

245. Bolz, S.S.; Pohl, U. Indomethacin enhances endothelial NO release–evidence for a role of PGI2 in the autocrine control of calcium-dependent autacoid production. *Cardiovasc. Res.* **1997**, *36*, 437–444. [CrossRef]
246. Sfikakis, P.P.; Papamichael, C.; Stamatelopoulos, K.S.; Tousoulis, D.; Fragiadaki, K.G.; Katsichti, P.; Stefanadis, C.; Mavrikakis, M. Improvement of vascular endothelial function using the oral endothelin receptor antagonist bosentan in patients with systemic sclerosis. *Arthritis Rheum.* **2007**, *56*, 1985–1993. [CrossRef]
247. Gupta, N.; Zhao, Y.Y.; Evans, C.E. The stimulation of thrombosis by hypoxia. *Thromb. Res.* **2019**, *181*, 77–83. [CrossRef]
248. Xu, Z.; Shi, L.; Wang, Y.; Zhang, J.; Huang, L.; Zhang, C.; Liu, S.; Zhao, P.; Liu, H.; Zhu, L.; et al. Pathological findings of COVID-19 associated with acute respiratory distress syndrome. *Lancet Respir. Med.* **2020**, *8*, 420–422. [CrossRef]
249. Paranjpe, I.; Fuster, V.; Lala, A.; Russak, A.; Glicksberg, B.S.; Levin, M.A.; Charney, A.W.; Narula, J.; Fayad, Z.A.; Bagiella, E.; et al. Association of Treatment Dose Anticoagulation with In-Hospital Survival Among Hospitalized Patients with COVID-19. *J. Am. Coll. Cardiol.* **2020**. [CrossRef]
250. Basu, A.; Kanda, T.; Beyene, A.; Saito, K.; Meyer, K.; Ray, R. Sulfated homologues of heparin inhibit hepatitis C virus entry into mammalian cells. *J. Virol.* **2007**, *81*, 3933–3941. [CrossRef]
251. Lee, E.; Pavy, M.; Young, N.; Freeman, C.; Lobigs, M. Antiviral effect of the heparan sulfate mimetic, PI-88, against dengue and encephalitic flaviviruses. *Antiviral. Res.* **2006**, *69*, 31–38. [CrossRef] [PubMed]
252. Walker, S.J.; Pizzato, M.; Takeuchi, Y.; Devereux, S. Heparin binds to murine leukemia virus and inhibits Env-independent attachment and infection. *J. Virol.* **2002**, *76*, 6909–6918. [CrossRef] [PubMed]
253. Connell, B.J.; Lortat-Jacob, H. Human immunodeficiency virus and heparan sulfate: From attachment to entry inhibition. *Front. Immunol.* **2013**, *4*, 385. [CrossRef] [PubMed]
254. Nahmias, A.J.; Kibrick, S. Inhibitory effect of heparin on herpes simplex virus. *J. Bacteriol.* **1964**, *87*, 1060–1066. [CrossRef]

Permissions

All chapters in this book were first published by MDPI; hereby published with permission under the Creative Commons Attribution License or equivalent. Every chapter published in this book has been scrutinized by our experts. Their significance has been extensively debated. The topics covered herein carry significant findings which will fuel the growth of the discipline. They may even be implemented as practical applications or may be referred to as a beginning point for another development.

The contributors of this book come from diverse backgrounds, making this book a truly international effort. This book will bring forth new frontiers with its revolutionizing research information and detailed analysis of the nascent developments around the world.

We would like to thank all the contributing authors for lending their expertise to make the book truly unique. They have played a crucial role in the development of this book. Without their invaluable contributions this book wouldn't have been possible. They have made vital efforts to compile up to date information on the varied aspects of this subject to make this book a valuable addition to the collection of many professionals and students.

This book was conceptualized with the vision of imparting up-to-date information and advanced data in this field. To ensure the same, a matchless editorial board was set up. Every individual on the board went through rigorous rounds of assessment to prove their worth. After which they invested a large part of their time researching and compiling the most relevant data for our readers.

The editorial board has been involved in producing this book since its inception. They have spent rigorous hours researching and exploring the diverse topics which have resulted in the successful publishing of this book. They have passed on their knowledge of decades through this book. To expedite this challenging task, the publisher supported the team at every step. A small team of assistant editors was also appointed to further simplify the editing procedure and attain best results for the readers.

Apart from the editorial board, the designing team has also invested a significant amount of their time in understanding the subject and creating the most relevant covers. They scrutinized every image to scout for the most suitable representation of the subject and create an appropriate cover for the book.

The publishing team has been an ardent support to the editorial, designing and production team. Their endless efforts to recruit the best for this project, has resulted in the accomplishment of this book. They are a veteran in the field of academics and their pool of knowledge is as vast as their experience in printing. Their expertise and guidance has proved useful at every step. Their uncompromising quality standards have made this book an exceptional effort. Their encouragement from time to time has been an inspiration for everyone.

The publisher and the editorial board hope that this book will prove to be a valuable piece of knowledge for researchers, students, practitioners and scholars across the globe.

List of Contributors

Beata Olas
Department of General Biochemistry, Faculty of Biology and Environmental Protection, University of Lodz, Pomorska 141/3, 90-236 Lodz, Poland

Anne-Marie Galow and Andreas Hoeflich
Institute of Genome Biology, Leibniz Institute for Farm Animal Biology, 18196 Dummerstorf, Germany

Tom Goldammer
Institute of Genome Biology, Leibniz Institute for Farm Animal Biology, 18196 Dummerstorf, Germany
Molecular Biology and Fish Genetics Unit, Faculty of Agriculture and Environmental Sciences, University of Rostock, 18059 Rostock, Germany

Alexander Akhmedov
Center for Molecular Cardiology, Schlieren Campus, University of Zurich, 8952 Schlieren, Switzerland

Luca Liberale
Center for Molecular Cardiology, Schlieren Campus, University of Zurich, 8952 Schlieren, Switzerland
First Clinic of Internal Medicine, Department of Internal Medicine, University of Genoa, 16132 Genoa, Italy

Erik W. Holy, Fabian Nietlispach and Frank Ruschitzka
Department of Cardiology, University Hospital Zurich, 8091 Zurich, Switzerland

Christian M. Matter
Center for Molecular Cardiology, Schlieren Campus, University of Zurich, 8952 Schlieren, Switzerland
Department of Cardiology, University Hospital Zurich, 8091 Zurich, Switzerland

Nicole R. Bonetti and Jurg H. Beer
Center for Molecular Cardiology, Schlieren Campus, University of Zurich, 8952 Schlieren, Switzerland
Department of Internal Medicine, Cantonal Hospital of Baden, 5404 Baden, Switzerland

Francois Mach
Department of Cardiology, Hopital Universitaire de Geneve, 1206 Geneve, Switzerland

Fabrizio Montecucco
First Clinic of Internal Medicine, Department of Internal Medicine, University of Genoa, 16132 Genoa, Italy
IRCCS Ospedale Policlinico San Martino Genoa—Italian Cardiovascular Network, 16132 Genoa, Italy

Francesco Paneni and Giovanni G. Camici
Center for Molecular Cardiology, Schlieren Campus, University of Zurich, 8952 Schlieren, Switzerland
Department of Cardiology, University Hospital Zurich, 8091 Zurich, Switzerland
Department of Research and Education, University Hospital Zurich, 8001 Zurich, Switzerland

Peter Libby
Division of Cardiovascular Medicine, Department of Medicine, Brigham and Women's Hospital, Harvard Medical School, 02115 Boston, MA, USA

Thomas F. Luscher
Center for Molecular Cardiology, Schlieren Campus, University of Zurich, 8952 Schlieren, Switzerland
Royal Brompton and Harefield Hospitals and Imperial College, London SW3 6NP, UK

Sandra Guaita-Esteruelas
Vascular Medicine and Metabolism Unit, Research Unit on Lipids and Atherosclerosis, Sant Joan University Hospital, Universitat Rovira i Virgili, IISPV, 43201 Reus, Spain

Josefa Girona, Cèlia Rodríguez-Borjabad, Daiana Ibarretxe, Joan-Carles Vallvé, Raimon Ferré, Mercedes Heras, Ricardo Rodríguez-Calvo, Neus Martínez-Micaelo, Núria Plana and Lluís Masana
Vascular Medicine and Metabolism Unit, Research Unit on Lipids and Atherosclerosis, Sant Joan University Hospital, Universitat Rovira i Virgili, IISPV, 43201 Reus, Spain
Spanish Biomedical Research Centre in Diabetes and Associated Metabolic Disorders (CIBERDEM), 28029 Madrid, Spain

En-Young N. Wagner
Department of Psychiatry, University of California, San Diego, CA 92093, USA
Department of Consultation-Liaison Psychiatry and Psychosomatic Medicine, University Hospital Zurich, 8091 Zurich, Switzerland
Department of BioMedical Research, Inselspital, Bern University Hospital, 3010 Bern, Switzerland

Piero Pollesello
Critical Care, OrionPharma, 02101 Espoo, Finland

Roland von Kanel
Department of Consultation-Liaison Psychiatry and Psychosomatic Medicine, University Hospital Zurich, 8091 Zurich, Switzerland
Department of BioMedical Research, Inselspital, Bern University Hospital, 3010 Bern, Switzerland

Suzi Hong, Kathleen L. Wilson and Paul J. Mills
Department of Psychiatry, University of California, San Diego, CA 92093, USA
Department of Family Medicine and Public Health, University of California, San Diego, CA 92093, USA

Karen J. Calfas and Cheryl L. Rock
Department of Family Medicine and Public Health, University of California, San Diego, CA 92093, USA

Laura S. Redwine
College of Nursing, University of South Florida, Tampa, FL 33612, USA

Chien-Ning Hsu
Department of Pharmacy, Kaohsiung Chang Gung Memorial Hospital, Kaohsiung 833, Taiwan
School of Pharmacy, Kaohsiung Medical University, Kaohsiung 807, Taiwan

Guo-Ping Chang-Chien and Sufan Lin
Center for Environmental Toxin and Emerging-Contaminant Research, Cheng Shiu University, Kaohsiung 833, Taiwan
Super Micro Mass Research and Technology Center, Cheng Shiu University, Kaohsiung 833, Taiwan

Chih-Yao Hou
Department of Seafood Science, National Kaohsiung University of Science and Technology, Kaohsiung 811, Taiwan

Pei-Chen Lu
Department of Pediatrics, Kaohsiung Chang Gung Memorial Hospital and College of Medicine, Chang Gung University, Kaohsiung 833, Taiwan

You-Lin Tain
Department of Pediatrics, Kaohsiung Chang Gung Memorial Hospital and College of Medicine, Chang Gung University, Kaohsiung 833, Taiwan
Institute for Translational Research in Biomedicine, Kaohsiung Chang Gung Memorial Hospital and Chang Gung University, College of Medicine, Kaohsiung 833, Taiwan

Iginio Colaiori and Jozef Bartunek
Cardiovascular Research Center Aalst OLV Hospital, 9300 Aalst, Belgium

Giuseppe Di Gioia
Cardiovascular Research Center Aalst OLV Hospital, 9300 Aalst, Belgium
Department of Advanced Biomedical Sciences, University of Naples Federico II, 80100 Napoli, Italy

Raffaele Izzo, Emanuele Barbato, Danilo Franco, Antonio Rapacciuolo, Costantino Mancusi, Maria Angela Losi, Teresa Strisciuglio, Maria Virginia Manzi, Giovanni de Simone, Bruno Trimarco and Carmine Morisco
Department of Advanced Biomedical Sciences, University of Naples Federico II, 80100 Napoli, Italy

Giuseppina Gambino and Nicola Ferrara
Department of Translational Medical Sciences, University of Naples Federico II, 80100 Naples, Italy

Anne Lise Ferrara and Amato de Paulis
Department of Translational Medical Sciences, University of Naples Federico II, 80100 Naples, Italy
Center for Basic and Clinical Immunology Research (CISI), University of Naples Federico II, 80100 Naples, Italy
World Allergy Organization (WAO), Center of Excellence, 80100 Naples, Italy

Gilda Varricchi, Stefania Loffredo and Gianni Marone
Department of Translational Medical Sciences, University of Naples Federico II, 80100 Naples, Italy
Center for Basic and Clinical Immunology Research (CISI), University of Naples Federico II, 80100 Naples, Italy
World Allergy Organization (WAO), Center of Excellence, 80100 Naples, Italy
Institute of Experimental Endocrinology and Oncology "G. Salvatore" (IEOS), National Research Council (CNR), 80100 Naples, Italy

Leonardo Bencivenga
Department of Translational Medical Sciences, University of Naples Federico II, 80100 Naples, Italy
Department of Advanced Biomedical Sciences, University of Naples Federico II, 80100 Naples, Italy

Giuseppe Rengo
Department of Translational Medical Sciences, University of Naples Federico II, 80100 Naples, Italy
Istituti Clinici Scientifici Maugeri SpA Società Benefit, Via Bagni Vecchi, 1, 82037 Telese BN, Italy

Damiano Magrì, Giovanna Gallo, Dario Giordano, Camillo Autore and Beatrice Musumeci
Department of Clinical and Molecular Medicine, Sapienza University, 00100 Rome, Italy

Vittoria Mastromarino
Department of Clinical and Molecular Medicine, Sapienza University, 00100 Rome, Italy
Unit of Pediatric Cardiology and Cardiac Surgery, Sant'Orsola Hospital, 40100 Bologna, Italy

Fotios Konstantinou and Dimitrios Mikroulis
Department of Cardiothoracic Surgery, Democritus University of Thrace, 68100 Alexandroupolis, Greece

Piergiuseppe Agostoni
Centro Cardiologico Monzino, IRCCS, 20100 Milan, Italy
Department of Clinical Sciences and Community Health, University of Milan, 20100 Milan, Italy

Speranza Rubattu and Massimo Volpe
Department of Clinical and Molecular Medicine, Sapienza University, 00100 Rome, Italy
IRCCS Neuromed, 86077 Pozzilli (IS), Italy

Maurizio Forte and Maria Cotugno
IRCCS Neuromed, 86077 Pozzilli (IS), Italy

Maria Rosaria Torrisi, Simona Petrucci, Aldo Germani and Maria Piane
Department of Clinical and Molecular Medicine, Sapienza University, 00100 Rome, Italy
UOC Medical Genetics and Advanced Cell Diagnostics, S. Andrea University Hospital, 00100 Rome, Italy

Camilla Savio
UOC Medical Genetics and Advanced Cell Diagnostics, S. Andrea University Hospital, 00100 Rome, Italy

Antonello Maruotti
Department of Scienze Economiche, Politiche e delle Lingue Moderne—Libera Università SS Maria Assunta, 00100 Rome, Italy
Department of Mathematics, University of Bergen, 5052 Bergen, Norway
School of Computing, University of Portsmouth, Portsmouth PO1, UK

Elena Grossini and Serena Farruggio
Laboratory of Physiology, Department of Translational Medicine, UPO, 28100 Novara, Italy

Daniele Pierelli and Carolina Monaco
Cardiothoracic Intensive Care Unit, AOU, 28100 Novara, Italy

Virginia Bolzani and Lidia Rossi
Cardiology Division, AOU, 28100 Novara, Italy

Ioannis Drosos, Maria Del Pilar Ortega Carrillo, Rajinikanth Gogiraju, Thomas Munzel and Katrin Schafer
Center for Cardiology, Cardiology 1, University Medical Center of the Johannes Gutenberg University Mainz, 55130 Mainz, Germany

Maria Pavlaki, Adriani Kourkouli, Georgios Chalikias, Christos Tortopidis and Dimitrios Tziakas
Department of Cardiology, Democritus University of Thrace, 68100 Alexandroupolis, Greece

Katja Buschmann and Christian F. Vahl
Department of Cardiothoracic and Vascular Surgery, University Medical Center of the Johannes Gutenberg University Mainz, 55130 Mainz, Germany

Federica Re and Elisabetta Zachara
Cardiac Arrhythmia Center and Cardiomyopathies Unit, San Camillo—Forlanini Hospital, 00100 Rome, Italy

Magdalena L. Bochenek
Center for Cardiology, Cardiology 1, University Medical Center of the Johannes Gutenberg University Mainz, 55130 Mainz, Germany
Center for Thrombosis and Hemostasis, University Medical Center of the Johannes Gutenberg University Mainz, 55130 Mainz, Germany

Stavros Konstantinides
Department of Cardiology, Democritus University of Thrace, 68100 Alexandroupolis, Greece
Center for Thrombosis and Hemostasis, University Medical Center of the Johannes Gutenberg University Mainz, 55130 Mainz, Germany

Ivana Škrlec
Histology, Genetics, Cellular, and Molecular Biology Laboratory, Department of Biology and Chemistry, Faculty of Dental Medicine and Health, Josip Juraj Strossmayer University of Osijek, Crkvena 21, HR-31000 Osijek, Croatia

Jakov Milić
Faculty of Medicine, Josip Juraj Strossmayer University of Osijek, Josipa Huttlera 4, HR-31000 Osijek

Robert Steiner
Faculty of Medicine, Josip Juraj Strossmayer University of Osijek, Josipa Huttlera 4, HR-31000 Osijek, Croatia
Clinical Department of Cardiovascular Diseases and Intensive Care, Clinic for Internal Medicine, University Hospital Osijek, Josipa Huttlera 4, HR-31000 Osijek, Croatia

Tuvia Ben Gal
Heart Failure Unit, Rabin Medical Center, Tel Aviv University, Petah Tikva 4941492d, Israel

Dominique Bettex
Institute of Anaesthesiology, University Hospital of Zurich, University of Zurich, 8091 Zurich, Switzerland

Vladimir Cerny
Department of Anesthesiology, Perioperative Medicine and Intensive Care, Masaryk Hospital, J.E. Purkinje University, 400 96 Usti nad Labem, Czech Republic

Josep Comin-Colet
Heart Diseases Institute, Hospital Universitari de Bellvitge, 08015 Barcelona, Spain

Alexandr A. Eremenko
Department of Cardiac Intensive Care, Petrovskii National Research Centre of Surgery, Sechenov University, 119146 Moscow, Russia

Dimitrios Farmakis
Department of Cardiology, Medical School, University of Cyprus, 1678 Nicosia, Cyprus

Francesco Fedele
Department of Cardiovascular, Respiratory, Nephrology, Anesthesiology and Geriatric Sciences, La Sapienza' University of Rome, 00185 Rome, Italy

Cândida Fonseca
Heart Failure Clinic of S. Francisco Xavier Hospital, CHLO, 1449-005 Lisbon, Portugal

Veli-Pekka Harjola
Emergency Medicine, Department of Emergency Medicine and Services, Helsinki University Hospital, University of Helsinki, 00014 Helsinki, Finland

Antoine Herpain
Department of Intensive Care, Experimental Laboratory of Intensive Care, Erasme Hospital, Université Libre de Bruxelles, 1050 Bruxelles, Belgium

Matthias Heringlake
Department of Anesthesiology and Intensive Care Medicine, University of Lubeck, 23562 Lubeck, Germany

Leo Heunks
Department of Intensive Care Medicine, Amsterdam UMC, Location VUmc 081 HV, The Netherlands

Trygve Husebye
Department of Cardiology, Oslo University Hospital Ullevaal, 0372 Oslo, Norway

Visnja Ivancan
Department of Anesthesiology, Reanimatology and Intensive Care, University Hospital Centre, 10000 Zagreb, Croatia

Kristjan Karason
Transplant Institute, Sahlgrenska University Hospital, 413 45 Gothenburg, Sweden

Sundeep Kaul
Intensive Care Unit, National Health Service, Leeds LS2 9JT, UK

Jacek Kubica
Department of Cardiology and Internal Medicine, Nicolaus Copernicus University, 87-100 Torun, Poland

Alexandre Mebazaa
Department of Anaesthesiology and Critical Care Medicine, AP-HP, Saint Louis and Lariboisière University Hospitals, Université de Paris and INSERM UMR-S 942-MASCOT, 75010 Paris, France

Henning Molgaard
Department of Cardiology, Arhus University Hospital, 8200 Arhus, Denmark

John Parissis
Emergency Department, Attikon University Hospital, National and Kapodistrian University of Athens, 157 72 Athens, Greece

Alexander Parkhomenko
Emergency Cardiology Department, National Scientific Center M.D. Strazhesko Institute of Cardiology, 02000 Kiev, Ukraine

Pentti Põder
Department of Cardiology, North Estonia Medical Center, 13419 Tallinn, Estonia

Gerhard Polzl
Department of Internal Medicine III, Cardiology and Angiology, Medical University of Innsbruck, 6020 Innsbruck, Austria

Bojan Vrtovec
Advanced Heart Failure and Transplantation Center, Department of Cardiology, Ljubljana University Medical Center, SI-1000 Ljubljana, Slovenia

Mehmet B. Yilmaz
Department of Cardiology, Dokuz Eylul University Faculty of Medicine, 35340 Izmir, Turkey

Zoltan Papp
Division of Clinical Physiology, Department of Cardiology, Faculty of Medicine, University of Debrecen, H-4032 Debrecen, Hungary
HAS-UD Vascular Biology and Myocardial Pathophysiology Research Group, Hungarian Academy of Sciences, 4001 Debrecen, Hungary

Raffaele Marfella
Department of Advanced Medical and Surgical Sciences, University of Campania "Luigi Vanvitelli", 80100 Naples, Italy

Celestino Sardu
Department of Advanced Medical and Surgical Sciences, University of Campania "Luigi Vanvitelli", 80100 Naples, Italy
Department of Medical Sciences, International University of Health and Medical Sciences "Saint Camillus", 00131 Rome, Italy

Jessica Gambardella
Department of Advanced Biomedical Sciences, International Translational Research and Medical Education Academic Research Unit (ITME), "Federico II" University, 80131 Naples, Italy
Department of Medicine, Division of Cardiology, Albert Einstein College of Medicine, Wilf Family Cardiovascular Research Institute, New York, NY 10461, USA

Xujun Wang
Department of Medicine, Division of Cardiology, Albert Einstein College of Medicine,Wilf Family Cardiovascular Research Institute, New York, NY 10461, USA

Marco Bruno Morelli
Department of Medicine, Division of Cardiology, Albert Einstein College of Medicine, Wilf Family Cardiovascular Research Institute, New York, NY 10461, USA
Department of Molecular Pharmacology, Fleischer Institute for Diabetes and Metabolism (FIDAM), Montefiore University Hospital, New York, NY 10461, USA

Gaetano Santulli
Department of Advanced Biomedical Sciences, International Translational Research and Medical Education Academic Research Unit (ITME), "Federico II" University, 80131 Naples, Italy
Department of Medicine, Division of Cardiology, Albert Einstein College of Medicine, Wilf Family Cardiovascular Research Institute, New York, NY 10461, USA
Department of Molecular Pharmacology, Fleischer Institute for Diabetes and Metabolism (FIDAM), Montefiore University Hospital, New York, NY 10461, USA

Index

www.ingramcontent.com/pod-product-compliance
Lightning Source LLC
LaVergne TN
LVHW060602210926
848485LV00005B/1354